Neural Network Model: Applications and Implications

Series Editor
Theodore Wasserman, Wasserman & Drucker PA, Boca Raton, FL, USA

Theodore Wasserman • Lori Drucker Wasserman

Apraxia: The Neural Network Model

Springer

Theodore Wasserman
Wasserman & Drucker PA
Boca Raton, FL, USA

Lori Drucker Wasserman
Wasserman & Drucker PA
Boca Raton, FL, USA

ISBN 978-3-031-24104-8 ISBN 978-3-031-24105-5 (eBook)
Neural Network Model: Applications and Implications
https://doi.org/10.1007/978-3-031-24105-5

This Springer imprint is published by the registered company Springer Nature Switzerland AG
The registered company address is: Gewerbestrasse 11, 6330 Cham, Switzerland

Introduction: Why Apraxia

There are many ways that can inspire in writing a book. One way, we suppose, is that the book results from a long-standing desire to explore a particular concept or idea. Another is that the book represented a continuation of a theme that was being developed over a period of time and across several books. In the current instance, both ways could be considered accurate. This book, about apraxia, is the continuation of a series of works on how the idea of the neural network organization of the way the human brain processes information can impact what we understand about the disorders practitioners confront when something goes wrong. This book is the third in our series on human neural network characteristics of the brain and disorders thereof. In that vein, we will raise themes we have been developing over the series of works that include two additional works the preceded the current series. Among these themes is the idea that the current diagnostic nosology, the Diagnostic and Statistical Manual of Mental Disorders and the behavioral grouping model upon which it is based, is inadequate to the task and probably injurious to the development of advancement of the true nature of most disorders of mental health. Another theme is the ongoing pathologizing of behaviors and groups of behaviors that may, in fact represent, normal, if atypical, variations of human behavior. Some examples of this phenomenon include the recently added to the DSM 5, namely, social engagement disorder and caffeine withdrawal disorders. Obviously, behavior in the extreme in these areas can be problematic but where the line gets drawn in practice will be an interesting process to observe.

One of the most striking things that stood out for us in preparing the material for this book is how little things have changed regarding the understanding of apraxia over the last 30 years. For the most part, apraxia remains described as the inability to make purposeful movement of one part of the body or another. The various types of apraxic conditions are essentially names of the part of the body or function that is impacted. The major theme for us, of course, is that once you understand how the neural network model explains the information processing of the brain and once you understand what can go wrong with those networks that form the basis of information processing, the basic understanding of disorders related to this system must change. The change in understanding must accompany a change in awareness of what it means for the system to be disordered. This inevitably leads to a change in understanding that nature and characteristics of the disorders themselves. What we described for disorders of mental health and for difficulties in motivation will also be very true for apraxia. We believe that it is long past time for a new understanding of this very large group of disorders. We hope that this new understanding leads to the formulation of newer and more neurologically accurate diagnostic categories and the development of more efficient treatment approaches.

While the motivation described above is sort of accurate, that isn't really what happened. What happened was that good friends of ours had a grandchild with delayed speech development and asked us for an opinion regarding etiology, potential treatment, and long-term prognosis. The youngster was about 18 months old and speech development was not occurring in the anticipated manner. Both of us have extensive experience in the assessment of children in the 0–3 age range, so this request was well within our capability. After a thorough assessment and developmental history, it was fairly clear that a diagnosis of developmental apraxia was appropriate and the parents and grandparents were informed. Referral was made to the local early intervention program to begin treatment, consisting of intensive speech and language therapy. The family was able to supplement the treatment provided through the program, so the child received treatment several days a week from providers who had experience in the area. So far, so good.

We have known this family for many years and had permission from the parents to discuss the case with the grandparents, who were very involved and worried about what the future may hold. As might be expected, one grandparent asked one of us and the other asked the other of us. Then one night we all went out to dinner and were chatting and trying to be supportive when it became obvious that the grandparents did not receive exactly the same information regarding impact and prognosis. One of us had described developmental apraxia as an issue of motor dysregulation emphasizing the development of speech with a good prognosis, albeit after a long and intensive program of treatment. The other of us, using neural network modeling, had described a more far-reaching disorder, impacting many areas of development and provided a more circumspect prognosis.

As you might imagine, there was a rather long discussion after we got home, and we realized that what was true for many things in the world of mental health was true for developmental apraxia. There wasn't agreement on what it was other than a description of behavior, and there were many different opinions about etiology, comorbidity, and outcome. We began to wonder if what was true about developmental apraxia was true for the many other acquired apraxias as well. What we have learned in line with the answers to those questions led to the creation of this book. To preview what we have found, we would tell you that developmental apraxia is a very different phenomena from the apraxia acquired during adulthood and perhaps should be in a separate category by itself. We would also tell you, what husbands have learned since the beginning of time, that perhaps it is better to listen to the wife and not argue in the first place.

There were many questions to be answered and many ideas to consider. Some of these were:

In the instance of an acquired apraxia, Where a lesion to a network component was the clear culprit, was the site of the lesion important?
Given the fact the apraxia is a complex behavioral dysfunction, usually resulting from the disruption of a network consisting of interrelated components, it is logical to assume that the downstream impact would be partially dependent on where in the system the messaging was disrupted. While all cases of oral motor apraxia would have the same core central behavior, might there be subtypes with different comorbidities dependent on the lesion site? It seemed to us that there might be.

Specifically, as we shall see, lesions to the brain which impair the ability to carry out simple oral gestures on imitation include the frontal and central opercula, the anterior insula, and a small area of the first temporal convolution of the left hemisphere. All these areas contribute to the various components of a rather complex oral motor movement related to speech. The disruption of speech is evident in all the affected individuals but it is not all that happens. A lesion to the frontal opercula produces comorbidities of disrupted function different to those that were produced by a lesion to the anterior insula. Depending on the subnetworks involved, it seemed likely that there would be numerous subtypes of oral motor apraxia, each with different complexities and with different impact and prognosis.

If one of the issues with developmental apraxia is the absence of an identifiable lesion, and no observable muscle weakness, what else might happen to produce the outcome?
What exactly caused developmental apraxia and was it just one thing, which we considered unlikely, or was it a collection of things? What other issues affect the ability of a neural network to carry information? What are the factors that impact the development of a neural network in the first place? Is the prognosis for a network that never develops at all different from one with only a focal point of damage in an otherwise fully developed and functional system? For example, human speech surely is one of the most complex tasks that we humans do and likely involves numerous networks in its creation, development and expression. Disruption to any one of those networks might produce the ultimate apraxic condition. The ongoing question is whether the failure to develop one component of this system would be more or less disruptive to language functioning as compared to damage to the same component after the system had been fully functional.

Would a disrupted developmental unfolding of skills imply more complex and far-reaching comorbidities that a localized lesion in an adult brain?
This question has been around for some time and we are not sure that the argument about which is better or worse has been settled. We probably won't settle it either, but we intend to take a look at it.

How does resiliency and plasticity factor into the equation for developmental apraxia and acquired apraxia?
Related to the question above, how do resilience and plasticity impact recovery of function (or development of function)? Are there some areas of the brain that have the ability to recover or adapt at a better rate than others?

Would the idea of cognitive reserve be an important consideration in adult acquired apraxia?

Is damage that occurs later in life more impactful because of all the previous life course incidents that have transpired? What is the impact of a lesion in an already compromised brain and are some brains more capable of recovering than others? What factors contribute to the ability to recover?

We will explore these issues and more. We realized that apraxia would be an ideal way of showing the power of a neural networking model to contribute to the understanding of a complex disorder. Given our backgrounds, and the circumstances surrounding the genesis of the book, it would be fair to say that we will have a heavy emphasis on developmental apraxia of speech. This is probably fair, as it seems to be the most complex of the issues to discuss. We will discuss in detail the other, significant numbers of apraxic conditions. You will be excused if you think our biases are showing, because they are. So, come along and find out why the wife was right and basing our response on a neural networking model as explained to the grandparents was the right way to go.

Contents

Chapter 1
Apraxia, Dyspraxia, and Motor Coordination Disorders: Definitions and Confounds

Providing the reader with a cogent and agreed-upon definition of apraxia would seem to be a valuable way to start any discussion of apraxia. We have discovered however, as is the case for other diagnoses, that goal is elusive when discussing apraxia and particularly so when addressing developmental coordination disorder or childhood/developmental apraxia of speech. This is not simply a matter of "Let's agree to disagree." The implications are significant. For those readers familiar with our other work, they will be aware of our concerns with the state of diagnostic specificity and sensitivity. The implications reach the worlds of clinical psychological practice, medical practice, neuropsychology, and neurology. Specifically, if we do not agree about what we are defining, how are we defining, treating, and researching it?

Before we begin our discussion of apraxia and its various forms, we wish to highlight that we include developmental coordination disorder (DCD) in our discussions and by extension, what is now a subcategory of DCD as listed in the DSM 5 (APA, 2013), childhood apraxia of speech (CAS). We do this because of the extensive contribution of the motor networks that these disorders share. We do this to demonstrate how disruption of motor networks is an integral part of what are currently considered discrete disorders but may in fact represent disruption of a unified motor system with pervasive implications. We do this because if we can understand the brain through its development, we should be better able to understand the implications of a disruption somewhere along the neural network pathways. Therefore, we start at the beginning, that is, the childhood development of motor-based disorders. The field has begun to understand this position as it has, in the DSM 5, grouped DCD as a motor disorder. In addition, CAS is a further subcategory of DCD; both are under the category of motor disorders falling under the larger umbrella of neurodevelopmental disorders.

Although somewhat less so for an *acquired* apraxia, the definition of what constitutes a given apraxia is often elusive and poorly defined. This may be even more

T. Wasserman, L. D. Wasserman, *Apraxia: The Neural Network Model*, Neural Network Model: Applications and Implications,
https://doi.org/10.1007/978-3-031-24105-5_1

so with regard to the etiology. Perhaps a better way to explain the problem is that there are multiple problems. With regard to specificity, the definitions of apraxia are largely behaviorally descriptive, but sometimes too confined. And sometimes they are too ambiguous secondary to a phenotype. Often there is phenotypical overlap across disorders. In addition, some disorders are based upon the magnitude of effect (dyspraxia), sometimes.

As you will see, there is a multitude of apraxia, all ostensibly delineated by the primary area of impact. Traditionally the diagnosis and treatment of apraxia focused on a highly behaviorally segregated symptom. This is clearly understandable as from a historical perspective it reflects the early observations of those noting and then studying these phenomena which became known as apraxia. Early contributions were foundational; however, they also had a cortical and somewhat modular bias. It is understood and appreciated that from a current perspective it allows clinicians to speak in short hand to each other about what is observable, impacted, and where to begin intervention. But from a neural network model-based perspective, there is a different reality: there is a multitude of potential areas of impact and impacted processes, often treated as dissociable entities, complicated further by questions about etiology being trauma based, genetic, or developmental. Hence, if we consider this component, then does a diagnostic label, lacking in specificity, and often sensitivity, *really tell us with what we are dealing*, and how to best intervene?

Further confusing the picture is how some of these identified apraxia or dyspraxia associate with other disorders. This greatly muddles the designs and/or outcomes of research. For example, it often results in confounds in population samples which can produce "dubious" findings. An interesting, and we believe important, observation of the current authors is that research papers often include a section on "limitations of the study." We believe that sometimes what is described as the study's limitations, rather than being confounds and limitations, are actually a reflection of the diversity of the disorder, its phenotypical presentations, and manifestations across subjects rather than a limitation of the study itself. This point is elaborated upon as we go through diagnostic research across chapters.

In summary, while the current state of definition might lead one to assume that the impact is highly specific, in order to diagnose or treat a person impacted by an apraxia, we must understand that it is not an isolated clinical finding. Humans are much more sophisticated and the systems much more complicated. Neural network modeling would have us understand that the impact of the network damage has implications far in excess of the most obvious symptomology.

History and Current State of the Study of Apraxia

This is an area that has been under study for a long time. Looking at the history, we can see that the definition of apraxia has evolved. Based upon observed behavior and conjecture about underlying neurological functioning, the presumed mechanisms initially were really quite different than that of our current understanding.

Assessment of this area began as early as the 1860s with a description of apraxia, although not labeled as such, provided by John Hughlings Jackson (Pearce, 2009). In 1871, Steinthal coined the term apraxia from the Greek term apraxia, meaning inaction. It was assumed that the reason a person may fail to correctly perform purposeful movements was that they were unable to recognize the object/tool associated with the desired movement (Pearce, 2009). In 1905, Arnold Pick introduced the concept that the movement failure in apraxia was assumed to result from motor "agnosia," or motor manifestations of asymbolia.

Hugo Liepmann presented his first paper on the topic of apraxia in 1900 (Gonzales-Rothi & Heilman, 1996; Pearce, 2009). The paper described deficits of motor function in a 48-year-old German imperial councilor whose initial presentation appeared to be dementia. The patient had difficulty with initiation and copying of gestures, although spontaneous movements, such as using utensils while eating, were normal. Liepmann suggested a disconnect of the visual, auditory, and somatosensory areas from the area of motor cortex, a disconnection of the hemispheres. He predicted cortical lesions which were confirmed upon autopsy and presented in a report in 1907. Liepmann's work led to the conclusions that apraxia was a defect dependent on lesions in the left hemisphere which contained the memory of skilled movements. He believed that plan of movement is stored in the dominant left parietal lobe. In order to execute a skilled movement, the space time plan had to be retrieved, and via cortical connections in the left sensorimotorium (precentral and postcentral gyri), the information was passed to the left primary motor areas and then transfer was made through the corpus collosum in order to activate the right motor cortex. He also concluded that lesions of the corpus callosum interrupted the process of movement located in the left hemisphere from the motor area located in the right hemisphere resulting in ideomotor apraxia of the left arm and hand. Liepmann created categories which included the distinguishing of ideomotor apraxia wherein the difficulty is with determining the nature of a single movement, from limb-kinetic apraxia wherein the movements are awkward and slowed, and ideational apraxia wherein the sequence of movements is disrupted. Liepmann's work was foundational, if not completely correct, in correlating cortical anatomy with behavior. Geschwind who largely supported Liepmann's ideas, believed the "analyses of the mechanisms underlying disturbances in motor performances (Geschwind, 1965) to be of greater importance than the listing of types of apraxia." He went on to create his own "disconnexion theory" for limb apraxia embracing Liepmann's work and Wernicke's foundational disconnection theory model for language.

Despite advances, Pearce (2009) points out that "Recent functional imaging studies correlated with neuropsychological deficits have not clarified the fundamental nature of the many different patterns of apraxia in relation to its varied anatomical lesions." He also posits that "brain diseases that damage the multiple parallel parieto-frontal circuits devoted to specific sensorimotor transformations cause different praxis deficits depending on the context in which the movement is preformed and the cognitive demands of the action."

Current Definitions

There are currently several definitions of apraxia in use. These definitions revolve around a couple of central themes. One medical definition of apraxia covers two aspects: (1) apraxia is a disorder of the brain and nervous system and (2) a disorder wherein a person is unable to perform tasks or movements when asked, even though the request or command is understood. They are willing to perform the task and the muscles needed to perform the task work properly (National Library of Medicine, 2022). However, people with apraxia cannot execute them. This definition goes on to provide more detail. Apraxia is caused by damage to the brain. When apraxia develops in a person who was previously able to perform the tasks or abilities, it is called acquired apraxia. The most common causes of acquired apraxia are:

Brain tumor
Conditions that cause gradual worsening of the brain and nervous system (neurodegenerative illness)
Dementia
Stroke
Traumatic brain injury
Hydrocephalus

There are similar definitions encompassing more or less specificity. For instance, "Apraxia which is a neurological disorder characterized by loss of the ability to execute or carry out skilled movements and gestures, despite having the desire and the physical ability to perform them." The term "dyspraxia" is used if the presentation is considered mild. "Apraxia results from dysfunction of the cerebral hemispheres of the brain, especially the parietal lobe, and can arise from many diseases or damage to the brain" (National Institute of Neurologic Disorders and Strokes, 2022). This casts a wider etiologic net by using the term dysfunction, which can refer to severity and/or etiology. This definition goes on to talk about difficulty coordinating complex muscle movements to produce an action. Other definitions concentrate only on the particular outcome behavior that cannot be performed.

Some other definitions are simpler and often leave out the idea of intentionality such as the following: "Apraxia is the loss or impairment of the ability to execute complex coordinated movements without muscular or sensory impairment" (Merriam-Webster, 2022). This definition leaves out etiology all together and focuses on phenotype. A similar definitional orientation is provided by the National Organization for Rare Diseases (2022): "Apraxia is a neurological disorder characterized by the inability to perform learned (familiar) movements on command, even though the command is understood and there is a willingness to perform the movement." Both the desire to move and the cognitive comprehension of the directive are present, but the person simply cannot execute the act.

None of these definitions cover the case of developmental apraxia or childhood apraxia of speech (CAS). Here, it is possible that a child has not yet developed speech and it is the development of speech that is being impeded. In addition, as we write this, the cause of most developmental apraxia conditions is unknown. For CAS, definitions like this example are common: "Childhood apraxia of speech (CAS) is an uncommon speech disorder in which a child has difficulty making accurate movements when speaking. In CAS, the brain struggles to develop plans for speech movement. With this disorder, the speech muscles aren't weak, but they don't perform normally because the brain has difficulty directing or coordinating the movements" (Mayo Clinic, 2022). This definition, while alluding to brain-based etiology, largely emphasizes the coordination of the *muscle* movement on speech.

Is childhood apraxia of speech a developmental disorder we should be defining based upon the expressed phonology? According to the American Speech-Language-Hearing Association apraxia may be developmental as in childhood apraxia of speech, or the result of a medical or traumatic event, which is then an acquired apraxia (ASHA, 2021; Diehl, 2022). With a concern that people not confuse developmental as implying a possibility of "outgrowing" the disorder, and stressing the need for intervention services, ASHA states "Neither disability is something a person will outgrow, or get over, but with careful instruction and hard work, it is both a hope and belief that people with either disability can learn to work through their challenges" (ASHA, 2021; Diehl, 2022).

Perhaps the most used definition of apraxia in the neuropsychological and medical literature was developed by Rothi and Heilman (1997). This definition defines apraxia "as a neurological disorder of skilled movement that is not explained by deficits of elemental motor or sensory system." In other words, apraxia is considered as being independent from other stroke comorbidity symptoms such as hemiplegia (loss of proprioception and motor control over limb on one side) or visual deficits such as hemianopia or neglect (Bieńkiewicz et al., 2014). Thus, to some extent, apraxia is a diagnosis of exclusion; you use it when you are not exactly sure what the specific etiology is.

Developmental coordination disorder (DCD) is another diagnostic category with much confusion about presentation and etiology. According to the American Psychiatric Association (APA, 2013), this disorder includes impairment in the development of motor coordination, wherein "the acquisition and execution of coordinated motor skills is substantially below that expected" with "difficulties manifested as clumsiness, as well as slowness and inaccuracy of performance of motor skills." This disorder is also referred to in the manual as dyspraxia. Additionally, these motor difficulties are not related to a medical condition or disease such as cerebral palsy. The disorder is listed in the DSM 5 under motor disorders, under the larger category of neurodevelopmental disorders. The World Health Organization (WHO, 1992) largely concurs with this overall definition and indicates that a child with DCD must score two standard deviations below the mean accompanied by academic and daily living impact. They note that there should not be neurological disorder. Of course, the exclusion of a neurological disorder as a prerequisite for being a neurodevelopmental disorder gives one pause.

Further complicating the picture, we should note that the terms apraxia and dyspraxia are not technically synonymous. Nor are they utilized consistently across the medical field and area of speech and language. Specifically,

1. In general, dyspraxia refers to the partial loss of the ability to coordinate and perform skilled, purposeful movements and gestures with normal accuracy. Apraxia is the term that is used to describe the complete loss of this ability. The terms are, however, often used interchangeably. In addition, dysfunction of a movement related to gross or fine motor movements, in isolation or a sequence, is referred to in the literature as apraxia.
2. In contrast, ASHA utilizes the term *dyspraxia* to define a developmental disability affecting gross and fine motor skills. ASHA utilizes the term *apraxia* to describe a speech disability affecting verbal planning. In summary then, according to ASHA "while dyspraxia is a broader term used to describe muscle planning developmental disabilities, apraxia is used to describe muscle planning needed especially for speech." Therefore, two professionals, a speech pathologist and a physical therapist, working together on an interdisciplinary team, would not agree as to the terminology for a child manifesting difficulty with, for example, independent ambulation or self-care behaviors.
3. And to highlight additional sources of confusion, the term *dyspraxia* is utilized in parts of Europe (Kirby, 2007) to describe children with what is generally known as developmental coordination disorder. In a recent "white paper" on guidelines for international practice (Blank, 2019), the consensus was for using the term DCD in countries which follow the DSM 5. In countries which adhere to the ICD, they recommend the term specific developmental disorder of motor function.

At this point the reader must be wondering how to follow if we are we talking about a motor problem or a speech problem, dyspraxia or apraxia? Rightly so. The current authors utilize the larger medically accepted definition of apraxia as it relates to gross and fine motor expression. As it relates to speech, the term childhood apraxia of speech will be utilized.

Finally, we would point out that the definitional distinction between apraxia and dyspraxia brings up some interesting issues for neural network modeling. At first glance, one might assume that because the networks involved in both types of problems are shared, the result should be the same functional deficit, identical as it is only the degree of disrupted function that is at issue. However, that is not the case because these networks are complex and disruptions can happen in a number of locations, thereby altering the final functional behavior and related comorbidities. To be clear, effect can be in magnitude and/or reach the area of impact.

Definitional Definitions and Confounds in Apraxia Research

While there are some commonalities between current definitions, there are also some striking differences. For example, consider this definition: "Apraxia designates the impaired ability to perform a gesture, in spite of preserved motor, somatosensory, and coordination functions in the limb engaged in the action" (De Renzi &

Faglioni, 1999). This definition represents a good example of a highly "confined" definition alluded to previously. It specifies motor-based movement issues for the research study currently referred to within a particular limb. There are even problems noted within this limited view as the authors state that "a unitary account of apraxia and aphasia runs into the same difficulty that undermines the theory of a common source for praxis skills and handedness, namely the occurrence of dissociations in either direction." This statement highlights difficulties in partitioning the symptomology.

Zadikoff and Lang (2005) also take issue with the definition of apraxia noting "The definition of apraxia specifies that the disturbance of performed skilled movements cannot be explained by the more elemental motor disorders typical of patients with movement disorders." These authors go on to point out that "the term 'apraxia' has also been applied to other motor disturbances, such as 'gait apraxia' and 'apraxia of eyelid opening', are perhaps misnomers, demonstrating the lack of a coherent nomenclature in this field" (pg. 1480). We concur with their concern.

The authors go on to highlight a common theme when considering apraxia in that it has a disease or injury emphasis. They note that diseases that cause the combination of apraxia and a primary movement disorder most often involve corticobasal degeneration. Corticobasal degeneration is characterized by various apraxia and particularly affects ideomotor and limb-kinetic apraxia (both of which are described further on in this chapter) as well as buccofacial and oculomotor apraxia (also described in this chapter). They point out that corticobasal syndrome may be caused by a variety of central nervous system disorders such as Alzheimer's disease, dementias, and supranuclear palsy. Of importance, supranuclear palsy and Parkinson's disease can result in differing or varying degrees of the expression of apraxia, particularly in those with more severe cognitive dysfunction. Is this then better described as dyspraxia? Germane to their position on definition and identification is that similar presentations of apraxia can involve a variety of cerebral cortical sites as well as basal ganglia structures. This implies that they consider apraxia and its movement components to possibly be dissociable and highlight the confounding that occurs in labeling something an apraxia when the etiology can be multidetermined or wherein various disorders can produce similar symptomology.

Cassidy (2016) also notes the confusion as a result of how apraxia is defined noting that it is "an inability to perform a motor task that cannot be adequately explained by motor weakness, sensory loss or a lack of understanding." This criterion has led to a plethora of motor disorders being described as forms of apraxia, despite many of these failing to capture the essence of what apraxia really is: a disorder of motor cognition. To rectify this situation, greater specificity is proposed leading to a definition of apraxia that reflects an impairment of the storage and transformation of motor representations in the brain, either through degradation of the semantic knowledge of gestures and tool use or through the inability to translate the neural representations of higher-level goals accurately into lower-level patterns of muscle activation and inhibition (Cassidy, 2016).

The above only represents the confused state of affairs as regards limb and other muscle movement disorders. It becomes even more confusing when developmental disorders are included.

There are definitions of apraxia that include speech difficulties. Some refer to speech, some to language. These are often regarded as a unique disorder in some ways. At one recent point, "Apraxia of speech (AOS) has emerged as the term to describe a motor speech disorder characterized by an impaired ability to coordinate the sequential, articulatory movements necessary to produce speech sounds" (Ogar et al., Apraxia of Speech An overview, 2005). Clearly, this definition requires deficiencies in the motor components of speech making the two elements nondissociable. The authors go on to point out that "confusion in the literature around AOS stems from the fact that terminology associated with this disorder has varied greatly. Also, symptoms associated with AOS often co-occur or overlap with those caused by neuromuscular deficits indicative of the dysarthrias and the linguistic errors associated with aphasia" (pg. 427). An example of the overlap is as follows: childhood dysarthria (CD) or childhood apraxia of speech (CAS) is suspected in children who, in addition to such errors, have imprecise and/or unstable spatiotemporal distortions of vowels and consonants, inappropriate prosody, and deficits in voice (Shriberg et al., 2019).Despite this, the authors insist that "AOS is, however, a distinct motor speech disorder." A careful inspection of this definition would note that there were disorders where speech was disrupted in exactly the same manner that it is with apraxia, making discriminating between the two conditions a matter of art as opposed to science. For example, they point out that "AOS is often confused with conduction aphasia, perhaps because sound level errors (substitutions, additions, transpositions or omissions) are prominent in both disorders. However, the nature of errors is *thought* to be different" (pg. 429). As with the other disorder definitions we have looked at, this definition is disease or insult based. The authors posit that while vascular lesions are the most common cause of AOS, the disorder also results from tumors and trauma.

To put a fine point on this discussion, we offer this from the online medical dictionary which, based on an article from the *American Journal of Speech-Language-Pathology* in 2003, provided the following description of the diagnostic problem: "The diagnostic criteria used to identify developmental apraxia of speech (DAS) have been at the center of controversy for decades. Despite the difficulty in determining the characteristics that differentiate DAS from other speech acquisition disorders, many children are identified with this disorder. The current report presents the criteria used by 75 speech-language pathologists to establish a diagnosis of DAS. Although 50 different characteristics were identified, 6 of these characteristics accounted for 51.5% of the responses. These characteristics included inconsistent productions, general oral-motor difficulties, groping, inability to imitate sounds, increasing difficulty with increased utterance length, and poor sequencing of sounds. These results are consistent with the general ambiguity of the diagnostic criteria of DAS and suggest that no single deficit is used among clinicians" (The Medical Dictionary, 2021).

This led to the following definition: "Childhood Apraxia of Speech (CAS) is a neurological childhood (pediatric) speech sound disorder in which the precision and consistency of movements underlying speech are impaired in the absence of neuromuscular deficits (e.g. abnormal reflexes, abnormal tone). CAS may occur as a result of known neurological impairment, in association with complex neurobehavioral disorders of known and unknown origin, or as an idiopathic neurogenic speech sound disorder. The core impairment in planning and/or programming spatiotemporal parameters of movement sequences results in errors in speech sound production and prosody" (ASHA, 2021).

"An understanding of developmental apraxia depends on consistent utilization of a group of symptoms for diagnosis so that data-based results can be used to generate inferences about the disorder" (Davis et al., 1998). This is a point which is also made and is relevant to the diagnosis of developmental coordination disorder. The criteria having been outlined above will not be repeated here. However, the current point, consistency in distinguishing symptoms, is clearly problematic across these two developmental disorders. In addition, as alluded to by Zadikoff and Lang (2005) in reference to limb and ideational apraxia, etc., there are problems with confounding variables including symptoms being *caused* by other disorders (etiology outside this diagnostic category) and symptoms clouded by other disorders, e.g., separating speech difficulties from other disorders, causing symptoms which may exacerbate or confound those of the "identified" neurodevelopmental disorder.

These issues of definition and explanation clearly and succinctly articulate many of the issues that motivated us to write this book. It suggests that what was called developmental apraxia, and is now referred to as childhood apraxia of speech, or developmental coordination disorder may well have been better described as developmental and, perhaps, represents a distinct and dissociable diagnostic entity.

Which brings us to what we consider a well-taken point, referred to previously by the current authors and elucidated by Geuze et al. (2015): "Clinical and research diagnostic criteria serve different purposes." Clinical issues include "decisions related to special education, treatment, remedial teaching, and reimbursement of costs related to services rendered." Research issues revolve around accurately identifying an entity, etiology, and presentation rather than a confounded construct. The current authors would argue that the latter, rather than the former, is critical for treatment. For example, the successful treatment of an attention-deficit disorder requires a greater understanding than just the involvement of attention. In fact, unless one understands the interplay of attention, motivation, reward circuitry, and attention being specific to task, one is not really possessing a therapeutic understanding of the diagnosis.

In summary, it should be apparent that there are multiple definitions of apraxia, all circulating around a central theme describing an inability to willfully move a specific muscle group. Within that wide net, there are those disorders that are clearly related to damage to the neurological integrity of the individual through either disease or insult and those disorders that are presumed to have damage, although no damage is identifiable. There is a third group which constitutes disorders for which there might not be damage from disease or insult at all. Arguably, there is yet a fourth group for whom the skill never developed and the lack of integrity of the neurological system is never clearly established.

Hypothetical Neural Mechanisms of Apraxia

Logically, apraxia is likely not a movement disorder with a solitary neurological or neurobiological etiology. This is because apraxia conditions variously affect behaviors in relation to their nature and the modality through which the instructions eliciting the appropriate motor responses are conveyed (De Renzi et al., 1982). This understanding is increasingly complicated when, by using network modeling, it is understood that a disruption of function can be caused by problems anywhere in the network. Apraxia can be modality-specific, that is, contingent upon the selective severing of a pathway or pathways linking one sensory association area with the integration center where the movement is constructed. Whether there is one such center or several is, as we shall see, a matter of conjecture, but it does seem logical to guess at the likelihood that there are multiple centers representing specific classes of output (limb movement, speech). It is understandable that in the majority of individuals, a lesion will result in apraxia appearing in every modality, either because it destroys the programming center or because it interrupts all the pathways connecting it with other sensory or motor areas. That, however, is not always the case. A highly discrete injury may isolate a programming center from one type of information and render the patient unable to execute the gesture when it is elicited by a given sensory center but capable of performing it under the guidance of other modalities.

Conceptually, there may be ways to think about apraxia based upon where the disruption originates. For example, is there a difference between apraxias which are caused by a disruption in pathways that supply specific elements of a complex movement before they are integrated into a whole, as opposed to disruptions for the pathways carrying the integrated whole to impact movement? What are the implications of each circumstance for remediation and recovery? Is there a way to conceptualize developmental apraxia in a way that does not imply brain injury or damage to the network system? There are many of these questions that we will attempt to address as we progress.

Double-Duty Neurons and Apraxia

Double-duty neurons are neurons that subserve more than one function or, to put it another way, participate in more than one network. For example, processing of spatial and object information is segregated into two discrete cortical visual pathways. These activities have to be integrated at some point, but it is unclear where this information is unified. Research demonstrates that, at least in monkeys, performing tasks that involve saccadic eye movements, neurons in the tail of the caudate nucleus (CDt) encode both object-specific and position-specific information of visual objects. In addition, weak electrical stimulation in the CDt induced saccades, and CDt neurons became active before saccades to particular positions and particular objects. These findings suggest that CDt neurons guide saccades to particular visual objects in particular locations (Tse, 2012). They do double duty. Clearly, injury to an area such as this would impact more than one function or skill. This would imply that if a double-duty neuron was injured, more than one function, such as apraxia, would be implicated. An injury to this area would be unlike an injury to any other part of the network. Thus, for a subgroup of people, with oral apraxia for example, the apraxia, even though impacting the same overall network, would be accompanied by other deficits.

Recognized Apraxia Conditions

There is no true consensus on all the different types of apraxia that have been identified in the literature. There are descriptions based on the dysfunction demonstrated and some descriptions based on the area of the brain that is damaged, for example, callosal apraxia (Watson & Heilman, 1983). The following is a list of some of the most common and well-known apraxic conditions depending on the area of the body or specific function affected.

Different types of apraxia affect the body in slightly different ways:

- Limb-kinetic apraxia
- Ideomotor apraxia
- Conceptual apraxia
- Ideational apraxia
- Buccofacial apraxia
- Constructional apraxia
- Oculomotor apraxia
- Verbal apraxia

Limb-Kinetic Apraxia

According to Liepmann (Liepmann & Mass, 1907), patients with limb-kinetic apraxia (LKA) had a loss of upper limb deftness or dexterity. Originally, limb-kinetic apraxia described a loss of the ability to make precise, independent, but coordinated finger and hand movements (Foki et al., 2016). The definition has expanded somewhat and now limb-kinetic apraxia indicates the inability to make precise or exact movements with a finger, an arm, or a leg. An example of this type of apraxia would be an individual who was familiar with the use of a wrench but could not, after a cerebral insult, demonstrate the use of the wrench even when one was placed in their hands. Limb-kinetic apraxia is frequently demonstrated in patients with advanced Parkinson's disease. It has to be delineated from the classical forms of apraxia, namely, ideomotor and ideational/conceptual apraxia (Zadikoff & Lang, 2005)

Ideomotor Apraxia

Ideomotor apraxia (IMA) is a disorder characterized by deficits in properly performing tool-use pantomimes (e.g., pretending to use a hammer) and communicative gestures (e.g., waving goodbye). These deficits are typically identified with movements made to verbal command or imitation (Wheaton & Hallet, 2007). The movements are spatially incorrect and may be abnormally slow and deliberate. It is a basic motor coordination deficit, not explainable by more elemental deficits implicating areas such as the cerebellum or corticospinal tract. The distinguishing factor is that people with the disorder are able to convey knowledge of how to perform a sequence task (e.g., making a ham sandwich), but they fail to properly order the elements of the task, for example, missing steps or doing steps out of order.

Conceptual Apraxia

Conceptual apraxia is the cousin of ideational apraxia. They both correspond to a disruption of the conceptual component of the praxis system (i.e., action semantic memory). The idea of conceptual apraxia was developed to describe content errors in single actions, exclusive of sequence errors in multistage actions with tools (Ochipa et al., 1992). For instance, Barbieiri and De Renzi (1984) report on a patient who demonstrated eating with a toothbrush and brushing their teeth with a spoon and a comb. Their inability to use tools could not be explained by a motor production deficit that would characterize ideomotor apraxia. Remarkably, although this person was able to name the tools and point to them on command, they could not match the tools with the purpose. This set of behaviors hence was considered suggestive of a loss of knowledge related to the use of tools.

Ideational Apraxia

Historically, ideational apraxia was defined as a disturbance in the conceptual organization of actions. People with ideational apraxia are not impaired in the action execution per se but demonstrate inappropriate use of objects and may fail in gesture discrimination and matching tasks. Ideational apraxia is regularly confused with conceptual apraxia. It is characterized as a failure to sequence task elements correctly. Conceptual problems are not the main issue. Ideational apraxia was first assessed by performing purposive sequences of actions that require the use of various objects in the correct order, such as starting a plant from a seed. This initial deficit was expanded when it was recognized that ideational apraxia is not only associated with complex actions but represented a larger deficit comprising the initiation of single actions. This circumstance is a theme to which we will return. Network modeling would imply, at least for several apraxia conditions, that there are far-reaching sequelae than the target and obvious motor movement.

Buccofacial Apraxia

Buccofacial apraxia (also called facial-oral apraxia) is characterized by the inability to coordinate and carry out facial and lip movements such as whistling, winking, coughing, etc. on command. Buccofacial apraxia is considered a specific form of verbal or speech developmental apraxia. As pertains to the thesis of this book, there is some interesting research regarding the network characteristics of those individuals with buccofacial apraxia. Specifically, individuals with buccofacial apraxia, who are by definition impaired in performing specific gestures as described above, are also impaired in recognizing sounds specifically linked to human actions (Pazzaglia et al., 2008). This finding supports research demonstrating that sound-producing actions are mapped on the same mirror circuits that are activated during the visual recognition and execution of actions (Tettamanti et al., 2005; Bangert et al., 2006).

Constructional Apraxia

Constructional apraxia is defined as an inability or difficulty to build, assemble, or draw objects. It has become increasingly obvious that constructional apraxia is a heterogeneous construct that can be assessed with very different tasks. These tasks are not assessing the same thing. The tasks themselves are quite disparate and are only mildly interconnected. These tasks tap various kinds of visuospatial, perceptual, attentional, planning, and motor mechanisms (Gainotti & Trojano, 2018). Once considered entirely reflective of parietal lobe functioning, it is now recognized that there is a plethora of constructional apraxia conditions reflecting both the nature of the task itself and the plurality of functions and of processing streams linking different parts of the parietal lobes to the occipital and frontal lobes (Fig. 1.1).

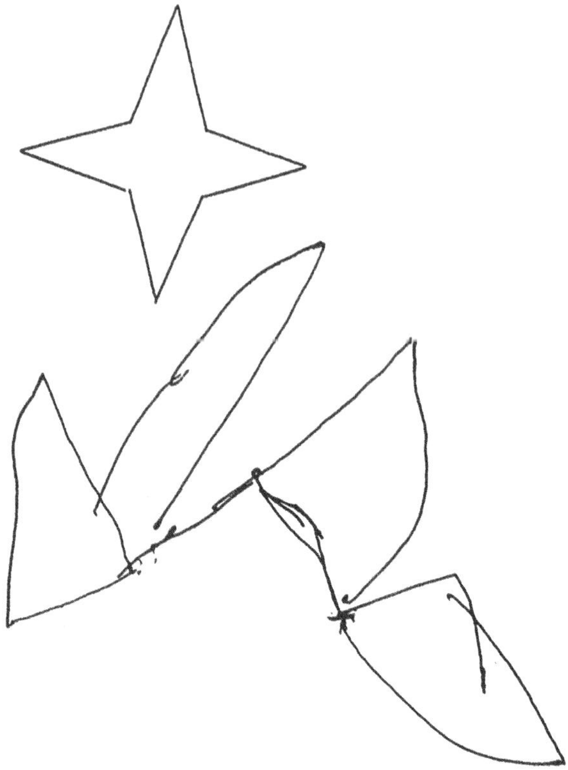

Fig. 1.1 Severe constructional apraxia demonstrated by the copy of a simple drawing. https://www.researchgate.net/profile/Gianluca-Floris-2/publication/221821714/figure/fig2/AS:619737000181761@1524768223720/Severe-constructional-apraxia-demonstrated-by-the-copy-of-a-simple-drawing.png

Oculomotor Apraxia

There are several different types of ocular motor apraxia, but all types have a core group of problems revolving around an inability to move the eyes in a coordinated fashion. Specifically, people with ocular motor apraxia have difficulty moving their eyes horizontally and/or quickly. The main difficulty is considered to be saccade initiation. There is also impaired cancellation of the vestibulo-ocular reflex (VOR). The vestibulo-ocular reflex stabilizes gaze during head movement, with eye movement due to activation of the vestibular system. The reflex serves to stabilize images on the retinas of the eye during head movement. Gaze is held steadily on a location by producing eye movements in the direction opposite that of the head movement.

Affected individuals have to turn their head in order to compensate for the lack of eye movement initiation to follow an object or see objects in their peripheral vision, but they often exceed their target. There is controversy regarding whether OMA should be considered an apraxia, since apraxia is the inability to perform a learned or skilled motor action to command, and saccade initiation is neither a learned nor a skilled action (Malkani & Zadikoff, 2011).

In Cogan-type ocular motor apraxia, there is a defect in side-to-side (horizontal) eye movements. The eyes do not move properly in response to stimuli or voluntarily. The disorder manifests in infancy. When impacted infants are asked to fixate on an object to the side, their eyes will lag and then move in the opposite direction. In order to compensate for this, the infants will sharply jerk their heads past the desired object in an effort to bring the eyes to a position where they can see the stimulus properly. When the eyes fixate on the object, the head will return to its normal position. These jerking head movements are the most recognizable sign of Cogan-type ocular motor apraxia. They are usually recognizable 3–4 months after birth. Before these jerking head movements occur, an infant's inability to fixate on an object may sometimes be mistaken for blindness (NORD, 2021).

Type 1

Ataxia-oculomotor apraxia type 1 (AOA1) in most instances has an onset of symptoms during childhood. It is an autosomal recessive cerebellar ataxia (ARCA) associated with hypoalbuminemia and hypercholesterolemia. Mutations in the APTX gene have been identified to be responsible for AOA1. Sensorimotor axonal neuropathy, as shown by nerve conduction velocity studies, is usually present. MRI studies have shown cerebellar atrophy, mild brainstem atrophy, and, in advanced cases, cortical atrophy associated with the disorder (Tarsy, 2012).

Ataxia-Oculomotor Apraxia Type 2 (AOA2)

This disorder is also known as spinocerebellar ataxia with axonal neuropathy type 2. It appears later in development, usually adolescence. It is characterized by cerebellar atrophy and peripheral neuropathy. Alterations in the SETX gene are responsible. AOA2 causes a constellation of difficulties including cerebellar atrophy, loss of Purkinje cells, and demyelination. In particular, there is a failure of the cerebro-cerebellar circuit in AOA2. This circuit impact numerous skills related to the coordination of complex cognitive functions such as working memory, executive functions, speech, and sequence learning.

Orofacial Apraxia

Orofacial apraxia (Gross & Grossman, Update on Apraxia, 2008) is characterized by an impairment of skilled movements involving the face, mouth, tongue, larynx, and pharynx (e.g., blowing a kiss). It seems synonymous with Buccofacial apraxia in most of its aspects. Research has associated orofacial apraxia with inferior frontal, deep frontal white matter, insula, and basal ganglia lesions. As in ideomotor limb apraxia, automatic movements of the same muscles are often preserved.

Usually, orofacial apraxia coexists with limb apraxia. Based on these observations, orofacial apraxia has been considered a subtype of ideomotor apraxia. However, orofacial and limb apraxia are dissociable, suggesting that the neural systems underlying these two disorders are at least partially separable.

Verbal Apraxia

Verbal apraxia is mainly described as an inability to respond properly to verbal commands to make certain movements. It covers a wide range of problems all related to motor-driven language output, although, as we shall see, there are motor components to thinking where no language is produced.

Other Apraxia Conditions

Other apraxia conditions have been described. Admittedly, some of these may be alternative names for other conditions. They are included here because they have appeared in the literature.

Verbal–Motor Dissociation Apraxia

Individuals with the disorder fail to respond to verbal commands to make movements and, at the same time, demonstrate inability to copy a gesture or posture demonstrated by an examiner (visual input) or to execute a verbal command (auditory input), even though that person could copy the position in which the examiner placed their arm (Luzzi et al., 2010). This phenomenon has also been called dissociation apraxia and has also been referred to as disassociation apraxia. Dissociation is the preferred term. This disorder may be more involved with speech processing than motor performance (Wheaton & Hallet, 2007). This is an issue to which we will return as it directly relates to the discussion of developmental apraxia. There are things that look like movement disorders but may in fact not be.

Tactile Apraxia

Tactile apraxia is a selective disturbance of active touch. Hand skills not related to object exploration and manipulation are left intact. The disruption of function is not specific for tool use but affects any use of the hand as a sense organ (Binkofsky et al., 2001). Tactile apraxia represents a deficit in the programming of exploratory finger movement-mediated network component located in the parietal lobe. The comparison with lesions of other regions participating in the cortical network for tactile exploration reveals that apraxia of exploratory movements in parietal lobe lesions represents a disturbance distinct from elementary motor or sensory abnormalities.

Of note, given the general orientation of this book, in the haptic domain, a double dissociation can be proposed on the basis of neurological deficits between tactile information for action, represented by tactile apraxia, and tactile information for perception, represented by tactile agnosia. This dissociation comes from different networks, both involving the anterior intraparietal area of the posterior parietal cortex (Binkofsky et al., 2007). We mention this here only to highlight that disruption anywhere in a group of interconnected networks can produce a separate and potentially dissociable disruption of behavior that can look like apraxia.

Acquired Apraxia of Speech (AOS)

AOS (Whiteside et al., 2015) is a motor speech disorder that affects the implementation of articulatory gestures and the fluency and intelligibility of speech. In AOS speech output is impacted by a range of disturbances that affect intelligibility. Speech often appears effortful and under conscious control with a corresponding loss of automaticity in the production of speech. There is often evidence of initiation difficulties and articulatory groping. Groping involves visible preparatory and sometimes audible speech movements and gestures. The temporal components of speech may also be disrupted and features such as the voice onset time patterns of plosives can be disturbed. A plosive denotes a consonant that is produced by a coordinated stopping of airflow using the lips, teeth, or palate, which is then followed by a sudden release of air.

Other temporal dimensions of speech can also be affected, with output displaying longer intersyllabic pauses, prolonged segment, and syllable durations. Disrupted prosody is also manifested. Prosody is the patterns of stress and intonation in a language. Furthermore, in AOS, the spatiotemporal dimensions of speech are affected, and substitutions and distortions of articulatory targets are perceived as a result of misdirected gestures. Finally, in AOS, the overlap of articulatory gestures is reduced, resulting in lower levels of coarticulation.

AOS is an example of the wide range of dysfunction that is usually associated with apraxia conditions. We believe that historically, only one main target symptom was identified and other symptoms were minimized or ignored. This has led to constricted research in this area.

Newer Models of Speech Production

Newer models of speech production may go a long way in clarifying the nature of apraxia of speech (Van Der Merwe, 2020). At the current time, the complexity of motor aspects of speech, particularly motor control, and the incomplete conceptualization of phases in the transformation of the speech code from linguistic symbols to a code amenable to a motor system tend to obscure the understanding of acquired apraxia of speech (AOS). Van Der Merwe proposes a four-level framework (FLF) of speech sensorimotor control which infers a differentiation between speech motor planning, programming and execution, and locating the locus of disruption in AOS in the motor planning phase. This suggests that AOS can occur with a disruption of any one of these phases. As it stands now, terminological confusion and uncertainty regarding phases in speech motor control still complicate the characterization of AOS.

This four-level model differentiates two pre-execution phases and an execution phase. The first pre-execution phase is controlled by a motor planner and involves a reverse model, an efference copy, and a forward model for each sound or over learned utterance. This phase also involves a forward predictive planner which enables the system to handle the planning of several sounds and to plan coarticulation of sounds. The motor planner is operating on an auxiliary forward model architecture. AOS is hypothesized as a breakdown at several possible points in the motor planning phase. The second pre-execution phase is driven by a motor program generator and predictive controller that is governed by an integral forward model architecture. The final execution phase is portrayed as being driven by closed loop control. As we shall see, models such as this correlate well with neural network modeling and have a lot of diagnostic utility potential.

Childhood Apraxia of Speech

Childhood apraxia of speech (CAS) is a speech disorder, of presumed organic etiology, characterized by deficits in planning verbal motor function with poor consistency of oral-motor movements (Iuzzini, Inconsistency of Speech in Children with Childhood Apraxia of Speech, Phonological Disorders, and Typical Speech, 2012). In addition to the articulation and phonation problems, children with CAS are known to have a high cooccurrence of developmental coordination disorder (DCD). Affected children often have learning problems leading to various developmental problems including cognitive impairment. Children with CAS also have a higher risk of persistent reading and spelling disabilities, which in turn affects learning abilities such as writing or reading. These developmental problems can cause significant depression and anxiety, and they often have a low quality of life and lack self-satisfaction even in adulthood (Yun et al., 2021).

Most apraxia has known network areas which, when damaged, produce the apraxic condition. CAS does not. It appears as the child develops and there are no certain indicators. This fact and the rationale that there is a high overlap with developmental coordination disorder play an important part of the story we intend to tell in this book. Network disruptions are far reaching and long lasting in their implications. Understanding this will dramatically alter the way we diagnose and treat these problems.

It could be argued that there are as many apraxia conditions as there are specific motor dysfunctions. It could also be argued that there are as many apraxia conditions as there are potential network sites to be lesioned. Clearly a case can be made for either of these points of view. What is most accurate to say is that apraxia emanates from a disruption of the motor circuitry in conjunction with circuitry related to task-specific behavioral responses or to the motor components of human functioning. That means that there are a lot of possibilities. In addition, the same type of disrupted functioning can occur from damage to a number of structures that are part of the responsible networks. Different lesion sites produce the same apraxia. Does this situation have relevance for treatment or diagnosis? It might or might not. As it stands now, most treatment for apraxia involves practice of the desired skill with the hope of compensation and the creation of new network capacity. Clearly that's more difficult to expect in cases where the cause is genetic mutation as opposed to specific lesion.

Given the fact that the motor components of networks are involved with apraxia conditions, it is also likely that the sequelae of apraxia are far more reaching than just the obvious observed movement disorders. We will examine this aspect of apraxia in more detail.

Neuropsychological Models of Apraxia

Over the years there have been several attempts at developing neuropsychologically based models that describe apraxia. The following is a brief summary of some of the major conceptualizations.

Liepmann (1920) hypothesized that the representation of an action, or what he termed a space-time plan, is retained in whole form, in the left parietal lobe. In order to execute the action, the space-time plan is retrieved from memory, and, via the left premotor cortex, plan information is carried to primary motor areas. For example, for the left arm to perform an action, information crosses via the corpus callosum to the right premotor areas. According to Liepmann, for patients with ideomotor apraxia, motor representations and limb kinetics are intact. Their inability to act is due to the disruption of frontoparietal connections. Ideational apraxia was thought to result from disruption of action representations in the left parietal lobe and limb-kinetic apraxia from disruption of "kinesthetic-innervatory engrams" in the left frontal lobe.

Geschwind (1965) described apraxia of speech as a disconnection between motor and more posterior language areas. The disruption was hypothesized to involve the superior longitudinal fasciculus that connects Wernicke's area to the left frontal cortex. A lesion in this white matter pathway would compromise performance of actions elicited by verbal command but not affect comprehension. To account for impaired gesture imitation (which does not require intact language function) in patients with apraxia, Geschwind proposed that visual association areas and premotor cortex are connected via the same white matter tracts running between language and motor areas, but this theory remains controversial (Gross & Grossman, Update on Apraxia, 2008).

Dual-component models of apraxic conditions have been proposed. Heilman and Rothi (2003) hypothesized anterior execution-production and posterior conceptual-representational components. Knowledge and representations of objects and actions are believed to be stored in the left parietal lobe, specifically the angular gyrus and supramarginal gyrus, and then transformed into a signal by the premotor cortex (including the supplementary motor area). This signal is then used by motor cortex to carry out the action. According to the model, damage to anterior regions causes a gesture production deficit. Individuals with posterior apraxia typically have impaired movement production as well as difficulty with gesture comprehension and discrimination of well- versus ill-formed gestures.

Buxbaum et al. provide a model where the left inferior parietal lobe and frontoparietal information processing system is proposed (Buxbaum et al., 2007). According to this model, the inferior parietal lobe processes internal representations of movements and body part position. The frontoparietal processing system is responsible for spatial-motor transformation. Damage to this component results in "dynamic apraxia" due to disruption of the process by which gesture representations, having incorporated information about current and intended body part positions, are transformed into motor programs for action.

Research on multiple pathways involved in apraxia has grown. Areas of the parietal lobe have been identified that are involved in higher-order information processing and integration. For example, object use involves information processed by the ventral (occipitotemporal) and dorsal (parietooccipital) streams and that these two types of information are integrated by the inferior parietal lobe (Gross & Grossman, Update on Apraxia, 2008). In addition, Goldenberg and Hagmann (1997) found evidence for impaired manipulation or elaboration of gesture representations in patients with left angular gyrus lesions.

Gross and Grossman (2008) point out that the discovery of mirror neurons represents a significant advance in the understanding of how the brain processes action. Neuronal populations have been identified that are activated when an action is produced and when an individual observes that same action. They note that these findings may pose a challenge for models stipulating separate structures specialized for action execution versus action recognition or comprehension. They speculate that perhaps a new model would have to account for the dissociations between gesture production and reception seen in individuals with a variety of underlying neuropathologies. The mirror neuron system thus may have a substantial impact on how we understand the relation between expressive and receptive praxis and how these are integrated into a larger praxis network.

More recently, multiple pathway models have been proposed (Sperber et al., 2019). They identified multiple areas that underlie high-order motor control and participate in the various neural networks involved. These areas include inferior parietal lobule, precentral gyrus, posterior parts of the middle temporal cortex, and insula. Further, long association fibers were involved, such as the superior longitudinal fascicle, inferior and superior occipito-frontal fascicle, and uncinated fascicle. This data suggests multiple networks acting simultaneously to produce the complex disruption of behavior associated with apraxia.

Dual-Stream Models and Types of Apraxia

The idea that an apraxic condition can arise from disruption of one of several pathways enables us to distinguish different etiologic factors in apraxia. For example, the dual-stream hypothesis (Goodale & Milner, 1992) has been used to explain separate categories of disruption depending on the neural network properties of the information flow. According to this model, ideational apraxia is thought to relate to a deficit in the concept of a movement (coded in the ventral stream). These patients have difficulty using objects, sequencing actions to interact with them or pantomiming their use. On the other hand, ideomotor apraxia is thought to arise from problems in the accurate implementation of movements within the dorsal stream. Extending on the knowledge, Rounis and Humpreys (2015) developed the affordance competition hypothesis as a way to explain certain apraxic conditions. They note that one of the limitations in understanding apraxia is the failure by the clinical literature to draw on knowledge of the factors determining actions in the environment. The cited work indicates that responses to stimuli are strongly influenced by the actions that the objects "afford," based on their physical properties and the intentions of the actor. The concept of affordance postulates that interactive behavior arises by a process of competition between possible actions elicited by the environment. "Affordance competition" plays a role in apraxia in that at least some aspects of apraxia may reflect an abnormal sensitivity to competition when multiple affordances are present and/or a poor ability to exert cognitive control over this competition occurs. We note that this model coincides nicely with the valuation and behavioral economic modeling we identify as an essential feature of neural network operation (Wasserman & Wasserman, 2019, 2020).

References

American Speech Hearing Association (ASHA). (2021). *Childhood apraxia of speech*. Retrieved from ASHA / Practice Portal / Clinical Topics /. https://www.asha.org/practice-portal/clinical-topics/childhood-apraxia-of-speech/

Bangert, M., Peschel, T., Schlaug, G., Rotte, M., Drescher, D., Hinrichs, H., et al. (2006). Shared networks for auditory and motor processing in professional pianists: Evidence from fMRI conjunction. *Neuroimage, 30*, 917–926.

Barbieiri, C., & De Renzi, E. (1984). THE Executive and ideational Components of Apraxia. Cortex, (1988) 24, 535–542.

Bieńkiewicz, M., Brandi, M. G., Hughes, C., & Hermsdörfer, J. (2014, April 23). The tool in the brain: Apraxia in ADL. Behavioral and neurological correlates of apraxia in daily living. *Frontiers in Psycholology*. https://doi.org/10.3389/fpsyg.2014.00353, online.

Binkofsky, F., Kunesch, E., Classen, J., Seitz, R., & Freund, H. (2001). Tactile apraxia: Unimodal apractic disorder of tactile object exploration associated with parietal lobe lesions. *Rain, 124*(1), 132–144. https://doi.org/10.1093/brain/124.1.132

Blank, R. b.-E. (2019). International clinical pactice guidelines on the definition, diagnosis, assessment, intervention, and psychosocial aspecs of developmental coordination disorder. Developmental Medicine and Child Neurology, 242–285. https://doi.org/10.1111/dmcn.14132

Buxbaum, L., Kyle, K., Grossman, M., & C. H. (2007). Left inferior parietal representations for skilled hand-object interactions: evidence from stroke and corticobasal degeneration. *Cortex, 43*, 411–423.

Cassidy, A. (2016). The clinical assessment of apraxia. *Practical Neurology, 16*, 317–322.

Davis, B., Jakielski, K., & Marquardt, T. (1998). Developmental apraxia of speech: Determiners of differential diagnosis. *Clinical Linguistics & Phonetics, 12*, 25–45. https://doi.org/10.3109/02699209808985211

De Renzi, E., & Faglioni, P. (1999). Apraxia. In G. Denes & L. Pizzamiglio (Eds.), *Handbook of clinical and experimental psychiatry*. Psychology Press. https://doi.org/10.4324/9781315791272

De Renzi, E., Faglioni, P., & Sorgato, P. (1982). Modality specific and supramodal mechanisms of apraxia. *Brain, 105*, 301–312.

Diehl, E. (2022). Dyspraxia vs. Apraxia. Retrieved from Study.com: https://study.com/academy/lesson/dyspraxia-vs-apraxia.html

Foki, T., Vanbellingen, C. T., Pirker, A. L., Bohlhalter, S., Nyffeler, T., Kraemmer, J., et al. (2016). Limb-kinetic apraxia affects activities of daily living in Parkinson's disease: A multi-center study. *European Journal of Neurology, 23*(8), 1301–1307. https://doi.org/10.1111/ene.13021

Gainotti, G., & Trojano, L. (2018). Chapter 16 - Constructional apraxia. In G. Vallar & H. Coslett (Eds.), *Handbook of clinical neurology* (Vol. 151, pp. 331–348). Elsevier. https://doi.org/10.1016/B978-0-444-63622-5.00016-4

Geschwind, N. (1965). Disconnexion syndromes in animals and man. Brain Disconnexion syndromes in animals and man, 237–294, 585–644.

Goldenberg, G., & Hagmann, S. (1997). The meaning of meaningless gestures: a study of visuo-imitative apraxia. *Neuropsychologia, 35*, 333–341.

Gonzales-Rothi, L., & Heilman, K. (1996). Liepmann (1900 and 1905): A definition of apraxia and a model of praxis. In C. Code, Y. Joanette, A. Roch-Lecours, & C. Wallesch (Eds.), *Classic cases in neuropsychology*. Psychology Press.

Goodale, M. A., & Milner, D. (1992). Seaparate visual pathways for perception and vision. *Trends in Neuroscience 15*, 20–25. https://doi.org/10.1016/0166-2236(92)90344-8

Gross, R., & Grossman, M. (2008). Update on apraxia. *Current Neurology and Neuroscience Reports, 8*(6), 490–496. https://doi.org/10.1007/s11910-008-0078-y

Hamilton, J., Haaland, K., Adair, J., & Brandt, J. (2003). Ideomotor limb apraxia in Huntington's disease: Implications for corticostriate involvement. *Neuropsychologia, 41*, 614–621.

Heilman, K., & Rothi, L. (2003). Apraxia. In K. Heilman, & E. Valenstein, Clinical Neuropsychology (pp. 215–235.). New York: Oxford University Press.

Iuzzini, J. (2012). *Inconsistency of speech in children with childhood apraxia of speech, phonological disorders and typical speech*. Indiana University ProQuest Dissertations Publishing.

Kirby, A. S. (2007). Children with developmental coordination disorders. *Journal of the Royal Society of Medicine*, 182–186.

Liepmann, S., & Mass, O. (1907). Fall von linksseitiger Agraphie und Apraxie bei rechtsseitiger Lahmung. *Journal of Psychology and Neurology, 10*, 14.

Luzzi, S., Piccirilli, M., Pessalacia, M., Fabi, K., & Provincialia, L. (2010). Dissociation apraxia secondary to right premotor stroke. *Neuropsychologia, 48*(1), 68–76. https://doi.org/10.1016/j.neuropsychologia.2009.08.010

Malkani, R., & Zadikoff, C. (2011). The apraxias in movement disorders. In N. Galvaez-Jimenez, P. Tuite, & K. Bhatia (Eds.), *Uncommon causes of movement disorders* (pp. 35–45). Cambridge University Press.

Mayo Clinic. (2022). Childhood apraxia of speech. Retrieved from Mayo Clinic: https://www.mayoclinic.org/diseases-conditions/childhood-apraxia-of-speech/diagnosis-treatment/drc-20352051

Morgan, A., & Webster, R. (2018). Aetiology of childhood apraxia of speech: A clinical practice update for paediatricians. *Journal of Paediatrics and Child Health, 54*, 1090–1095. https://doi.org/10.1111/jpc.14150

NORD. (2021). *Ocular Motor Apraxia, Cogan Type*. Retrieved from National Organization of Rare Disorders. https://rarediseases.org/rare-diseases/ocular-motor-apraxia-cogan-type/

Ochipa, C., Rothi, L. J., & Heilman, K. M. (1992). Conceptual apraxia in Alzheimer's disease. *Brain, 115*(Pt 4), 1061–1071.

Ogar, J., Slama, H., Dronkers, N., Amici, S., & Gorno-Tempini, M. (2005). Apraxia of speech: An overview. *Neurocase, 11*, 427–432. https://doi.org/10.1080/13554790500263529

Pazzaglia, M., Pizzamiglio, L., Pes, E., & Aglioti, S. (2008). The sound of actions in apraxia. *Current Biology, 18*(22), 1766–1772. https://doi.org/10.1016/j.cub.2008.09.061

Pearce, J. (2009). Hugo Karl Liepmann and apraxia. *Clinical Medicine*, 466–470.

Rothi, L., & Heilman, K. (1997). Apraxia: The Neuropsychology of Action. Hove, UK: Psychology Press.

Rounis, E., & Humpreys, G. (2015). Limb apraxia and the "affordance competition hypothesis". Frontiers Human. *Neuroscience, 28*, online, https://doi.org/10.3389/fnhum.2015.00429

Shriberg, L., Kwiatkowskil, J., & Mabie, H. (2019). Estimates of the prevalence of motor speech disorders in children with idiopathic speech delay. *Clinical Linguistics & Phonetics, 33*, 679–706. https://doi.org/10.1080/02699206.2019.1595731

Sperber, C., Weisen, D., Goldenberg, G., & Karnath, H. (2019). The network underlying human higher-order motor control: Insights from machine learning-based lesion-behaviour mapping inApraxia. Tübingen, Germany: bioRxiv https://doi.org/10.1101/536391

Tarsy, D. (2012). *Movement disorders: A video atlas*. Humana Press.

Tettamanti, M., Buccino, G., Saccuman, M., Gallese, V., Danna, M., Scifo, P., et al. (2005). Listening to action-related sentences activates fronto-parietal motor circuits. *Journal of Cognitive Neuroscience, 17*, 273–281.

The Medical Dictionary. (2021). *Apraxia*. Retrieved from The Medical Dictionary. http://the-medical-dictionary.com/apraxia_article_2.htm

Tse, M. (2012). Double duty of tail caudate nucleus neurons. *Nature Reviews Neuroscience, 13*, 11005–11016. https://doi.org/10.1038/nrn3342

Van Der Merwe, A. (2020). New perspectives on speech motor planning and programming in the context of the four- level model and its implications for understanding the pathophysiology underlying apraxia of speech and other motor speech disorders. Aphasiology, online, https://doi.org/10.1080/02687038.2020.1765306

Wasserman, T., & Wasserman, L. D. (2019). Therapy and the Neural Network Model. Wsitzerland: Springer.

Wasserman, T. W. (2020). Motivation, Effort and the Neural Network Model. Switzerland: Springer.

Watson, R., & Heilman, K. (1983). Callosal apraxia. *Brain, 106*(2), 391–403. https://doi.org/10.1093/brain/106.2.391

Wheaton, L., & Hallet, M. (2007). Ideomotor apraxia: A review. *Journal of the Neurological Sciences, 260*, 1–8. https://doi.org/10.1016/j.jns.2007.04.014

Whiteside, S., Dyson, L., Cowell, P., & Varley, R. (2015). The relationship between apraxia of speech and oral apraxia: Association or dissociation? *Archives of Clinical Neuropsychology, 30*(7), 670–682. https://doi.org/10.1093/arclin/acv051

WHO, W. H. (1992). World Health Organization Classification of Mental and Behavioural Disorders: Clinical Descriptions and Diagnostic Guidelines. Geneva.

Yun, J., Shin, S., & Son, S. (2021). Clinical utility of repeated urimal test of articulation and phonation for patients with childhood apraxia of speech. *Children, 8*(12), 1–7. https://doi.org/10.3390/children8121106

Zadikoff, C. L., & Lang, A. (2005). Apraxia in movement disorders. *Brain, 128*(7), 1480–1497. https://doi.org/10.1093/brain/awh560

Chapter 2
The Etiology of Apraxia

Apraxia can be caused by congenital or idiopathic means, by trauma such as stroke, as part of a neurodevelopmental disorder or associated with a neurodegenerative disorder. Left hemispheric brain damage caused by ischemic or hemorrhagic stroke is the most frequent neurological correlate of apraxia. Apraxia conditions can be also observed in numerous neurodegenerative disorders such as Parkinson's disease, Alzheimer's disease, or posterior cortical atrophy. Apraxic behavior is also known or occur as an effect of trauma such as anoxia and infection such as herpes encephalitis (Bieńkiewicz et al., 2014).

Thus, the etiology of apraxia can be understood as either network insult (stroke, penetrating wound, head injury, etc.) or genetic and related constitutional factors. Research has demonstrated that more than 33 percent of left hemispheric stroke patients in rehabilitation centers present some form of apraxia (Donkervoort & Deelman, 2000). Stroke or other brain injuries are the most frequent causes of apraxia of speech (Duffy, 2012). On face value it might seem that childhood apraxia of speech (not to be confused with apraxia of speech) would be the almost sole occupant of the genetic category, while almost every other apraxia would inhabit the insult category. To an extent that statement remains largely accurate, although not entirely so. As noted, apraxia also co-occurs with a number of genetically based neurodegenerative disorders although the frequency of apraxia in these genetic conditions is much lower than that of the brain insult category. These disorders produce numerous symptoms related to the degradation of the neural network. Among those symptoms are often apraxia. When movement disorders co-occur with known genetic movement disorder etiology, they are frequently labeled something other than apraxia.

What is true for movement disorders in general is also true of apraxia of speech. As it currently stands, the most current and widely accepted defining clinical features of apraxia of speech (AOS) are still not associated with any specific etiology. That being said, stroke is the most frequent cause of AOS and the most frequent

T. Wasserman, L. D. Wasserman, *Apraxia: The Neural Network Model*,
Neural Network Model: Applications and Implications,
https://doi.org/10.1007/978-3-031-24105-5_2

etiology reported in the vast majority of historic and recently published studies from which its diagnostic criteria have evolved (Duffy, 2012), Among nondegenerative etiologies, stroke is also more likely to induce AOS in a predominant or "pure" form, without the "contaminating" cognitive deficits or other motor speech disorders induced by diffuse or multifocal conditions such as infection or trauma.

Genetically Based Apraxia

Another useful distinction occurs when confronting apraxic conditions that arise in isolation, free of comorbidity from those apraxic conditions that occur because of some general neurodegenerative process or disease. Looking at these disorders might provide crucial details regarding the network components of many apraxic conditions. In this chapter we will look at the known etiologies of apraxia and discuss the network implications.

Non-stroke-Related Progressive Apraxia of Speech

It has been recognized that AOS can be caused by neurodegenerative conditions that emerge insidiously and progress slowly. In some cases, AOS is the only, or the most prominent, indicator of neurodegenerative disease, or, in the alternative, it is the major communication disorder when it coexists with primary progressive aphasia.

Progressive apraxia of speech (PAOS) is a neurodegenerative syndrome affecting spoken communication (Josephs et al., 2021). It was first described in 1967 (Darley, 1967) as a motor speech disorder characterized by varying combinations of slow speaking rate, abnormal prosody, speech sound simplifications, distorted sound substitutions, additions, repetitions, prolongations as well as segmentations between syllables and words, and groping and trial-and-error articulatory movements.

Stroke-related AOS is generally described as improving over time and will be discussed in a separate section. In the past three decades, a subtype of AOS has been identified that is very subtle in onset and progressive in nature (Deramecourt, 2010). This progressive AOS (PAOS) is frequently associated with progressive agrammatic aphasia (Ogar et al., 2007) (AOS-PAA) or occurs as a feature of a more widespread neurodegenerative syndrome, such as corticobasal syndrome (CBS) or amyotrophic lateral sclerosis. The term primary progressive apraxia of speech (PPAOS) was later developed to describe PAOS in the absence of aphasia and not embedded as a feature of a larger neurodegenerative syndrome (Duffy, 2006). The syndrome of PPAOS was later more fully characterized and shown to relate to degeneration of a network of regions that include the lateral premotor cortex and supplementary motor area (SMA) (Josephs et al., 2012). The prevalence of PAOS, which encompasses PPAOS, has been estimated to be about 4.4 per 100,000 individuals.

Two types of PAOS have been described (Josephs, 2014). Type 1, the phonetic subtype, is characterized by a predominance of articulatory distortions, distorted sound substitutions or additions, and articulatory groping. This is the subtype that is similar to what has been reported in patients with stroke. The second, type 2, the prosodic subtype, is characterized by a predominance of slow speech rate and segmentation within multi-syllabic words or across words. Type 2 has not been described in stroke patients and was not previously formally identified. Features supporting the validity of PAOS subtypes include the phonetic subtype being associated with a significantly younger age at onset and more likely accompanied by moderate to severe aphasia than the prosodic subtype. In fact, the literature describing PAOS accompanying aphasia, or AOS embedded in the context of a neurodegenerative syndrome, almost always reveals characteristics consistent with phonetic AOS. Structurally, PAOS subtypes involve degeneration of the lateral premotor and SMA, although the phonetic subtype appears to be more strongly linked to neocortex while the prosodic subtype has been linked to noncortical regions, such as the superior cerebellar peduncle (Utianski et al., 2018).

Research (Josephs et al., 2021) clearly indicates a genetic etiology for both PAOS subtypes. PAOS is most often associated with a 4R tauopathy when it exists in isolation or when it co-exists with aphasia. Four-repeat (4R-) tauopathies are a group of neurodegenerative diseases The spectrum of tauopathy encompasses heterogenous group of neurodegenerative disorders characterized by neural or glial deposition of pathological protein tau. Clinically they can present as cognitive syndromes, movement disorders, or motor neuron disease (Ganguly & Jog, 2020). On the contrary, when AOS accompanies behavioral dyscontrol, executive dysfunction, or features of motor neuron disease, the underlying pathology is heterogeneous, less commonly 4R tau, and may be related to a mutation in the GRN gene.

For our discussion here the point is that there is a heterogeneous group of hypothesized genetic disorders that produce these conditions. The disease leaves a discernable footprint in terms of tau deposition on white matter and the result is apraxia that on one hand replicates what is usually seen in brain injured patients and on the other hand is unique. These are serious degenerative disorders and cause progressive dysfunction which makes them very different from what is understood to be general apraxia. The disorders impact white matter functionality and resulting neural network operation.

In 1952, Cogan (1952) described an apraxia wherein the person was unable to initiate voluntary horizontal saccades. Head thrusts were utilized to facilitate the necessary ocular refixation. He termed this ocular motor apraxia (OMA). OMA may be congenital or acquired and idiopathic or associated with structural brain-based abnormalities (such as cerebellar hypoplasia or agenesis of the corpus callosum). In a study by Marr et al. (2005), a retrospective review of 34 children with OMA was conducted. The OMA was categorized into four categories outlined above. For three of the five children with acquired OMA, the impact was transitory and the conditions were resolved. For the other two children, progressive deterioration over time was noted. Twenty-nine children were diagnosed with congenital OMA. Fourteen of these children were diagnosed with isolated/idiopathic OMA (normal birth and early history). Of the 14 children with congenital OMA without associated abnormalities, all the children were found to have motor, language, educational, and/or behavioral problems. Fifteen of the twenty-nine children with congenital OMA were found to have associated abnormalities including seven with structural abnormalities, six with perinatal insult, and two with a neurodegenerative disorder. The most frequent finding was cerebellar hypoplasia. Historically, non-idiopathic OMA was associated with neurodevelopmental disorders, and so risk factors are associated with the underlying disorder, whereas children with idiopathic OMA were considered to carry a limited neurological risk prognosis. The current study, in contrast, concluded that for most, cerebellar involvement will be found. Additionally, irrespective of labeled domain, all groups run a substantial risk of neurodevelopmental disorders.

Advances in genetics have allowed for greater demarcation of some disorders. Oculomotor apraxia mapped to chromosome 2p13 is a dominant genetic trait. In this case, only a single copy of an abnormal gene, that is, from either the mother or the father, is necessary to cause the emergence of the disease.

Ataxia with ocular motor apraxia type 1 (AOA1) associated with cerebellar ataxia is an autosomal recessive cerebellar ataxia (ARCA) associated with oculomotor apraxia, hypoalbuminemia, and hypercholesterolemia. The gene *APTX*, which encodes aprataxin, has been identified (Le Ber et al., 2003). Apraxic dysfunction occurs in the vast majority, but not all, of affected individuals. This is one of a number of disorders which have apraxic dysfunction associated with it.

A related condition, ataxia with oculomotor apraxia type 2 (AOA2), is a relatively recently described autosomal recessive cerebellar ataxia (ARCA) defined by genetic location to 9q34. It is characterized by onset between the age of 10 and 22 years, cerebellar atrophy, peripheral neuropathy, and oculomotor apraxia. The original research described just six families sharing gait ataxia, oculomotor apraxia, and/or elevated α-foetoprotein (AFP) levels (Le Ber et al., 2004). Again, not all families with the genetic disruption produce an apraxia, so the exact nature of the process remains undetected. However, if Marr et al.'s (2005) data are predictive, undetected does not mean without consequence.

Apraxia Associated with Neurodevelopmental Disorders

Looking at white matter implications of neurodegenerative disease can provide a model to understand how a condition such as childhood apraxia might develop and help understand how specific damage to white matter produces apraxia.

One such disorder is Friedreich ataxia (FRDA). It is the most common autosomal recessive neurodegenerative disease among Europeans and people of European descent. Friedreich ataxia is characterized by an early onset (usually before the age of 25), progressive ataxia, sensory loss, absence of tendon reflexes, and pyramidal weakness of the legs (Date et al., 2001). It is linked to chromosome 9p13. Ocular motor apraxia is often associated with this disorder. In FRDA, the proprioceptive system appears to be affected early, with reduced number of dorsal root ganglion (DRG) cells mediating proprioception and of their large, myelinated axons in peripheral nerves, dorsal roots, and dorsal columns of the spinal cord. At the same time, the dorsal spinocerebellar tracts, relaying proprioceptive information to the cerebellum, are affected. Somewhat later in the disease, the dentate nucleus of the cerebellum and, to some degree, the corticospinal tracts degenerate.

Ataxia oculomotor apraxia-1 (AOA1) is a neurological disorder caused by mutations in the gene (APTX) encoding aprataxin (Ahel et al., 2006). It is also the apraxia most often associated with FRDA. As such, the white matter pathways would be the same. It is important to note that cases of oculomotor apraxia have been caused by both stroke and tumor although the foci of damage would arguably be the same.

Motor neuron disease (MND) is a neurodegenerative disease that typically affects the upper motor neuron (UMN) and lower motor neuron (LMN) systems, with subsequent symptoms and signs of spasticity and flaccid weakness. It usually begins with limb involvement, but in about one quarter of cases, dysarthria is its first manifestation. Its most serious representative disorder is amyotrophic lateral sclerosis (ALS) (Duffy et al., 2007). Apraxic symptomology usually involves poor initiation of speech or stuttering as part of the overall clinical picture.

Moebius syndrome is a rare congenital disorder that results from underdevelopment of the facial nerves that control some of the eye movements and facial expressions. The condition can also affect the nerves responsible for speech, chewing, and swallowing. Related symptoms can include severe congenital hypotonia, facial diplegia, jaw ankylosis, velopharyngeal incoordination, pyramidal tract signs, and ocular motor apraxia. Research demonstrates neuronal depletion of the IV, VII, VIII, and IX cranial nerve nuclei and intact morphology of the cerebral hemispheres. If the 7th nerve is involved, an individual with Moebius syndrome is unable to smile, frown, pucker the lips, raise the eyebrows, or close the eyelids. If the 6th nerve is affected, the eye cannot turn outward past the midline. Other abnormalities include underdevelopment of the pectoral muscles and defects of the limbs. When ocular motor apraxia is present, most of the nerve disruption occurs in the brain stem (Roig et al., 2003). A genetic etiology is suspected but not clearly established.

Childhood Apraxia of Speech (CAS)

The vast majority of cases of childhood apraxia of speech remain of uncertain etiology. There are, however, recently identified genetic anomalies that have been shown to produce the condition (Morgan & Webster, 2018). Among these are the following.

FOXP2/7q31.1 Deletion

FOXP2 was the first gene implicated in the absence of frank neurological lesion, intellectual impairment, or other overt neurodevelopmental conditions. There are de novo and inherited forms of the heterozygous FOXP2 mutations pathogenic for CAS. Both have been reported. Individuals with the underlying genetic alteration of "FOXP2-only" typically have a spared nonverbal intelligence compared to verbal intelligence, appropriate social abilities, and typical fine and gross motor skills. This being said mild cognitive impairment, mild motor impairments, autistic features (but not a formal autism spectrum disorder (ASD) diagnosis), and even mild dysmorphology (e.g., narrow palpebral fissures, mild finger pads, horizontal eyebrows, large ears) have recently been reported in some cases with FOXP2-only mutations. By contrast, individuals with FOXP2-plus genetic aberrations are more likely to have global developmental and behavioral issues with oral-motor deficits, global developmental delay, and ASD in addition to CAS. These additional phenotypes may relate to disruptions of other genes neighboring FOXP2 in that region of chromosome 7.

GRIN2A

GRIN2A has been long associated with speech and language disorders, particularly aphasia. Recently, mutations or very small deletions in GRIN2A have been identified in patients with both focal epilepsy and speech and language dysfunction (Carvill et al., 2013). In CAS, dysarthria and oral-motor impairments have been consistently reported across families regardless of the associated form of epilepsy. The speech phenotype may also occur in the absence of a seizure disorder, implying an important role for GRIN2A in speech-motor function or CAS.

SETBP1

Chromosomal deletions and truncating mutations in SETBP1 are associated with loss-of-function mutations with impaired expressive speech, relatively intact receptive language abilities, decreased fine motor skills, hyperactivity/ADHD, autistic traits, and subtle dysmorphism (Coe et al., 2014). The phenotype has been expanded to specify broader neurodevelopmental phenotypes in children seen with childhood apraxia of speech.

Microdeletions of BCL11A

Microdeletions of BCL11A have been reported in association with CAS, dysarthria, hypotonia, and general oral and gross motor dyspraxia. Associated features include intellectual disability (ID) with related poor expressive language, growth retardation, ASD, craniofacial and skeletal dysmorphic traits, internal organ defects, abnormal muscle tone, and gross motor delays.

KANSL1 or 17q21.31 Microdeletion Koolen-De Vries Syndrome (KdVS)

This is a rare multi-system disorder associated with developmental delay, ID, hypotonia, and facial dysmorphism. Speech development is impaired for children with KdVS, particularly early in the developmental course. Early history includes hypotonia, feeding difficulties, and delayed onset of first words, occurring between 2.5 and 3.5 years of age (Morgan & Webster, 2018). Almost all children with KdVS receive a diagnosis of CAS, which is often comorbid with dysarthria and additional articulation and phonological errors.

ELKS/ERC1 and 12p13.33 Deletion

This is a very rare deletion with a hypothetical relationship to CAS. Affected children display delayed first words (36–42 months), delayed walking, and prominent ear lobes. The primary study identified nine children with the deletion, five of which displayed CAS (Thevenon et al. 2013). To presage a later discussion, the children also demonstrated neurodevelopmental disorders beyond speech and language, including intellectual impairment (5/9), psychiatric manifestations (5/9), behavioral difficulties (7/9), ADHD (6/9), and ASD (2/9).

16p11.2 Deletion

The 16p11.2 is a relatively common deletion of about 1 in 5000 individuals. It can occur either de novo or in inherited variants. Associated features include moderate ID, ASD, poor cognitive and language ability, epilepsy, and macrocephaly. Other brain abnormalities such as Chiari type 1 malformations or cerebellar ectopia have been identified. Research have also confirmed the high penetrance of CAS in children with this deletion (Mei et al. 2018). Of note, other speech profiles have also been reported in 16p11.2 deletion in addition to CAS, including articulation and phonological disorders, dysarthria, and minimal verbal output.

Corticobasal Degeneration (CBD)

Ideomotor apraxia occurs in corticobasal degeneration (CBD), a neurodegenerative condition described as an asymmetric akinetic-rigid syndrome with cortical features such as apraxia as well as the alien-limb phenomenon and cortical sensory loss. Murray et al. (2015) showed that 40% of studied CBD patients had apraxia at disease onset, and 72% had apraxia at the time of death. Patients had predominantly ideomotor limb apraxia, and fewer exhibited orofacial apraxia. CBD is characterized by atrophy and decreased metabolism in the network of frontal, parietal, and basal ganglia structures thought to underlie apraxic conditions (Gross & Grossman, 2008).

In addition to CBD, apraxia is also a component of various movement disorders, Parkinson's disease (Soliveri et al., 2005), progressive supranuclear palsy (Soliveri et al., 2005), and Huntington's disease (Hamilton et al., 2003), All of these disorders compromise the basal ganglia. Proposed contributions of the basal ganglia to praxis include sequencing, fine tuning of movements, selection of competing motor programs, and performance of automatic or overlearned movements (Gross & Grossman, 2008). Interestingly, it is not clear that basal ganglia-specific dysfunction causes significant apraxia. Most cases of apraxia also involve the surrounding white matter tracts and frontoparietal cortex.

There is a syndrome of parkinsonism and prominent apraxia which have been designated as "corticobasal syndrome" (CBS). CBS may be occurring in a variety of other central nervous system pathologies including progressive supranuclear palsy (PSP), Alzheimer's disease, dementia with Lewy bodies, and frontotemporal dementias (Zadikof & Lang, 2005). In patients with left hemispheric stroke, for example, apraxia has been reported to be prevalent in approximately one-third of this population (Park, 2017).

Distinct from the CBS, Parkinson's disease can also demonstrate degrees of apraxia on selected tasks, especially in those patients whose cognitive functioning is also severely compromised. Diseases that cause the combination of apraxia and a primary movement disorder most often involve a variety of cerebral cortical sites as well as basal ganglia structures. Clinical-pathological correlates and functional imaging studies are confounded by both this diffuse involvement and the confusion experienced in the clinical evaluation of apraxia in the face of the additional elemental movement disorders. As far as a clear understanding of the apraxic elements of these disorders, it should be recalled that the definition of apraxia specifies that the disturbance of performed skilled movements cannot be explained by the more elemental motor disorders typical of patients with movement disorders. In many instances, this does not present a significant diagnostic problem when dealing with "higher-level" apraxic disturbances (e.g., ideational apraxia), but it can be a major confound in establishing the presence of limb-kinetic apraxia. The great majority of motor disturbances characteristic of extrapyramidal disorders, particularly bradykinesia and dystonia, will compromise the ability to establish the presence of loss of dexterity and deftness that constitutes this subtype. The term "apraxia" has also been applied to other motor disturbances, such as "gait apraxia" and "apraxia of eyelid opening," which, while clearly associated with parkinsonism, are perhaps misnomers (Zadikof & Lang, 2005). This situation again demonstrates the lack of a coherent nomenclature in this field, a situation we will review in detail later.

The above is not an exhaustive review. The sections and examples are presented to make the point that apraxia, or apraxia-like behavior, can and does occur when the white matter that controls related motor movement is disrupted. Any disorder that disturbs the related white matter has the potential to produce an apraxic condition. Of note, this same functional disorder, apraxia, may occur in a child born with a congenital disorder, resulting in damage to the child's central nervous system, as well as to the adult with a degenerative disorder, such as dementia. It leaves open the possibility that one day the term apraxia, as a free-standing diagnosis, will be unnecessary as we will understand all of the neurophysiological causes of the various movement disorders.

References

Ahel, I., Rass, U., El-Khamisy, S., Katyal, S., Celements, P., Mckinnon, P., et al. (2006). The neurodegenerative disease protein aprataxin resolves abortive DNA ligation intermediates. *Nature, 443|12*, 713-716. https://doi.org/10.1038/nature05164

Bieńkiewicz, M., Brandi, M. G., Hughes, C., & Hermsdörfer, J. (2014, April 23). The tool in the brain: Apraxia in ADL. Behavioral and neurological correlates of apraxia in daily living. *Frontiers in Psycholology.* https://doi.org/10.3389/fpsyg.2014.00353, online.

Carvill, G., et al. (2013) GRIN2A mutations cause epilepsy-aphasia spectrum disorders. *Nature Genetics, 45*, 1073–1076. https://doi.org/10.1038/ng.2727

Coe, B., Witherspoon, K., Rosenfeld, J., et al. (2014). Refining analyses of copy number variation identifies specific genes associated with developmental delay. *Nature Genetics, 46*, 1053–1017.

Cogan, D. (1952). A type of congenital ocular motor apraxia presenting jerky head movements. *Transactions of the American Academy of Ophthalmology and Otolaryngology, 56*, 579–588.

Darley, F. (1967). Lacunae and research approaches to them. In C. Miliken & F. Darley (Eds.), *Brain mechanisms underlying speech and language*. Grune & Stratton.

Date, H., et al. (2001). Early-onset ataxia with ocular motor apraxia and hypoalbuminemia is caused by mutations in a new HIT superfamily gene. *Nature Genetics, 29*, 184–188. https://doi.org/10.1038/ng1001-184

Deramecourt, V. (2010). Prediction of pathology in primary progressive language and speech disorders. *Neurology, 74*, 42–49.

Donkervoort, M.-S., & Deelman, B. (2000). Prevalence of apraxia among patients with a first left hemisphere stroke in rehabilitation centres and nursing homes. *Clinical Rehabilitation, 14*(2), 130–136.

Duffy, J. (2006). Apraxia of speech in degenerative neurologic disease. *Aphasiology, 20*, 511–527.

Duffy, J. R., Peach, R. K., & Strand, E. A. (2007). Progressive apraxia of speech as a sign of motor neuron disease. *American Journal of Speech and Language Pathology 16*, 198–298.

Duffy, J. J. (2012). The diagnosis and understanding of apraxia of speech: Why including neurodegenerative etiologies may be important. *Journal of Speech, Language and Hearing Research, 55*(5), S1518–S1522. https://doi.org/10.1044/1092-4388(2012/11-0309)

Ganguly, J., & Jog, M. (2020). Tauopathy and movement disorders—unveiling the chameleons and mimics. *Frontiers in Neurology: Movement Disorders, 11*, 599384. https://doi.org/10.3389/fneur.2020.599384

Gross, R., & Grossman, M. (2008). Update on apraxia. *Current Neurology and Neuroscience Reports, 8*(6), 490–496. https://doi.org/10.1007/s11910-008-0078-y
Hamilton, J., Haaland, K., Adair, J., & Brandt, J. (2003). Ideomotor limb apraxia in Huntington's disease: Implications for corticostriate involvement. *Neuropsychologia, 41*, 614–621.
Josephs, K. A., et al. (2012). Characterizing a neurodegenerative syndrome: primary progressive apraxia of speech. *Brain, 135*, 1522–1536.
Josephs, K. A. (2014). The evolution of primary progressive apraxia of speech. *Brain, 137*, 2783–2795.
Josephs, K., Duffy, J., & Whirwell, J., et al. (2021). A molecular pathology, neurobiology, biochemical, genetic and neuroimaging study of progressive apraxia of speech. *Nature Communications, 12*, 3452. https://doi.org/10.1038/s41467-021-23687-8
Le Ber, I., et al. (2003). Cerebellar ataxia with oculomotor apraxia type 1: clinical and genetic studies. *Brain, 126*(12), 2761–2772. https://doi.org/10.1093/brain/awg283
Le Ber, I., et al. (2004) Frequency and phenotypic spectrum of ataxia with oculomotor apraxia 2: a clinical and genetic study in 18 patients *Brain 127*(Pt 4), 759–767. https://doi.org/10.1093/brain/awh080. Epub 2004 Jan 21.
Marr, J., et al. (2005). Neurodevelopmental implications of ocular motor apraxia. Developmental Medicine. https://doi.org/10.1111/j.1469-8749.2005.tb01086.x
Mei, S., Montanari, A., Nguyen, P. (2018). A mean field view of the landscapre of two layer neural networks PNAS https://doi.org/10.1073/pnas.1806579115
Murray, E., McCabe, P., & Ballard, K. J. (2015). A randomized controlled trial for children with childhood apraxia of speech comparing Rapid Syllable Transition treatment and the Nuffield. *Journal of Speech, Language, and Hearing Research, 58*, 669–686. https://doi.org/5810.1044/2015_JSLHR-S-13-0179
Morgan, A., & Webster, R. (2018). Aetiology of childhood apraxia of speech: A clinical practice. *Journal of Paediatrics and Child Health, 54*, 1090–1095. https://doi.org/10.1111/jpc.14150
Ogar, J. M., Dronkers, N. F., Brambati, S. M., Miller, B. L., & Gorno-Tempini, M. L. (2007). Progressive nonfluent aphasia and its characteristic motor speech deficits. *Alzheimer Disease and Associated Disorders, 21*, 523–530.
Park, J. (2017). Apraxia: Review and update. *Journal of Clinical Neurology, 13*(4), 317–324. https://doi.org/10.3988/jcn.2017.13.4.317
Roig, M., Gratacòs, M., Vazquez, E., del Toro, M., Foguet, A., Ferrer, I., & Macaya, A. (2003). Brainstem dysgenesis: Report of five patients with congenital hypotonia, multiple cranial nerve involvement and ocular motor apraxia. *Developmental Medicine & Child Neurology, 45*, 489–493.
Soliveri, P., Piacentini, S., & Girotti, F. (2005). Limb apraxia in corticobasal degeneration and progressive supranuclear palsy. *Neurology, 64*, 448–453.
Thevenon, J., et al. (2013). Higher risk of death among MEN1 patients with mutations in the JunD interacting domain: a Groupe d'étude des Tumeurs Endocrines (GTE) cohort study. *Human Molecular Genetics, 22*(10), 1940–1948. https://doi.org/10.1093/hmg/ddt039
Utianski, R. L., et al. (2018). Prosodic and phonetic subtypes of primary progressive apraxia of speech. *Brain and Language, 184*, 54–65.
Zadikof, C., & Lang, A. (2005). Apraxia in movement disorders. *Brain, 128*(7), 1480–1497. https://doi.org/10.1093/brain/awh560

Chapter 3
The Human Connectome: An Overview

Before we get into the specifics of brain connectivity and apraxia, it is probably useful to provide an overview of the playing field. The human brain is frequently referred to as the most intricate object in the world, if not the universe. The brain is a network of nerve cells, regions, interconnected regions, and systems whose interconnections remain largely unmapped. Indeed, exploration of how these neural interconnections are established has only fairly recently begun. To understand how these networks are connected, it is critically important to understand how neural elements exchange signals and influence each other dynamically, encode statistical regularities present in the sensory environment, coordinate movement and behavior, retain traces of the past, and predict future outcomes (Sporns, 2013). This task is further complicated by the fact that these networks are, in many ways, unique to each human being in terms of mapping their functional properties. While it is true that the physiology and biochemistry of their operation are the same, the neural components of each individual's network is to some extent idiosyncratic. For example, it is accurate to say that both Broca's and Wernicke's areas are involved in human speech. How they are associated with each other and to other recruited network components varies slightly from person to person.

Therefore, to understand the functioning of this network, it is important to understand its elements and their interconnections. To understand the foundation of a neural network, it is absolutely essential to understand the concept of the human connectome (Sporns et al., The human connectome: A structural description of the human brain, 2005). Conceptualizing the connectome allows one to better conceptualize the complexities of the multitude of potential associations between regions of the brain and, by extension, their functional output.

T. Wasserman, L. D. Wasserman, *Apraxia: The Neural Network Model*,
Neural Network Model: Applications and Implications,
https://doi.org/10.1007/978-3-031-24105-5_3

The Connectome and Neural Networks

As a point of both interest and clarification, the term neural network comes from the work on artificial intelligence where networks are created to mimic the functioning of the human brain. The concept is most helpful when considering research. It is a term we generally now use to refer to the human brain proper as well.

A human neural network is composed of a group of chemically connected or functionally associated neurons. A single neuron may be connected to many other neurons, and the total number of neurons and connections in a network may be extensive. Connections, called synapses, are usually formed from axons to dendrites, though dendrodendritic synapses and other connections are possible. The reason that these neurons are connected to each other is to allow the brain to plan and carry out behaviors designed to reach goals.

Neural network models assume that neural circuit function arises from the activation of groups or ensembles of neurons. According to these models, these ensembles generate emergent functional states that, by definition, cannot be identified by studying one neuron at a time. In fact, it is thought that the brain, unlike other body organs, could be specifically built to generate emergent functional states (Yuste, 2015).

The term "neural network" refers to models of distributed neural circuits in which neurons are abstracted into nodes and linked by connections that change through learning rules. Typically, neurons in neural networks are connected in an all-to-all or a random fashion and integrate inputs linearly, leading to a threshold nonlinearity that causes the cell to fire and activates its outputs.

The term "connectome" was defined by Sporns et al. (2005) as a "comprehensive structural description of the network of elements and connections forming the human brain." Sporns et al. called for a compilation of the connectome based upon structural and functional mapping. The idea of "connectomic maps" was introduced by Jeff Lichtman et al. also in 2005 (Sporns, 2013) wherein these connectivity maps were defined as "connectivity maps in which multiple, or even all, neuronal connections are rendered." Clearly, the notion was centered on recognizing the importance of understanding the structure and function of the human brain. At its core, the human connectome is still largely hypothetical in its comprehensive map of all of the neural connections in the human brain. Conceptually, it represents what is a "wiring diagram" of the brain's organization. Fundamentally, the human brain/nervous system is made up of neurons which communicate through synapses. A connectome map is constructed by tracing the neuron in a nervous system and mapping where neurons are connected through synapses. A connectome model of a human brain remains a hypothetical construct because each human brain, while following general principles of physiological connectivity, establishes these connections idiosyncratically. No two human brains are "wired" in exactly the same fashion. Human brains accomplish the same function across the population, but how they do that is accomplished by a unique connectome for each human being (Sato et al., 2021). The combinations and patterns of various brain structures and their connections exhibit significant variations between individuals, at every level of organization. These individual variations can be due to genetic differences, others the result of developmental and experiential history, gender differences, pathologies, or responses to injury. Incorporating individual variations and developmental stages is absolutely crucial in understanding the connectome in operation.

The Importance of Understanding the Connectome

Understanding how the connectome is organized leads to critical understanding about how information, stimuli, and emotions are processed by the system it represents. This understanding is critically important because the significance of the connectome stems from the knowledge that the structures and functions of the human brain are intricately linked, through multiple levels and hubs of brain connectivity. There are, of course, strong natural constraints on which neurons or neural populations can interact, or how strong or direct their interactions are. A connectome model posits that the foundation of human cognition lies in the pattern of dynamic interactions shaped by the connectome. This is not a direct linear relationship.

The emphasis on structure as the foundation of connectomics is important for several reasons. Perhaps most importantly, the actual structure of the brain represents a true baseline. This is because these anatomical connections, whether they are individual synapses or interregional pathways, define a large but finite set of relations among neural components that can be objectively verified and reliably mapped. That is because anatomical connections either exist or don't.

This anatomical certainty stands in sharp contrast to functional connections that describe the operation and outcome of the systems operation. By and large these outcomes are described as statistical dependencies derived from observations of behaviors. These behaviors can be the firing of a single neuron or a complex sequence of behaviors. The most functional connections demonstrate significant temporal fluctuations, may or may not disclose true causal relations between neural elements, and are highly dependent on measurement and analysis technique (Sporns, 2013). This is compounded by the fact that, for complex behaviors at a minimum, the outcome can be obtained by similar but not identical networks that interconnect the same brain regions using different neural connection maps.

Hubs

Essentially, network modeling of brain function implies that all domains of cognitive function require the integration of distributed neural activity. As part of this model, analysis of human brain network connectivity has regularly identified sets of regions that are vitally important for supporting efficient neuronal signaling and communication. The central embedding of these candidate regions or "brain hubs" in anatomical networks supports their diverse functional roles across a broad range of cognitive tasks and widespread dynamic coupling within and across functional networks. The essential core of brain hubs also implies that they are points of vulnerability that are susceptible to disconnection and dysfunction in brain disorders such as apraxia (van den Heuvel & Sporns, 2013).

Several different types of hubs have been described. Connector hubs filter and route information between brain regions. They coordinate and integrate the flow of data so that brain networks dedicated to specific roles, such as vision and movement, can focus on their jobs while at the same time integrate with other networks to develop complex functional behaviors. More than two dozen connector hubs have been identified. These play a key role in complex cognitive tasks and are also vulnerable to brain damage and dysfunction. Provincial hubs facilitate coordinated action within a specific region of the brain. They facilitate a subset of skills such a visual or processing (Sporns et al., 2007). There are many more of these hubs distributed throughout the brain.

Networks and Connectomics

Numerous studies have reported on the relation of synaptic connectivity in neuronal circuits and observed patterns in neural dynamics, especially the correlations observed in large neuronal populations (Sporns, 2013). Similar research has demonstrated a strong and robust relationship between large-scale patterns of long-distance connections between brain regions and their functional connectivity. It is clear that these white matter systems are the "highways" along which information travels between areas of the brain responsible for different behavioral components of coordinated and complex action. Data indicate that the presence and strength of a structural connection partially predicted the strength of a functional connection between various brain nodes (Honey et al., 2009). This same line of research also demonstrated strong network connectivity between certain brains nodes that did not appear functionally connected. This implies that there are, in place, potential brain resources for future connectivity should the situation arises. This also suggests that merely identifying connectivity patterns will not clearly establish functional properties of a specific brain. What remains clear is that anatomic architecture conditions do not determine the functional neural network dynamic. The functional connectivity of a human brain cannot be explained only considering the anatomical substrate (Batista-García-Ramó & Fernández-Verdecia, 2018). More specifically, anatomic architecture determines, but not strictly, network dynamics, meaning that part of functional connectivity cannot be explained by considering only anatomical connectivity. Other factors are at work.

Scaling

Sporns (2013) discussed the idea of scaling. It is the idea that many complex systems are themselves composed of subscales. "This mode of organization implies that the system can be partially decomposed into coherent functional components at different spatial scales" (Sporn, 2013). When discussing brain behavior functional relationships, this implies that there can be hypothetically almost and unlimited amount of subcomponent scales that contribute to a complex behavior, each impacted by degeneracy and plasticity. This can extend down from a functional network to a component consisting of one neuron. "Consider, for example, a full description of the human cerebral cortex at cellular or system levels. Given current best estimates for the number of neurons and number of synaptic connections (on the order of 1010–1011 and 1014–1015, respectively), the microscale connectome map would be extremely sparse: fewer than one in a million (less than one ten thousandth of a percent) of all possible synaptic connections actually exist. However, at system scale tracing and imaging studies of structural anatomy of regions and their projections suggest that around 20–40% of all interregional pathways (and possibly up to 60%; can be found" (Sporns, 2013, pg. 56). This issue of scale is closely associated with the problem of "node definition" which is essential for understanding networks from human imaging data derived from either diffusion or fMRI data. Based upon small world hub models, node definition is critical for defining a network's basic elements. Research has shown that topological features of networks revealed by graph theory methods sensitively depend on how the brain is broken down or parcellated into components.

Degeneracy

Degeneracy (Edelman & Gally, 2001) has been defined as the ability of elements that are structurally different to perform the same function or yield the same output. Degeneracy means "many to one" in that many combinations of neurons can produce the same outcome. A high degree of degeneracy, as is the case with many outcomes of complex cognitive operations, makes it difficult to detect consistent underlying structure to function relations. Therefore, the wiring diagram of individual exemplars of neural circuits would not be sufficient for "reading out" or decoding how it actually functions. There are exceptions to this principle, for example, the more primitive and basic "always on" neural networks" display remarkable anatomical consistency.

It is important to note that the differences in wiring connectivity can and do produce sometimes subtle and sometimes significant differences in the functional properties of the outcome behaviors (Baldassare et al., 2012)

Structural Plasticity

All molecular and cellular components of the nervous system are being continually remodeled, replaced, resynthesized, and reconfigured. This of course includes all structural elements of the human connectome. These structural changes are underpinned by numerous mechanisms, from synaptic modifications to neuronal growth and structural plasticity, operating not only during early development but across the life span. Research suggests that the structural arrangement of neuronal circuits, including their connection topology, can undergo significant and rapid alterations in the adult brain on a regular basis (Holtmaat & Svoboda, 2009). There is a multiplicity of forces that cause these changes, most significantly the person's interaction with and feedback from the environment. Even essentially similar networks at the beginning of life will demonstrate considerable degeneracy as the individual's life experiences diverge. The chapters on childhood apraxia of speech and motor coordination disorder provide an understanding of the significant implications when considering the impact of developmental apraxia on the development of the child. It is one of the many reasons that developmental apraxia cannot be understood utilizing an adult "damage" model. In the damage model, the already developed functional system is disrupted. Therefore, that impact may be mitigated. In the developmental situation, that functional system has not yet developed, is not developing appropriately, and through its aberrant development will disrupt all downstream operations dependent upon it.

Neurons grow and extend out to connect to other neurons, thereby establishing connections. One neuron can connect to many other neurons should the *necessity* arise. This is called neuroplasticity. Neuroplasticity allows new connections to be created or areas to move and change function. The same neuron can participate in several different functions. This is particularly true of motor neurons, which participate in most cognitive functions (Koziol et al., 2012). Synapses may strengthen or weaken based on their importance. The adage neurons that fire together, wire together may not be totally accurate but nevertheless represent the idea that neurons involved in the completion of a particular task will have connections that strengthen. Learning involves building on information that is already stored in the brain. As our knowledge deepens by repetition and during sleep, tasks that once required a focus can be executed automatically once mastered. Humans rely on this automaticity for much of their everyday functioning.

Challenges to Understanding the Connectome

Conceptualizing the human connectome faces two unique significant challenges. First, the human brain is a highly complex organ with a great number of structurally distinct, heterogeneous components. As discussed, these components are interconnected in a generally similar, yet idiosyncratic pattern. Conceptually, the connectome is a structural substrate for understanding the basis of human cognitive function. Each connectome is unique and brain areas of importance are interconnected in slightly different ways, rendering the making of an authoritative, static reference map impossible.

In addition to the individualized white matter connectivity patterns, human brains demonstrate structural variability in mass and volume. Folding patterns of cortical surfaces, and the absolute and relative sizes of brain regions and projections, have all been shown to differ across individuals. It is still unclear how these differences affect connectivity and function as they are influenced by individual differences, age, gender, environmental influences, and sometimes pathologies.

A second challenge is that basic structural elements of the human brain, in terms of network nodes and connections, are difficult to define and standardize. Different kinds of structural descriptions could target at least three rather distinct levels of organization ranging from single neurons and synapses (microscale) to the level of anatomically distinct brain regions and interregional pathways (macroscale). Between these two levels is the level of neuronal groups or populations (mesoscale) (Sporns et al., The human connectome: A structural description of the human brain, 2005). Moving forward, understanding how these levels interact with each other will be essential for understanding how a network model informs our understanding of human cognitive and emotional functioning (Wasserman & Wasserman, 2017, 2019a, b).

The Relationship of Connectome to Clinical Diagnosis

Much of what modern psychiatry and psychology do is to attempt to understand how our developed model of psychopathology conforms to the operation of this network. We make a diagnosis based on behavioral clusters and then make connectome-based hypotheses concerning their etiology. The neurotransmitter models of depression and obsessive-compulsive disorder are examples of this practice. For example, as we have written about (Wasserman & Wasserman, 2016), much of the current behaviorally based understanding and classification of human psychopathology do not conform to the operation of the human connectome. A recent finding (Moncrieff, 2022) invalidate the long-held belief that depression was the result of serotonin abnormalities, specifically low levels. This can be problematic as demonstrated by the facts that prescriptions for antidepressants have risen dramatically in the past three decades with people being administered a medication under the belief that it speaks to the etiology of their disorder. In fact, it does not. When it comes to apraxia, the parallel is largely the same. While it is accurate to say that in the case of stroke an area of connectomic disruption can readily be identified, there are apraxias, childhood apraxia of speech being the primary example, where no specific connectomic disruption has been identified and alternate areas of disruption may cause the same functional outcome. As we shall see, even in the case of the acquired apraxia, the connectomic implications are often overlooked.

The study of developmental apraxia, specifically, offers unique insight into the relationship between the properties of the connectome and the development of disorders related to it. It illuminates a feedforward model of the effects of development/aberrant development on the connectome. Research suggests that damage to topologically central brain regions is associated with widespread effects on network function. The functional impact of these effects will vary depending on the topological role of the affected region. For example, dysfunction of provincial hubs is expected to produce specific deficits, whereas dysfunction of connector hubs is proposed to impair multiple behavioral domains. As we shall see, this finding has significant implications for the development of children with developmental apraxia.

The sequelae of dysfunctional neural pathway operation are rarely confined to a single locus. Rather, they often spread via axonal pathways to influence other regions that share the operational network pathway. Patterns of such disordered development are, to a degree, constrained by the extraordinarily complex, yet highly organized, topology of the underlying neural architecture. Thus, network organization fundamentally influences brain disease, and a connectomic approach grounded in network science is integral to understanding neuropathology (Fornito et al., 2015). This necessity can be easily conceptualized when considering disorders such as schizophrenia, attention-deficit disorder, autism, and diseases such as Huntington's and dementias (Fig. 3.1).

Neural Response to the Disruption of Pathway Function

In line with our discussion, we think it bears mentioning that a disruption at any level of network integrity could produce a disruption of complex, integrated, function, such as is experienced in apraxia. While the functional outcome disruption could look the same, the underlying connectome causes could be very different. We believe that these connectome differences, although potentially producing functional disorders which on the surface appear indistinct, actually do produce distinct and dissociable disorders, each with its own unique sequelae and associated comorbidities. There are several reasons for this belief, even when only considering acquired apraxia. Disruption of functional outcomes can be understood by identifying and understanding the various responses of the brain to a traumatic event and how neural network topology constrains these responses. Knowledge of these processes can inform our understanding of the impact of brain injury on the developing constellation of problems associated in acquired apraxia.

Diaschisis

Diaschisis is a temporary interruption of function in an interconnected region that is remote from an injured site. Diaschisis is now a well-established phenomenon, particularly following stroke. It has been observed in the forebrain after damage to the

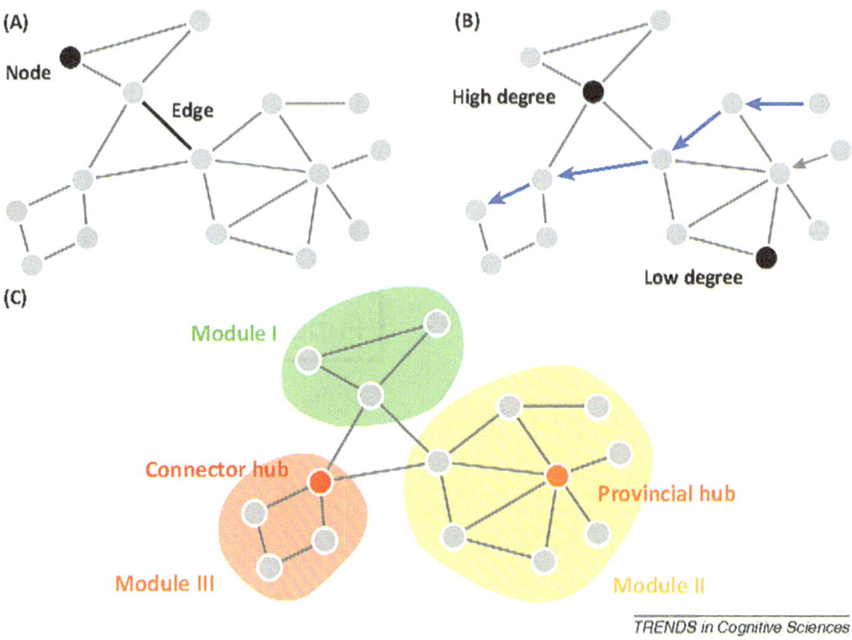

Fig. 3.1 Basic network attributes. (**a**) Brain networks can be described and analyzed as graphs comprising a collection of nodes (describing neurons/brain regions) and a collection of edges (describing structural connections or functional relationships). The arrangement of nodes and edges defines the topological organization of the network. (**b**) A path corresponds to a sequence of unique edges that are crossed when traveling between two nodes in the network. Low-degree nodes are nodes that have a relatively low number of edges; high-degree nodes (often referred to as hubs) are nodes that have a relatively high number of edges. (**c**) A module includes a subset of nodes of the network that show a relatively high level of within-module connectivity and a relatively low level of intermodule connectivity. "Provincial hubs" are high-degree nodes that primarily connect to nodes in the same module. "Connector hubs" are high-degree nodes that show a diverse connectivity profile by connecting to several different modules within the network (van den Heuvel & Sporns, 2013)

brainstem or cerebellum, in cortical regions following subcortical infarction, and in contralesional cortex following focal cortical insult (Fornito et al., 2015; Rehme & Grefkes, 2012). These distributed changes seem to be circuit specific. Brain modeling has indicated that highly specific lesions can have a diffuse effect on interregional synchronization dynamics that extend well beyond the impacted site and in a way that critically depends on the connection topology of the damaged region (Honey & Sporns, 2008). Research suggests that the severity of behavioral dysfunction that follows focal neural damage often correlates with the extent of activation and connectivity changes in regions remote from the site of the lesion. These associations between behavior and altered network functional connectivity occur even if anatomical connectivity between damaged and undamaged regions is intact (van

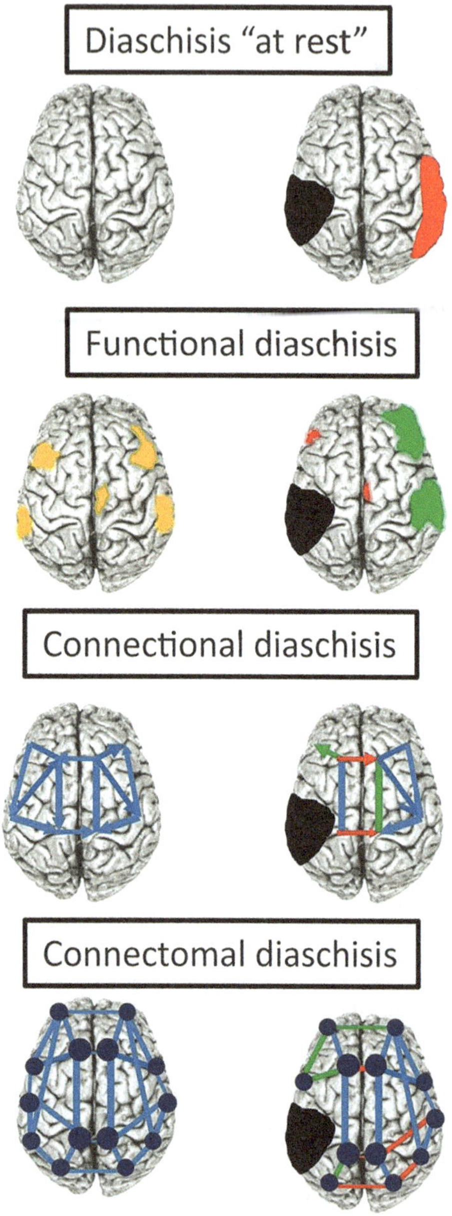

Fig. 3.2 Types of diaschisis. Types of diaschisis before (*left*) and after (*right*) a focal brain lesion (black). Diaschisis at rest: a focal lesion induces a remote reduction of metabolism (red). Functional diaschisis: normal brain activations (yellow) during a selected task may be altered, either increased (green) or decreased (red) after a lesion. Connectional diaschisis: distant strengths and directions of connections in a selected network may be increased (green) or decreased (red). Connectomal diaschisis: a lesion of the connectome induces widespread changes in brain network organization including decrease (red) or increase (green) in connectivity (Carrera & Tononi, 2014, https://doi.org/10.1093/brain/awu101)

Meer et al., 2010). This finding implies that a "functional deafferentation" of remote sites may be sufficient to impair behavior. Nonetheless, damage to anatomical pathways linking the lesioned area to unaffected regions seems to compound the severity of behavioral impairment (He et al. 2007) (Fig. 3.2).

All of this would, of course, imply associated dysfunction related to acquired apraxia. One mechanism identified with such a possibility is the research suggesting functional depression of the cerebellum which, in turn, causes reduced excitatory drive from the damaged cerebellum to associated down/upstream networks (Gold & Lauritzen, 2002).

Transneuronal Degeneration

While diaschisis is an interruption of function in a region that is remote from a lesion, it is presumed that that region remains intact and undamaged. It is a connectivity problem. Transneuronal degeneration represents actual structural deterioration of regions downstream from the area of initial insult. This damage occurs over time. Transneuronal degeneration can be either anterograde (damage or dysfunction of one neuron causes the degeneration of its postsynaptic target) or retrograde (a presynaptic neuron deteriorates because of reduced trophic support from an injured or necrotic postsynaptic target). The form of degeneration can vary and encompasses changes such as neuronal shrinkage, reductions in dendrite and synapse number, alterations of axonal myelin content and fiber number, and neuronal death. Both anterograde and retrograde degeneration have been identified in numerous neural circuits (Fornito et al., 2015).

Several mechanisms can cause transneuronal degeneration. Pathology in any single area can disrupt interactions with other regions, causing irregular firing and metabolic stress in the connected site (Saxena & Caroni, 2011). Degeneration of remote regions may also result from diminished excitatory input or a loss of trophic support from damaged presynaptic neurons.

Dedifferentiation

Dedifferentiation is the widespread, nonspecific recruitment of unnecessary brain regions to perform a task. It occurs as a result from a breakdown of usually specialized and segregated neural activity and is associated with aberrant neural plasticity or by a focal cortical pathology that disrupts the balance between excitation and inhibition within a specific neural system. Persistence of a dedifferentiated state is associated with poorer recovery of motor function following stroke (Fornito et al., 2015).

All of the above provide clear theoretical possibilities for the idea that acquired apraxia (of speech) is probably not only a speech dysfunction but is also related to other impairments in associated motor driven networks. This clarity is absent for developmental apraxia because there is no clear evidence of specifically damaged networks. We will discuss the implications of this dichotomy in some detail later on.

There are some important properties of these networks that have implications for the study of apraxia. For example, in neural network models, action is an emergent collective property, carried out by the assembly of neurons rather than by single cells. Individual neurons can participate in different functional groups, flexibly reorganizing themselves. This flexibility is a natural consequence of synaptic plasticity, and it also allows the modular composition of small assemblies into larger ones. Because of this flexibility, neural circuits may never be able to be in the same functional state twice, responding slightly differently even if the exact same sensory stimulus is presented. Many of these circuits are task dependent and created in the moment. They "cease to exist" as soon as the task is completed. They, of course, can be recreated if the same or similar task arises again, although the components, at the neuronal level, are likely never exactly the same.

The Neural Networks of Apraxia

The motor-based praxis system is comprised of component functions associated with particular brain regions and related structures. The brain regions work together to process action. This network of structures underlying praxis includes the frontal and parietal cortex, basal ganglia, and white matter tracts containing projections between these areas (Gross & Grossman, 2008). Indeed, white matter-based dysconnectivity between brain regions has recently been identified in gesture difficulty related to limb apraxia (Rosenzopf et al., 2022). They found pathological white matter alterations in a densely connected fronto-temporo-parietal network of short and long association fibers. This indicated involvement of middle and superior temporal lobe disconnection, including temporo-temporal short association fibers suggesting strong involvement of the temporal lobe in the praxis network.

The basal ganglia also play an essential role in praxis, via connections with frontal and parietal cortices (Zadikoff, 2005). Specific functions of the basal ganglia related to praxis include sequencing, fine tuning of movements, selection of competing motor programs, and performance of automatic or overlearned movements. It is important to note that isolated basal ganglia dysfunction by itself does not seem to cause significant apraxia. Most apraxias also involve surrounding white matter tracts and frontoparietal cortex.

Apraxia represents a disruption of a complex behavior, and as a result praxis depends on a complex, large-scale network of structures recruited collectively to accomplish the desired task. Imaging studies involving connectivity analysis revealed two coherent circuits: one involving the parietal cortex, supplementary motor area, and motor cortex and the other involving the parietal, lateral premotor, and motor areas involved in many apraxic conditions (Wheaton et al., 2005).

All of the above has significant implications for the study of apraxia. A complex output such as speech is dependent on multiple networks and their subserving networks. Many of these networks are involved in the product of other complex behaviors. Motor networks are involved in most human activities. Damage to a motor network would have implications far in excess of one particular outcome. Clinically speaking, this implies that if the clinician "sees" apraxia, it is very, very likely that there will be comorbid conditions that are directed related to, and caused by, the disruption causing the apraxia.

All of this indicates that while we may be able to understand how connectivity and network properties of the human brain contribute to the problems associated with apraxia, we will never be able to, on a case-by-case basis, identify how a specific connectivity problem causes a particular individual to manifest apraxia. This statement is probably much truer for those children with development apraxia as compared to those adults that demonstrate apraxia secondary to a traumatic brain insult. We will explore the implications of this hypothesis in some detail later. Suffice it to say here that, as we have indicated, the nature of dysfunction in the developing network would have significantly greater impact on a multiplicity of systems and behaviors that rely upon a typical and uninterrupted developmental progression. Simply stated, we would expect a far wider range of disrupted and dysfunctional behavior associated with developmental apraxia.

We can no longer think that a person that has apraxia just has apraxia. Damage anywhere in the complex integration of networks that produce an outcome has the possibility of impacting the production of the outcome. We can no longer be sure that we know where the lesion is by knowing what is not working. Damage to the same area of a network can produce a different pattern of comorbidities depending on the pattern of connectivity unique to that individual.

References

Baldassare, A., Lewis, C., Committeri, G., Romani, G. L., & Corbetta, M. (2012). Individual variability in functional connectivity predicts performance of a perceptual task. *Proceedings of the National Academy of Sciences of the United States of America, 109*, 3516–3521.

Batista-García-Ramó, K., & Fernández-Verdecia, C. (2018). What we know about the brain structure–function relationship. *Behavioral Science, 8*(39), 1–14. https://doi.org/10.3390/bs8040039

Carrera, E., & Tononi, D. (2014). Diaschisis: Past, present, future. *Brain, 137*(9), 2408–2422. https://doi.org/10.1093/brain/awu101

Edelman, G., & Gally, J. (2001). Degeneracy and complexity in biological systems. *Proceedings of the National Academy of Sciences of the United States of America, 98*(24), 13763–13768.

Fornito, A., Zalesky, A., & Breakspear, M. (2015). The connectomics of brain disorders. *Nature Reviews Neuroscience, 16*, 150–172.

Gold, L., & Lauritzen, M. N. (2002). Neuronal deactivisation explains decreased cerebellar blood flow in response to focal cerebral ischemia or suppressed neocortical function. *Proceedings of the National Academy of Sciences of the United States of America, 99*, 7699–7704.

Gross, R., & Grossman, M. (2008). Update on apraxia. *Current Neurology and Neuroscience Reports, 8*(6), 490–496. https://doi.org/10.1007/s11910-008-0078-y

He, B. J. (2007). Breakdown of functional connectivity in frontoparietal networks underlies behavioral deficits in spatial neglect. *Neuron, 53*, 905–918.

Holtmaat, A., & Svoboda, K. (2009). Experience-dependent structural synaptic plasticity in the mammalian brain. *National Review Neuroscience, 10*, 647–658.

Honey, C. J., & Sporns, O. (2008). Dynamical consequences of lesions in cortical networks. *Human Brain Mapping, 29*, 802–809.
Honey, C., Sporns, O., Cammoun, G. X., Thiran, J., et al. (2009). Predicting human resting-state functional connectivity from structural connectivity. *Proceedings of the National Academy of Sciences of the United States of America, 106*, 2035–2040.
Koziol, L., Budding, D., & Chidekel, D. (2012). From movement to thought: Executive function, embodied cognition, and the cerebellum. *Cerebellum, 11*(2), 505–525. https://doi.org/10.1007/s12311-011-0321-y
Moncrieff, J. C. (2022). The serotonin theory of depression: A systematic umbrella review of the evidence. *Molecular Psychiatry*. https://doi.org/10.1038/s41380-022-01661-0
Rehme, A. K., & Grefkes, C. (2012). Cerebral network disorders after stroke: Evidence from imaging-based connectivity analyses of active and resting brain states in humans. *Journal of Physiology, 591*, 17–51
Rosenzopf, H., Wiesen, D., Basilakos, A., Yourganov, G., Bonilha, L., Fridriksson, J., . . . Sperber, C. (2022). Mapping the human praxis network: An investigation of white matter disconnection in limb apraxia of gesture production Brain Communications 4 (1) https://doi.org/10.1093/braincomms/fcac004, 1–14.
Sato, J., Biazoli, C. E., Zugman, A., Pan, P., Bueno, A., Moura, L., & Affon, R. (2021). Long-term stability of the cortical volumetric profile and the functional human connectome throughout childhood and adolescence. *European Journal of Neuroscience*, 6187–6201. https://doi.org/10.1111/ejn.15435
Saxena, S., & Caroni, P. (2011). Selective neuronal vulnerability in neurodegenerative diseases: From stressor thresholds to degeneration. *Neuron, 71*, 35–48.
Sporns, O. (2013). The human connectome: Origins and challenges. *NeuroImage, 80*, 53–61. https://doi.org/10.1016/j.neuroimage.2013.03.023
Sporns, O., Tononi, G., & Kötter, R. (2005). The human connectome: A structural description of the human brain. *PLoS Computational Biology*. https://doi.org/10.1371/journal.pcbi.0010042
Sporns, O., Honey, C., & Kotter, R. (2007). Identification and classification of hubs in brain networks. *PLoS ONE, 2*(10), e1049. https://doi.org/10.1371/journal.pone.0001049
van den Heuvel, M., & Sporns, O. (2013). Network hubs in the human brain. *Trends in Cognitive Sciences, 17*(12), 683–696. https://doi.org/10.1016/j.tics.2013.09.012
van Meer, M. P., et al. (2010). Recovery of sensorimotor function after experimental stroke correlates with restoration of resting-state interhemispheric functional connectivity. *Journal of Neuroscience, 30*, 3964–3972.
Wasserman, T., & Wasserman, L. (2016). *Depathologizing psychopathology*. Springer.
Wasserman, T., & Wasserman, L. (2017). *Neurocognitive learning therapy: Theory and practice*. Springer.
Wasserman, T., & Wasserman, L. (2019a). *Neural networks series, therapy*. Springer.
Wasserman, T., & Wasserman, L. (2019b). *Therapy and the neural network model*. Springer.
Wheaton, L., Nolte, G., Bohlhalter, S., et al. (2005). Synchronization of parietal and premotor areas during preparation and execution of praxis hand movements. *Clinical Neurophysiology*, 1382–1390.
Yuste, R. (2015). From the neuron doctrine to neural networks. *Nature Reviews Neuroscience, 16*, 1-11. https://doi.org/10.1038/nrn3962
Zadikoff, C. L. (2005). Apraxia in movement disorders. *Brain*, 1480–1497.

Chapter 4
Neuronal Populations, Neural Nodes, and Apraxia

Population coding is a method to represent signals by the joint activities of a number of neurons. In population coding, each neuron has a distribution of responses over some set of inputs, and the responses of many neurons may be combined to determine the value about the inputs. Biologically, the idea of neuronal populations references nodes within a network that are connected to multiple other nodes. We are going to look at this level of brain organization, nodes, in detail because understanding this modeling is important in understanding the potentially far-reaching consequences of any one of a number of apraxia conditions (Fig. 4.1).

An important thing to remember is that any one node may participate in an almost unlimited number of specific networks. This is particularly true to nodes involved in motor activity. Since each of these population centers participates in multiple types of motor responses, damage to any one of them affects all of the downstream activities emanating from them. This implies that an individual with apraxia will experience potentially numerous disruptions in behavior related to the area of neuronal population that is dysfunctional. The resultant disrupted behavior will not only be the "apraxic" motor movement" that originally brought the individual to clinical attention but other impacted behaviors anywhere along the motor circuit as well. This disruption, by association, can also lead to disruption of cognitive functions.

Apraxia and Neural Pathways

Historically, researchers have ascribed independent encoding functions to the activity of single neurons (Evarts, 1868) or groups of neurons (Humphrey & Thompson, 1970). Research reflective of this line of thinking searched for correlations between

T. Wasserman, L. D. Wasserman, *Apraxia: The Neural Network Model*,
Neural Network Model: Applications and Implications,
https://doi.org/10.1007/978-3-031-24105-5_4

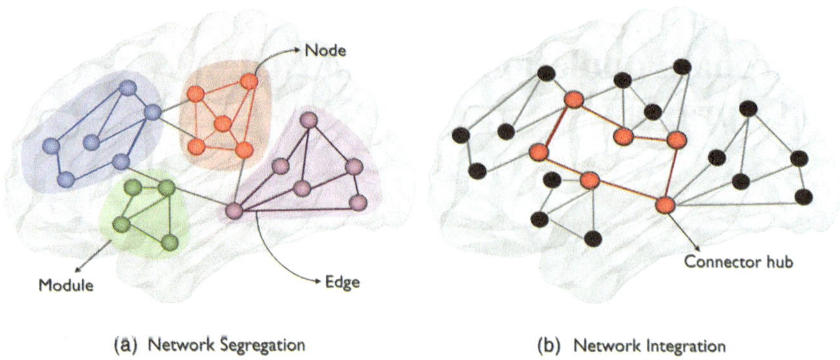

Fig. 4.1 Neural nodes. In the context of brain networks in this study, every anatomical region of interest is a node, whereas the connection between nodes is termed as an edge. (Handiru et al., 2021)

specific neural activity and specific movement parameters. The belief was that neural activity would encode particular parameters in a consistent and highly predictable manner. There were some problems with this logic. For example, research demonstrated considerable variability in the activity patterns across neurons (Churchland & Shenoy, 2007) and instability of movement parameter encoding by single neurons across different conditions (Scott & Kalaska, 1997).

More recent research has not been based on the independent modulation of single neurons but rather activities performed at the population level by networks of interconnected neurons. This is likely to be the place to look when considering the etiology of many apraxia conditions.

Populations of cortical neurons flexibly perform different functions; for the primary motor cortex (M1), this means they are involved in a rich repertoire of motor behaviors (Gallego et al., 2018). While each specific motor-involved task requires different patterns of muscle and single unit activity, there are considerable similarities at the neural population level among the areas involved for different tasks. In sum, research has demonstrated that the structure and activity of the neural nodes are largely preserved across tasks.

What Is the Neural Population Level?

The brain contains many millions of neurons that are organized in different brain areas. Within any specific brain area are different subregions. Each of these subregions is composed of different layers and inside each layer are various cell types.

The neuron doctrine (Yuste, 2015) held that the neuron was the structural and functional unit of the nervous system. However, multineuronal recording methods have now revealed that it ensembles of neurons, rather than individual cells, which can form physiological units which serve to generate emergent functional properties and states. This new paradigm creates neural network models which potentially better understand how emergent functional states generate behavior and cognition. By extension, this understanding of normal development and function can also then be applied to understanding disease and the results of trauma.

While much research then has historically focused on the operation of a single neuron, these populations of neurons, at the subregion level (neuronal populations), have characteristic properties that are derived from their working collaboratively. Theory suggests a relationship between neuron responses and psychophysical decisions which may prove useful for identifying cell populations underlying specific perceptual capacities (Zohary et al., 1994). That allows for modeling that includes the unique response properties of these specific populations.

For example, rather than looking at the response time of a single neuron which belongs to a certain cell class at a certain level, a number of questions might be reasonably asked. So, for example, supposing a human brain receives a certain type of stimulus, what is the activity of all the cells in a particular layer of the subregion processing the response? What is the activity of the population class of cells in that layer of the subregion? Finally, what is the response of this subregion as a whole? This of course leads to the question, what is the response of a brain area? In other words, at any of the scales of spatial resolution, it is productive to look at the response of the neuronal population as a whole rather than the activities of an individual neuron (Gerstner et al., 2014) (Fig. 4.2).

Integrating Neural Populations into a Coherent Neural Network

Now that we understand that there are groups of neurons that essentially operate together as part of a larger network to produce behavior and cognition, how can we integrate that knowledge into a network model that would help explain what the clinician is seeing in apraxia? How these neuronal populations are related to the well-established hub and node model is critical for understanding how neural networks operate.

Effectively every domain of cognitive function in the human brain requires the integration of distributed neural activity. Network analysis of human brain connectivity has routinely identified sets of regions that are essential for enabling efficient neuronal signaling and communication. These areas have been termed brain hubs or nodes. The central embedding of these candidate "brain hubs" in anatomical networks supports their diverse functional roles across a broad range of cognitive tasks and widespread dynamic coupling within and across functional networks. The high level of centrality and importance of these brain hubs also makes them points of vulnerability that are susceptible to disconnection and dysfunction in brain disorders (van den Heuvel & Sporns, 2013). The relationship between a neural node, neural population, and neural hub can be defined as follows. A neural node can be as small as a single neuron and is a network component that has one or more input

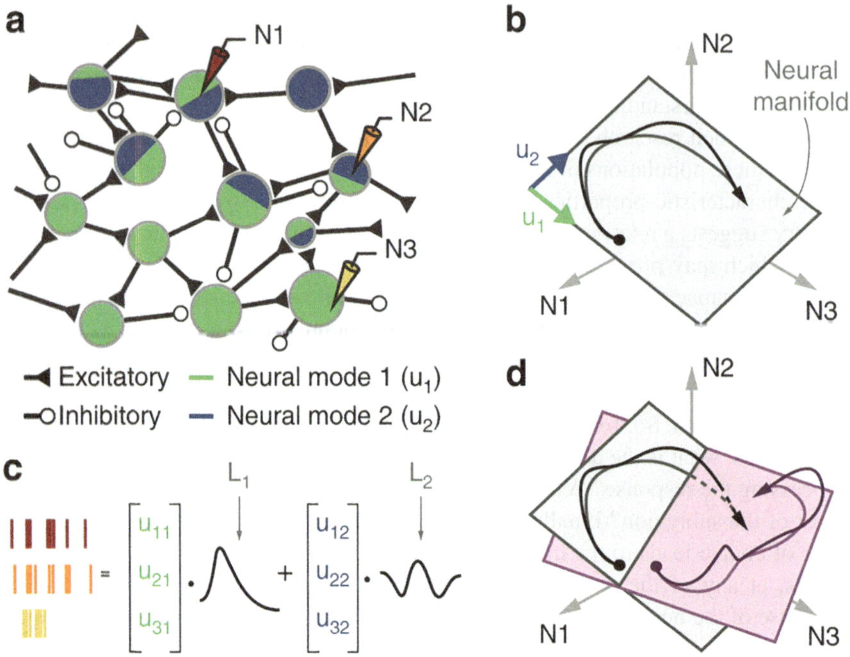

Fig. 4.2 Cortical population activity within a preserved neural manifold underlies multiple motor behaviors. Hypothesis: Varied motor behaviors are caused by the flexible activation of combinations of neural modes. (**a**) The connectivity of the cortical network results in neural modes whose combined activity explains the specific activity of individual neurons. (**b**) The neural space for the three neurons recorded in (**a**). The time-dependent population activity is represented by a trajectory (in black, arrow indicates time direction) mostly confined to a two-dimensional neural manifold (gray plane) spanned by two neural modes (green u_1 and blue u_2 basis vectors). (Gallego et al. (2018). https://doi.org/10.1038/s41467-018-06560-z)

connections, a transfer function that combines the inputs in some way, and an output connection. In the context of a network, a hub is a node with a large number of connections with many other nodes. A neural population is essentially a highly integrated complex hub consisting of a large number of individual neurons operating in a synchronized manner. As regards our current discussion, damage or disruption of any of these components will impact the network of which they are a part.

There are a good number of terms that are associated with this modeling, and we are providing the reader with a glossary of these terms. This glossary was generated by van den Heuvel and Sporns (2013):

Glossary

Brain connectivity:	description of structural or functional connectivity between brain network elements (i.e., brain regions, neurons).
Centrality:	measures of the relative importance of a node or edge within the overall architecture of a network. Several centrality metrics have been proposed, including (among many others) degree, betweenness, closeness, eigenvector, and PageRank centrality.
Clustering:	the tendency of small groups of nodes to form connected triangles. Many triangles around a central node imply that the connected neighbors of the node are also neighbors of each other, forming a cluster or clique.
Community:	in networks, communities refer to modules, densely interconnected sets of nodes.
Connection matrix:	a summary of all pairwise associations (connections) between network nodes, rendered in the form of a square matrix.
Connection:	expresses the existence and/or strength of a relationship, interaction, or dependency between two nodes in the network. Connections can be binary or weighted and they can be directed or undirected. Connections are also referred to as edges.
Connectome:	a comprehensive network map of the anatomical connections of a species' nervous system.
Connector hub:	a high-degree network node that displays a diverse connectivity profile across several different modules in a network.
Core:	a group of nodes that share a large number of mutual connections, rendering them resistant to damage. Cores are identified by using a recursive procedure that prunes away weakly connected nodes.
Degree:	the number of edges attached to a given node.
Directed network:	a network comprising directed connections (edges).
Edge:	a term for a network connection.
Functional connectivity:	measured as the statistical dependence between the time series of two network nodes (e.g., brain regions, neurons).
Graph:	a mathematical description of a network, comprising a collection of nodes and a collection of edges.
Hub:	a node occupying a central position in the overall organization of a network.

Module: a group of nodes that maintain a large number of mutual connections and a small number of connections to nodes outside their module.

Parcellation: a subdivision of the brain into anatomically or functionally distinct areas or regions.

Participation coefficient: a graph-theoretical measure that expresses the distribution of edges of a node across all modules in a network.

Provincial hub: a high-degree network node that mostly connects to nodes within its own module.

Resting-state network: a set of brain regions that show coherent functional connectivity during task-free spontaneous brain activity.

Rich-club organization: the propensity of a set of high-degree nodes in a network to be more densely interconnected than expected on the basis of their node degree alone.

Scale-free organization: a network with a degree distribution that follows a power-law function.

Shortest path length: the shortest path length between two nodes reflects the minimal number of links that have to be crossed to travel from one node to another node in the network.

Small-world organization: a network that shows a level of clustering higher than that observed in random networks and an average shortest path length that is equal to that observed in random networks.

Structural connectivity: a description of the anatomical connections between network nodes (i.e., brain regions, neurons), for example, reconstructed anatomical projections derived from diffusion MRI, directed anatomical pathways derived from neural tract tracing, or synaptic connections between individual neurons.

Undirected network: a network comprising undirected connections (edges) (Fig. 4.3).

How the Neural Substrate Enables Integration of Distributed Neural Information and Thus the Emergence of Coherent Mental and Cognitive States

Two aspects of brain organization appear essential in the understanding of how the brain generates complex action or thought. First, integration depends on neural communication among specialized brain regions, unfolding within a network of interregional projections (Fuster, 1997), which gives rise to large-scale patterns of

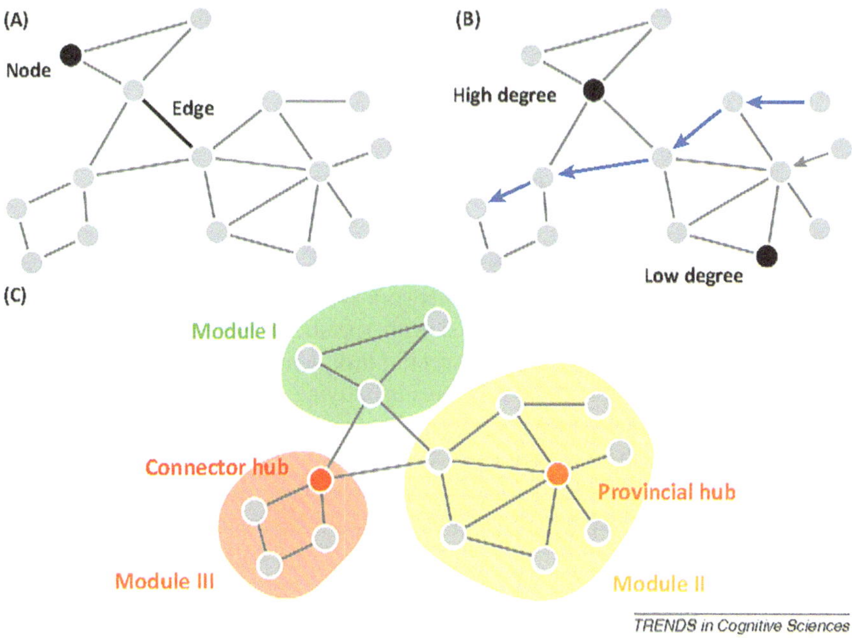

Fig. 4.3 Basic network attributes. (**a**) Brain networks can be described and analyzed as graphs comprising a collection of nodes (describing neurons/brain regions) and a collection of edges (describing structural connections or functional relationships). The arrangement of nodes and edges defines the topological organization of the network. (**b**) A path corresponds to a sequence of unique edges that are crossed when traveling between two nodes in the network. Low-degree nodes are nodes that have a relatively low number of edges; high-degree nodes (often referred to as hubs) are nodes that have a relatively high number of edges. (**c**) A module includes a subset of nodes of the network that show a relatively high level of within-module connectivity and a relatively low level of intermodule connectivity. "Provincial hubs" are high-degree nodes that primarily connect to nodes in the same module. "Connector hubs" are high-degree nodes that show a diverse connectivity profile by connecting to several different modules within the network. (Published in Trends in Cognitive Sciences 2013 Network hubs in the human brain M. V. D. Heuvel, O. Sporns)

coordinated activity (Singer, 1993) between connected elements of the network. Second, important integrative functions are performed by a specific set of brain regions and their anatomical connections. These regions are capable of complex and diverse responses and represent focal points of convergence or divergence of more specialized neural information ("confluence zones") (Meyer & Damasio, 2009).

Very recently, research has suggested that some of this integration happens at the subcortical level. For instance, subcortical visual areas such as the dorsal lateral geniculate nucleus (dLGN) or the superior colliculus (SC) have long been held as basic structures responsible for a stable, integrated, and defined function. The dLGN can be considered as a relay for visual information traveling from the retina to cortical areas and the SC as a sensory integrator orienting body movements toward visual targets. Findings suggest that both dLGN and SC neurons express functional plasticity, adding unexplored layers of complexity to their previously attributed functions (Duménieu et al., 2021).

What Is the Interface of Network Structure and Praxis?

Praxis is defined as an accepted practice or custom, or an idea translated into action. It is widely understood that the praxis network system of the human brain is made up of component functions associated with specific brain regions. These brain regions are recruited in response to specific task demands and work together to produce action. The network of structures underlying praxis is thought to include the frontal and parietal cortex, basal ganglia, and white matter tracts containing projections between these areas (Gross & Grossman, 2008). A disruption anywhere in that system, cortical or subcortical, or anywhere in the variously recruited loops, has the potential to disrupt praxis and produce an apraxic condition.

Neural Pathways and Structures Implicated in Apraxia Conditions

Now that we have an idea of the architecture of the neural network transmission system, let's look at what is known and accepted as the various network structures implicated in the forms of apraxia we have already reviewed. We will emphasize the common elements in bold when identified. For the purposes of the discussion at this point, we will omit apraxia conditions caused by genetic abnormalities as they tend to cause more widespread disruption in the various network systems.

Limb-Kinetic Apraxia

Please note that these areas cover a lot of cortical ground and that the literature is not talking about specific areas within these structures. Limb-kinetic apraxia (limb apraxia is often associated with left frontal and parietal brain damage than with right brain damage) (Pazzaglia et al., 2008b). Limb-kinetic apraxia is not explained by elemental motor or sensory systems or by defects in language comprehension. It typically affects both the ipsilesional and the contralesional limbs. *Conceptual and production components of gestural organization may be differentially affected* and may lead to ideational and ideomotor apraxia. We highlight the idea that within the category of limb-kinetic apraxia, the symptomology is not identical and the downstream effects differ. We would suggest that it is because the site of the damage to the network is different and the resultant downstream impact unique.

There is some data to suggest that this is the case. The discovery in the monkey frontal and parietal cortices of complex double-duty neurons that are activated during both action execution and observation (mirror neurons) suggests very strong connections between the perceptual and the motor components of an action (Fogassi et al., 2005). Additionally, early studies in patients with limb-kinetic apraxia reported an association between the inability to perform gestures and understand their meaning and left parietal lesions (Heilman et al., 1982).

Ideomotor Apraxia

An analogous situation arises when looking at the data of ideomotor apraxia (IMA). "If we consider the map of lesions in patients with ideomotor apraxia, we find something approximating to the classical notion of apraxia localization within the *left hemisphere*-namely, in the anterior, central, and suprasylvian retrorolandic areas disconnection of which from the central executor region has been regarded as responsible for apraxia" (Basso et al., 1980). Here again, it is not one specific area but several. It is also highlighted that it is the disconnection of these areas from the network that is the critical component of the problem.

A wider review of ideomotor apraxia highlights the numerous and diverse areas that have been noted to produce the condition. Studies of IMA and lesion location suggested that subcortical damage to white matter tracts was most critical (Wheaton & Hallet, 2007). This finding has occurred in the face of research on white matter lesions in general which indicated that white matter lesions are not more common in IMA patients than in others. In fact, lesions in deeper brain areas (e.g., white matter, thalamus, and basal ganglia) are more common in nonapraxia groups. This is not a surprising discrepancy as regards white matter because of both the amount and multiple functions of white matter, not all of which subserves motor functioning. It is clear that *white matter damage is found in studies showing that subcortical disconnection of the parietal and premotor areas may cause apraxia* (Kertes & Ferro, 1984). In addition, damage to cortical structures, particularly the angular gyrus or the supramarginal gyrus, has been observed in cases of apraxia.

Conceptual Apraxia

Conceptual deficits can be seen in patients with dementia and have been associated with lesions of posterior regions of the *left hemisphere* (Ochipa et al., 1992). There is research that suggests that conceptual apraxia is a subset of ideational apraxia, where the ability to conceptualize is impaired (Gross & Grossman, 2008). This would again suggest that it depends where in the underlying shared networks the difficulty was.

Ideational Apraxia

Ideational apraxia is usually demonstrated in people with extensive *left hemisphere damage*, dementia, or delirium (Heilman & Rothi, 2003). It is possible that the difficulty sequencing actions demonstrated by individuals impacted with this disorder may not represent a higher-order motor programming deficit, but rather, this deficit may be due to a combination of executive, language, and memory limitations (Weintraub, 2000) or to a general limitation in cognitive resources (Giovannetti et al., 2002)].

Buccofacial Apraxia

In buccofacial apraxia, the lesion is usually in or near area 44 or *Broca's area* as it is commonly known. Broca's area, located in the *frontal cortex*, plans the process of speech by interacting with the temporal cortex, where sensory information is processed, and the motor cortex, which controls movements of the mouth.

Oral Motor and Verbal Apraxia

The insula has been established as the area that is significantly impaired in both forms of oral and verbal apraxia and different severities and prominent forms of both of these apraxias. *Broca's area* was involved, but to a slightly less extent, than insula in two forms of apraxia (Yadegari et al., 2014). The insular (also known as insula and insular lobe) is a portion of the cerebral cortex folded deep within the lateral sulcus (the fissure separating the temporal lobe from the parietal and frontal lobes) within each hemisphere of the brain.

Constructional Apraxia

Constructional apraxia is thought to be caused by lesions in *the parietal lobe* following stroke. Its appearance may also serve as an indicator for Alzheimer's disease. Constructional apraxia occurs after injury to either cerebral hemisphere. Most, but not all, lesions are parietal. The nature of constructional apraxia differs according to the hemisphere injured. Individuals with left-sided lesions improve their drawings when aided by visual cues, whereas patients with right-sided lesions do not (Sharma & Wong, 2022).

We can see, as discussed, that most apraxic conditions arise from damage somewhere in the frontal, left temporal, or parietal lobes and to a lesser extent Broca's area. We suggest that "somewhere" is the operative word and that where the disruption occurs is essential in determining the downstream impact of the lesion. What is very likely is that there will always be associated disruption of function in addition to the primary motor impact, or apraxia.

This group of disorders is clearly dissociable from the apraxia condition of unknown etiology or those with genetic deficiencies where the impact is more specific, or in some instances more global. It is likely that there are considerably more sequelae for these disorders. We hope to show this to be especially true in childhood apraxia of speech whose etiology remains poorly understood. It should be clear that disruption in the motor network produces most acquired apraxic conditions. We will explore if that holds true for congenital or developmental apraxias.

Childhood Apraxia of Speech

As we have seen, childhood apraxia of speech (developmental apraxia) is different. In this case it is different because in contrast, most adult apraxias are the result of damage, injury, or insult to a specific brain area that produces specific and predictable functional deficits. Even though the specific network or group of networks cannot be demonstrated, the general area of damage usually predicts to some degree the type of dysfunction to follow. This is not the case for childhood apraxia of speech as to date, there is no evidence that unilateral damage can result in apraxia of speech or that left hemisphere lesions are more likely to result in dysarthria than lesion to the right. There are relatively few studies looking at the issue of etiology based on network principles. Those that do report on childhood apraxia of speech coalesced toward morphological, structural, metabolic, or epileptic anomalies affecting the basal ganglia, perisylvian, and rolandic cortices bilaterally. On a related note, persistent dysarthria was commonly reported in individuals with syndromes and conditions affecting these same structures bilaterally. In sum, the research suggests that long-term and severe childhood speech disorders result predominantly from bilateral disruption of several neural networks involved in speech production and could be caused by disruption anywhere in this network (Liégeoisa & Morgan, 2012).

Couple this research with the definition of childhood apraxia of speech and further difficulties arise. Childhood apraxia of speech (CAS) is an impairment in the programming and realization of intact motor units of speech (American Speech-Language-Hearing Association., 2007). Further, differential diagnosis of apraxia of speech is based on perceptual judgment (based on observation) of specific speech symptoms in the *absence of fundamental neuromuscular, cognitive, or linguistic impairments* (McNeil, 2011). In other words, there is no diagnostic emphasis regarding the involvement of neural networks, or any other brain-related area necessary for the diagnosis of childhood apraxia of speech. All that is necessary is that the requisite behavioral symptoms be present. There are three core symptoms used to differentiate apraxia of speech from other speech sound disorders: (a) prolongation of speech sounds including increase in segment and intersegment duration, (b) inconsistent distortion of speech sounds, with consistency in distortion type, (c) and abnormal prosody, characterized by inappropriate stressing of syllables and sounds (Murray et al., 2015).

Interestingly, while the literature is somewhat sparse on the network properties of CAS, there is research to suggest several single genes and copy number-variant conditions are associated with CAS either in relative isolation, as in the case of FOXP2 variants, or most typically in association with other neurodevelopmental conditions, such as epilepsy, intellectual disability, motor impairment, and autism (Morgan & Webster, 2018). This is not to say that these genetic differences do not impact network functioning; they probably do. The extant research is just not clear on the issue.

In this chapter we have taken a tour of the brain structures and network properties of the neural network system associated with the various forms of apraxia. It should be clear that historically, and as a consequence of a cortical bias, much of the extant research and conceptualization of apraxia has focused on large-scale, gray matter brain regions or specific smaller regions associated with speech (Broca's area, Wernicke's area). It should be clear that the historical research has not focused on white matter connectivity issues associated with the various apraxic conditions despite the fact that a very persuasive case can be made for a white matter contribution to the etiology of the various disorders. Current and emerging neuroimaging techniques, coupled with connectome models, are facilitating the establishment of this cortico-subcortical model as the standard.

Our point of view would express the belief that an apraxia is a functional end stage of a complex integrated network-based response. As such it could be produced by a disruption anywhere in one of the networks that contribute to the final behavior. Take, for example, the multiple pathways associated with apraxia of eyelid opening. In general, the pathogenesis of apraxia of eyelid opening and blepharospasm remains poorly understood. There are a few hypotheses based on animal model studies that suggest multiple etiologies dependent on the neural pathways involved. Among these are nigrostriatal basal ganglia pathways that seem to project to the premotor control of eyelid coordination. Therefore, it is associated with dysfunction in the corticothalamic, basal ganglia, and focal cranial nerve circuitry. Structures involved include sensorimotor cortical regions, substantia nigra pars reticulata, and brainstem motor nuclei (Cabrero & De Jesus, 2021).

In addition, depending on where the disruption is, other behaviors, which are dependent on the same connectivity patterns, would logically be impacted as well. In other words, for most apraxic conditions there would be several associated behavioral and perhaps emotional problems. The is clearly demonstrated in developmental apraxia where the research demonstrates that the most prevalent functional problems in addition to communication were attention (focus), vestibular function, temperament, fine hand use, maintaining attention, and learning to write. In addition, cognitive and learning problems, social communication difficulties, behavioral dysregulation, and other oral motor problems have been identified. More than 50% had health, mental health, and developmental conditions (Teverovsky et al., 2009).

Given the rather broad nature of the network disruption in CAS, these findings are not surprising. It is likely that the adult apraxic conditions, given an already established connectome, with possibly more restricted damage, have considerably less associated functional behavioral disruption related to the locus and severity of the damage causing the problem in the first place.

References

American Speech-Language-Hearing Association. (2007). *Childhood apraxia of speech (Position Statement)*. Retrieved from American Speech-Language-Hearing Association. www.Asha.org/policy

Basso, A., Luzzatti, C., & Spinler, H. (1980). Is ideomotor apraxia the outcome of damage to well-defined regions of the left hemisphere? *Journal of Neurology, Neurosurgery, and Psychiatry, 43*, 118–126.

Cabrero, F., & De Jesus, O. (2021, August 30). *Apraxia of lid opening*. Retrieved from National Library of Medicine: https://www.ncbi.nlm.nih.gov/books/NBK560542/

Churchland, M. M., & Shenoy, K. V. (2007). Temporal complexity and heterogeneity of single-neuron activity in premotor and motor cortex. *Journal of Neurophysiology, 97*, 4235–4257.

Duménieu, M., Marquèze-Pouey, B., Russier, M., & Debanne, D. (2021). Mechanisms of plasticity in subcortical visual areas. *Cell, 10*(11), 3162. https://doi.org/10.3390/cells10113162

Evarts, E. V. (1868). Relation of pyramidal tract activity to force exerted during voluntary movement. *Journal of Neurophysiology, 31*, 14–27.

Fogassi, L., Ferrari, P., Gesierich, B., Rozzi, S., Chersi, F., & Rizzolatti, G. (2005). Parietal lobe: From action organization to intention understanding. *Science, 308*, 662–667.

Fuster, J. (1997). Network memory. *Trends in Neuroscience, 20*(10), 451–459. https://doi.org/10.1016/S0166-2236(97)01128-4

Gallego, J., Perich, M., Naufel, S., Ethier, C., Solla, S., & Miller, E. (2018). Cortical population activity within a preserved neural manifold underlies multiple motor behaviors. *Nature Communications, 9*, 4233. https://doi.org/10.1038/s41467-018-06560-z

Gerstner, W., Kistler, W., Naud, R., & Paninsk, L. (2014). Neuronal populations. In W. Gerstner, W. Kistler, R. Naud, & L. Paninsk (Eds.), *Neuronal dynamics from single neurons to networks and models of cognition* (pp. 291–322). Cambridge University Press.

Giovannetti, T., Libon, D., Buxbaum, L., & Schwartz, M. (2002). Naturalistic action impairments in dementia. *Neuropsychologia, 40*, 1220–1232.

Gross, R., & Grossman, M. (2008). Update on apraxia. *Current Neurology and Neuroscience Reports, 8*(6), 490–496. https://doi.org/10.1007/s11910-008-0078-y

Handiru, V., Alivar, A., Hoxa, A., Saleh, S., Suviseshamuthu, E. S., Yue, G., & Allexandre, D. (2021). Graph-theoretical analysis of EEG functional connectivity during balance perturbation in traumatic brain injury: A pilot study. *Human Brain Mapping, 14*(42), 4427–4447. https://doi.org/10.1002/hbm.25554

Heilman, K., Rothi, L., & Valenstein, E. (1982). Two forms of ideomotor apraxia. *Neurology, 32*, 342–346.

Heilman, K., & Rothi, L. (2003). Apraxia. In K. Heilman & E. Valenstein (Eds.), *Clinical neuropsychology* (pp. 215–235). Oxford University Press.

Humphrey, D. R., & Thompson, W. D. (1970). Predicting measures of motor performance from multiple cortical spike trains. *Science, 170*(7), 758–762.

Kertes, A., & Ferro, J. (1984). Lesion size and location in ideomotor apraxia. *Brain, 107*(92), 1–33.

Liegeoisa, F., & Morgan, A. (2012). Neural bases of childhood speech disorders: Lateralization and plassticity for seech functions during development. *Neuroscience & Behavioral Reviews, 36*(1), 439–458. https://doi.org/10.1016/j.neubiorev.2011.07.011

McNeil, M. (2011). *Clinical management of sensorimotor speech disorders*. Thieme.
Meyer, K., & Damasio, A. (2009). Convergence and divergence in a architecture for recognition and memory. *Trends in Neuroscience, 32*(7), 376–382. https://doi.org/10.1016/j.tins.2009.04.002
Morgan, A., & Webster, R. (2018). Aetiology of childhood apraxia of speech: A clinical practice update for paediatricians. *Journal of Paediatrics and Child Health, 54*, 1090–1095. https://doi.org/10.1111/jpc.14150
Murray, E., McCabe, P., & Ballard, K. J. (2015). A randomized controlled trial for children with childhood apraxia of speech comparing rapid syllable transition treatment and the Nuffield. *Journal of Speech, Language, and Hearing Research, 58*, 669–686. https://doi.org/10.1044/2015_JSLHR-S-13-0179
Ochipa, C., Rothi, L., & Heilman, K. (1992). Conceptual apraxia in Alzheimer's disease. *Brain, 115*(4), 1061–1071. https://doi.org/10.1093/brain/115.4.1061
Pazzaglia, M., Smania, N., Corato, E., & Aglioti, S. (2008b). Neural underpinnings of gesture discrimination in patients with limb apraxia. *The Journal of Neuroscience, 28*(12), 3030–3041. https://doi.org/10.1523/JNEUROSCI.5748-07.2008
Scott, S. H., & Kalaska, J. F. (1997). Reaching movements with similar hand paths but different arm orientations. I. Activity of individual cells in motor cortex. *Journal of Neurophysiology, 77*, 826–852.
Sharma, V., & Wong, L. (2022). Middle cerebral artery disease. In J. Grotta, G. Albers, J. Broderick, S. Kasner, R. Sacco, A. Day, et al. (Eds.), *Stroke (seventh edition) pathophysiology, diagnosis, and management* (pp. 317–346). Elsevier. https://doi.org/10.1016/B978-0-323-69424-7.00024-7
Singer, W. (1993). Synchronization of cortical activity and its putative. *Annual Review of Physiology, 55*, 349–374.
Teverovsky, E., Bickel, J., & Feldman, H. (2009). Functional characteristics of children diagnosed with childhood apraxia of speech. *Disability and Rehabilitation, 31*(2), 94–102. https://doi.org/10.1080/09638280701795030
van den Heuvel, M., & Sporns, O. (2013). Network hubs in the human brain. *Trends in Cognitive Sciences, 17*(12), 683–696. https://doi.org/10.1016/j.tics.2013.09.012
Weintraub, S. (2000). Neuropsychological assessment of mental state. In I. M. Mesulam (Ed.), *Principles of behavioral and cognitive neurology* (pp. 135–136). Oxford University Press.
Wheaton, L., & Hallet, M. (2007). Ideomotor apraxia: A review. *Journal of the Neurological Sciences, 260*, 1–8. https://doi.org/10.1016/j.jns.2007.04.014
Yadegari, F., Azimian, M., Rahgozar, M., & Shekarchi, B. (2014). Brain areas impaired in oral and verbal apraxic patients. *Iranian Journal of Neurology, 13*(2), 77–82.
Yuste, R. (2015). From the neuron doctrine to neural networks. *Nature Reviews. Neuroscience, 16*, 487–497. https://doi.org/10.1038/nrn3962
Zohary, E., Shadlen, M., & Newsome, W. (1994). Correlated neuronal discharge rate and its implications for psychophysical performance. *Nature, 370*, 140–143.

Chapter 5
It Is Not Only Apraxia

If the network model, for the functional impact of the damage that causes apraxia, based on white matter connectivity problems is plausible, then it stands to reason that disruption of a network pathway would not only produce a localized functional disruption but also produce problems with other functional behaviors dependent on (downstream from) that pathway for their operation. In apraxia caused by brain injury or damage due to stroke, it is likely that any behavior directly reliant on the affected pathway would be impacted. In apraxia of speech, where there are likely numerous etiologic agents, it is likely there would be numerous potential comorbid conditions. Understanding how those interconnections originate and develop would be critical for understanding the functional impact of apraxic conditions.

The Structural Beginnings of Brain-Based Behavioral and Cognitive Connections: A Theoretical Basis

At the general practice level, much of what we talk about in the fields of neuropsychology, adult occupational therapy and physical therapy and related fields, most often is our attempt to assess and remediate damage. In order to facilitate this discussion, we offer this section as a theoretical basis for understanding the sophistication and complexity of human communication. It is our hope that by doing so we can move the discussion from "you have apraxia, and you need therapy to address the sole sequelae of that disorder" to a more comprehensive understanding of the potential impact apraxia might entail.

Communication in humans recruits all areas of the brain depending upon the task and how familiar with the task we are (novel vs. automaticity). We recruit language, but, at the same time, we also recruit pathways associated with attention, memory, and executive function as part of the complicated communication process. As

T. Wasserman, L. D. Wasserman, *Apraxia: The Neural Network Model*,
Neural Network Model: Applications and Implications,
https://doi.org/10.1007/978-3-031-24105-5_5

mentioned elsewhere in this book, motor behavior and motor-sensory development predates cognitive language and also comprises an integral part of communication.

If the premise that disruption of a neural pathway would, as a rule, cause disruption further down the pathway, then it would stand to reason that those pathways would develop in an interconnected manner. In addition, structures within the pathway would be recruited for multiple other functional outcomes. By extension, damage to the earlier structures, developed earlier ontogenically, would cause disruption to the development of multiple functional outcomes.

The Development of Networks

A developmental perspective is invaluable for understanding how functional brain networks come into existence. The current imaging studies are providing insight into how these functional brain networks develop from childhood. We have talked about how brain networks start out as locally segregated small world hubs. The basic anatomical structure is largely in place by 2 years of age (Menon, 2013). This is not to imply that nothing goes on before that time because that is not the case. It is accurate to say that by age of 2, the basic structure of future network operations is in place. As we develop, the shorter-range connections in children evolve between these segregated hubs, becoming, with practice and repetition, stronger long-range connections, ultimately creating a large-scale connectome. There is a body of evidence indicating that while gray matter changes over the course of development, the development of white matter actually undergoes a more intensive change than gray matter (Menon, 2013). This maturation then includes cortical subcortical reconfigurations. This vertical brain model, from a developmental perspective, allows us to consider how microstructural changes in white matter and changes from local to long-range white matter development impact both the integrity and reach of these neural network connections. By understanding how intensively neural pathways are associated, we can better understand how maturation involves broad regions of the brain and how multiple regions must be incorporated on a task-specific (functional) basis. And by extension, we can also understand how disruption to any part of the connectome will impact the larger connectome, or functional outcomes.

Feedforward Impact

The principle of a feedforward impact in the face of disruption applies to developmental and trauma-based impact. A feedforward neural network is a computerized network model wherein node connections do not form a loop. Feedforward neural networks are so named because information flows in a forward manner only. These networks develop across domains such as motor, cognitive, working memory, language, and functionally to academic and daily living skills. In summary, "A thorough characterization of the development of large-scale brain networks requires the integration of multiple structural and functional measures. The complexities of this effort, including linking brain structure, anatomical connectivity, task and context specific functional connectivity and characterizing their dynamic maturation with age" (Menon, 2013) is all to be considered.

The Cerebral Cortex and Basal Ganglia

"The cerebral cortex is a six layered structure that performs a wide range of highly specialized operations" (Koziol & Budding, 2009, pg. 41). "These operations can be divided into two broad categories. First, posterior cortices are involved in sensory perceptual information processing and storage. These cortical areas are the occipital, parietal, and temporal lobes. Second, the anterior cortices, or the frontal lobes, are involved in the processing or programming and retention of movement and action patterns. The products of the information processing computations performed by the cortex remain represented within the cortex" (pg. 41).

The basal ganglia receive afferents from nearly all cortical regions while sending efferent signals back to those same cortical regions through the thalamic nuclei (Middleton & Strick, 2000). The basal ganglia do not directly participate in the computations performed by the cortex. They are involved in gating or selecting the representations that are processed by the cortex so that these representations become active or can be expressed. Hence, the basal ganglia are the gatekeepers which enable the frontal cortex to execute the appropriate motor plan at the appropriate time (Frank et al., 2001).

As part of this process, we can extrapolate how this cortical-subcortical process impacts working memory. Let us first state that working memory, a cognitive task, may be considered the mainstay of executive function. Koziol and Budding (2009) ask and answer: How can an activity that seems so uniquely cognitive be analogous to motor behavior in any way? For the business of the basal ganglia, motor functioning and cognition are similar or even parallel processes. They further state that they believe that the basal ganglia interact in the same way with the presentation of plans and goals that reside in the prefrontal cortex. In this way, the processes that guide motor functioning have much in common with the cognition of working memory that ultimately guides behavior. The processes that guide movement manage many of the same requirements that are essential for manipulating the contents of working memory. "The cognitive control system is likely and evolutionary extension of the frontal basal ganglia motor control system" (Hazy, 2007) which includes working memory or "the set of cognitive processes for holding goals and subgoals in mind in the service of planning and executing complex behaviors. In other words, the basal ganglia select and gate movement, and they also gate cognitions: they do the same things for cognition that they do for movement. Koziel (2009) highlights that this is the underpinning of self-directed, controlled behavior.

The same modeling applies to speech as well. Koziol and Budding (2009) note that just as gesturing requires movements to be expressed in a certain order, vocal sound sequences also rely on an organized sequence to express a particular meaning. This ties the connection between motor sequencing and verbal sequencing. In fact, this also ties into the subcortical-cortical nature of the process with basal ganglia-cortical loops providing a unique neural architecture for the necessary foundations for sequencing the structure, or rules across gestures and vocalizations. From an evolutionary standing, these structures already existed and were specialized over time so that the result is that language is dependent upon the basal ganglia for sequential learning and upon the frontal cortex for the necessary motor programming.

In fact, the current authors wish to remind the reader that intention predates language development. During the motor-sensory period, infants demonstrate the innate reflex of curiosity (Wasserman & Wasserman, 2020), the expression of which results in the execution of intent through motor movement. This movement is reinforced and thereby found to be rewarding to the infant-seeking behavior. We also know that categorization precedes language (Rakison, 2010), setting the stage for language development. We should also remember that this exploration involves the salience network and, by inclusion, attention. In this way we can see that attention, intent (goal-directed behavior), working memory, motivation, language, and motor movement are inexorably linked in human development and remain interconnected in more complex human cognition. The potential exists for these interconnected systems to be disrupted by a brain insult that produces an apraxic event with impact to a potential multitude of functional areas.

For example, with respect to speech, Hickok et al. (2011) proposed a model incorporating the dorsal stream, emphasizing the role of internal forward models in speech motor control. They posited that these relevant neural systems make forward predictions about the future state of the motor articulators and the sensory consequences of the predicted actions in order to control desired functional action. The predictions are generated by an internal model that receives efferent copies of motor commands and integrates them with information being received about the current state of the system. This allows for a mechanism for detecting and correcting motor errors, that is, motor actions that fail to hit their sensory targets. The ability to suppress errors, whether motor or language based, is very important. This process, which requires defining a target and implementation of corresponding behavior, whether this is behavioral or speech based, requires inhibition of attention or attempts of other behaviors, that is, monitoring and necessary inhibition. It is likely within the cerebellum that this constant and highly sophisticated computational monitoring takes place. It is within the basal ganglia that inhibition is initiated, strengthening the inter-association of the motor areas acting in concert with the cerebellum and basal ganglia loops (Hickok, 2012). The reader will note the expansion of the originally cortical centric model to a cortical subcortical model incorporating constant modulation and monitoring of the inhibition and expression of behaviors.

Changes to this excitatory-inhibitory process then, at some phase of development, not only impacts the local circuit excitability but can also alter large-scale brain connectivity resulting in atypical development of functional neural associations and process (Menon, 2013). This then provides the physiological hypothesis for deviant neural development and that this imbalance underlies aberrant brain connectivity in many developmental psychopathologies (Menon, 2013).

Aberrations in the neurodevelopment of the cortico-subcortical process has been linked to multiple neurodevelopmental disorders including autism, attention-deficit disorder, emotional disorders, schizophrenia (Menon, 2013), and sensory integration disorder (Koziol, 2009). A large focus of multiple chapters of this volume is to emphasize that abnormal neurodevelopment is the base of developmental coordination disorder and childhood apraxia of speech, with implications going far beyond what might be assumed if limiting ourselves to the nomenclature of the diagnostic label.

All of the above is reported so that the reader understands that, looking at both neurodevelopmental disorders and apraxias which occur as a result of trauma, the basis of the disorder is complex reflecting highly integrated and associated areas of both cortex and subcortex. Damage, whether from a developmental source or as the result of acquired trauma, will impact these systems in multiple and complex ways. Both the integrity of the system and their associated functional behaviors will be negatively affected.

Neural Pathways Are Recruited for Multiple Functional Outcomes

There is research that indicates that recruitment of network and network-related systems is the rule rather than the exception, and this makes sense. For example, dopamine (DA)-producing neurons are critically involved in the production of motor behaviors in multiple circuits that are conserved from basal vertebrates to mammals (Barrios, Weng, England, Reifenberg, & Douglass, 2020). Similarly, exposure to drug-related cues in human addicts results in drug craving and localized activation of central circuits that are known to mediate cue-induced reinstatement of drug-seeking behavior in animal models of relapse. Similar regional activation patterns occur in humans in response to cues associated with foods (Kelley, Shiltz, & Landry, 2005).

Similar examples of shared network working are found in motor circuits. For example, numerous muscle groups would be common among a variety of related functional behaviors. There is clear evidence that the modular control of muscles in groups, often referred to as muscle synergies, provides a motor repertoire of actions for the robust control of movement. This research demonstrates that a common pool of spatially fixed locomotor muscle synergies is recruited by different neural pathways, including the central pattern generator for walking, brainstem pathways for balance control, and cortical pathways mediating voluntary gait modifications. These muscle synergies provide a repository of motor subtasks that can be flexibly recruited by parallel descending pathways to generate a variety of complex natural movements in the upper and lower limbs (Chvatal & Ting, 2012). Similarly, phrenic motor neurons are recruited across a range of motor behaviors. These motor units are recruited in a fixed order across a range of motor behaviors. These motor neurons were recruited for different motor behaviors, i.e., eupnea, hypoxia-hypercapnia, deep breaths, sustained airway occlusion, and sneezing (Seven, Mantilla, & Sieck, 2014).

Other research may also have direct implication for apraxia as well as conditions such as tic disorder and obsessive compulsive disorder. Research has clearly indicated that unexpected events recruit a fronto-basal-ganglia network for stopping. Elements of this network include specific prefrontal cortical nodes and is thought to project to the subthalamic nucleus, with a putative global suppressive effect on basal-ganglia output. This is a global suppressive network. Its existence provides a common mechanistic basis for different types of unexpected events; links the literatures on motor inhibition, performance monitoring, attention, and working memory; and is relevant for understanding clinical symptoms of distractibility and mental inflexibility (Wessel & Aron, 2017).

In fact, we have already had a hint as to the impact of shared networks in cases of childhood apraxia of speech (CAS) where the research has shown numerous functional problems in addition to communication. We know CAS affects phonetic-motoric planning of speech. What is now clear is that the motor control impairment of CAS and apraxia of speech (AOS) extends beyond speech and is manifest in nonspeech movements of the oral structures (Kirrie, Granier, & Robin, 2008). Associated problems include difficulty with attention (focus), vestibular function, temperament, fine hand use, maintaining attention, and learning to write. In addition, cognitive and learning problems, social communication difficulties, behavioral dysregulation, and other oral motor problems have been identified. More than 50% of AOS patients had health, mental health, and developmental conditions (Teverovsky, Bickel, & Feldman, 2009). Estimates suggest that approximately only 4% of individuals diagnosed with an acquired neurological communication disorder present with AOS as the primary disorder and individuals with stroke-induced AOS as their only communication impairment are rarely reported in the literature. In patients with AOS, there is an estimated co-occurrence of aphasia in 81%, dysarthria in 29–47%, and nonverbal oral apraxia in 48–75% of cases (Moser, Basilakos, Fillmore, & Fridriksson, 2016).

It could be argued that both AOS and CAS clearly have significant discrepancies from the other forms of apraxia so that they represent outliers. It would be, therefore, beneficial to see whether other forms of acquired apraxia, that is, apraxia caused by brain insult or injury, would demonstrate the same properties regarding the implications of shared neural networks. There is striking evidence that the properties of disrupted neural network activity are quite different.

Disruption of Early Domains Are Not Just Domain Specific

Again, returning to a developmental framework, we must ask how these functional trajectories work by association. In a study of the developmental relationship between language and motor behavior (Wang, 2014b), multiple important questions were asked. The first is how is research impacted by looking at a single variable rather than associated developmental domains. The second are the trajectories and cross-associations for these domains. Wang (2014a) attempted to look at three perspectives, namely, co-occurrence of difficulties, stability of each domain across time, and the predictive power of each across time. They found that language at 3 years of age was a better predictor of later language skills than gross motor skills, indicating stability within the domain. However, they also found an increase over time for shared variance with both fine and gross motor development with language development. Language at 3 years of age was significantly associated with later fine and gross motor performance. They conclude that these findings support the hypothesis that motor and language are developmentally associated trajectories. Also important was the combining of their earlier study (Wang, 2014a, b) with the current study for a greater longitudinal perspective. They found that language did not predict motor development from 18 months to 3 years of age; however, from 3 to 5 years of age, this association was found to be significant. In contrast, there was a significant association from 18 months of age to 3 years of age between motor skill development and later language performance, although neither gross motor nor fine motor development at 3 years of age was predictive for late language development (age 5). These are important findings for many reasons. First, it demonstrates stability within domains. Second, it highlights a difference in development at different stages of development for domains with associations greater and lesser at different ages. Specifically, language was not predictive of motor skills early on (18 months to 3 years) but was found to be more highly associated between ages 3 and 5. In contrast, early motor skills (18 months to 3 years) were found predictive of later language skills, although the predictive power of gross and fine motor skills dropped off for language development for the 3–5-year-old age group. Therefore, early motor development and later language development were significantly associated. For the older age group, motor development did not predict language development, although for the 3–5 age group, the association was significant.

These findings also suggest that a disorder, such as developmental coordination disorder, can be assessed earlier on, and should be, as aberrant motor development can affect language development. The findings also suggest that by age 3, development in one domain is highly associated with development in the second domain supporting the idea that disruption at that point can impact more than one area of development. Given what we have discussed with respect to early architecture being in place by age 2, with following connectivity alterations, the call for early intervention becomes all the clearer.

As we have just seen, it is likely that apraxic conditions are associated with other dysfunctions, so let's take a look at what is known.

Limb-Kinetic Apraxia and Associated Conditions

Limb-kinetic apraxia seems to be particularly relevant for activities of daily living especially those requiring dexterity skills (Foki, et al., 2016). Limb apraxia is primarily classified by the nature of the errors made by the individual and the pathways through which these errors are elicited. It is based on a two-system model for the organization of action: a conceptual system and a production system (Leiguarda & Marsden, 2000). These systems are dissociable, and each has its own constellation of downstream effects. Deficits include, but are not limited to, visual and somatosensory transformations for reaching; transformation of information about the location of body parts necessary for the control of movements; somatosensory transformation for posture; visual transformation for grasping; and internal representation of actions. Problems with sensory motor integration have been noted.

Ideomotor Apraxia and Associated Conditions

As we have seen, ideomotor apraxia (IMA) is a disorder of skilled, purposeful movement, characterized by spatiotemporal deficits during a variety of actions. Historically, these deficits have been attributed to damage to, or impaired retrieval of, stored representations of learned actions, especially object-related movements. This however is not the only available possibility. These same deficits might be caused by impaired visuomotor transformation mechanisms that operate in parallel to or downstream from mechanisms for storage of action representations. These transformation processes convert extrinsic visual information into intrinsic neural commands appropriate for the desired motion. These processes are essential for movement planning process and performance errors due to inadequate transformations. If this model is correct, we could predict that patients with ideomotor apraxia would demonstrate planning deficits when reaching to visual targets, especially when the coordination and/or dynamic requirements of the task increase. This is indeed the case (Mutha, Sainburg, & Haaland, 2010).

In addition, much research has demonstrated that spatiotemporal deficits in apraxia are not limited to object-use movements. For example, apraxic patients make errors that are consistent with impaired integration of spatial and temporal features of movements during reaching and sequencing. Apraxic patients also make more errors than non-apraxic patients and healthy subjects when asked to imitate meaningless movements, such as touching the nose, and also intransitive gestures, such as saluting. Overall, research results have demonstrated that deficits in ideomotor apraxia are present during movements made in a variety of contexts and are not simply limited to object-use actions. Finally, there is research to suggest that a central deficit in IMA may be impaired postural representation causing inability to solve the problem of how to manipulate objects where neither affordance nor memory can dictate action (Sunderland & Shiner, 2007).

Conceptual Apraxia and Associated Conditions

Conceptual apraxia has two domains: associative knowledge (tool-action associations such as hammer pound; tool-object associations such as hammer nail) and mechanical knowledge such as knowing the advantage that tools afford (Heilman, Maher, Greenwald, & Rothi, 1997). It is likely that these two domains share some network components but are nevertheless dissociable from each other. Problems in either of these very broad domains are different from one another.

While it is known that conceptual praxis representations are stored in the left hemisphere, analysis of lesion sites in various research studies fails to clearly establish where in the left hemisphere they may be stored. This can be due to a number of reasons not the least of which is the possibility that these representations are not stored as integrated constructs but are reintegrated at the time the task demand is presented. Conceptual apraxia has been associated with problems with semantic memory (Dumont, Ska, & Joanette, 2000).

Ideational Apraxia and Related Conditions

There is some evidence to suggest that ideational apraxia, like conceptual apraxia, is related to semantic memory and may not be a disorder of defective motor control at all (De Renzi & Lucchelli, 1988). It has also been argued that ideational apraxia reflects a generalized disturbance of object representations that are held to trigger action schemas (Cooper, 2007). The point here is that semantic memory deficits, at a minimum, accompany ideational apraxia. It is not clear where in the process of memory reconfiguration these semantic problems arise and that means that there might be more than one etiological factor.

Other problems have been regularly associated with ideational apraxia. The ability of ideational apraxic patients to perform simple tasks involving multiple objects is typically characterized by a variety of errors. Some of these errors concern the sequential organization of action through time; many others are related to the misuse of, or failure to use, necessary or appropriate tools.

Oral Motor and Verbal Apraxia and Related Conditions

This is a wide and poorly defined area, with the research often mixing childhood apraxia of speech and adult acquired oral motor apraxia. As we saw from the brief discussion of childhood apraxia of speech, there are numerous downstream effects that accompany CAS. In adults oral motor apraxia is frequently comorbid with aphasia (Conterno, et al., 2021) and other issues related to disrupted speech.

Apraxic Conditions Rarely Occur in Isolation

The point of this discussion is that it highlights the fact that apraxic conditions of all types rarely occur in isolation and are often accompanied by other forms of dysregulated behavior. From a network perspective, this makes sense. Research demonstrating that apraxia can be due to deep subcortical lesions, including damage to the basal ganglia or thalamus would clearly imply multiple potential downstream behavioral difficulties (Pramstaller & Marsden, 1996). What's more, far from being a disorder confined to discrete gray matter structures in the brain, apraxia can be caused by disruption of while matter located subcortically. Pramstaller and Marsden, in their research, indicated that apraxia was most seen when there were lesions in the lenticular nucleus or putamen with additional involvement of capsular, particularly of periventricular or peristriatal, white matter. While lesions of the globus pallidus or caudate nucleus rarely caused apraxia, the caudate lesions also had white matter involvement. Finally, involvement of periventricular or peristriatal white matter alone caused apraxia in their subject population. In other words, an unidentified subset of apraxic conditions resulted from white matter-based connectivity issues. On a functional behavioral level, these two causes (gray and white matter) produced similar if not identical disrupted outcome. The downstream effects from each etiology can be expected to be different. If a primary structure, such as Broca's area, was impacted, all downstream functions from Broca's areas would be impacted. If it were a white matter connectivity issue, then it could at least be anticipated that certain functional behavior would be impacted and other behavior spared.

How complicated can this get? Multiple overlapping white matter networks are involved in most higher-order cognitive functions.

If we are to conjecture that a disruption of a pathway, as can happen in acquired apraxia, can have far-reaching impact on the function outcome capacity of a person, it would require us to take a look at one system in detail to serve as the basis for a model. For example, communication in humans activates almost every part of the brain. Obviously, the known language gray areas predominate, but other cognitive functions associated with language, such as attention, memory, emotion, and executive processes, are also involved. In order to explain how our brain actually utilizes language to understand, speak, and write and in order to rehabilitate things like apraxic or aphasic disorders, neuroscience is just beginning to recognize that it must understand the responsible neural networks (Nasios, Dardiostis, & Messinis, 2019). Part of the recognition is that we cannot base our understanding of how this language system operates based upon an outdated model of the modular organization of the brain. Over the last three decades, neuroscience based on new imaging, recording, and manipulation techniques for brain research developed a new model of the functional neuroanatomy of language. The dual-stream model, consisting of two interacting networks ("streams")—one ventral, bilaterally organized, for language comprehension, and one dorsal, left hemisphere dominant, for language production—was identified.

These "streams" (network) are very complex and involve a multiplicity of structures. According to the dual-stream model, the dorsal pathway involves the left hemispheric structures in the posterior frontal lobe, the posterior dorsal temporal lobe, and the parietal operculum, including long white matter (WM) tracts connecting the frontal to the temporal and parietal lobes, specifically the articulate fasciculus (AF), and the indirect anterior and indirect posterior components of the superior longitudinal fascicle (SLF). The core anterior (frontal) hubs of the dorsal pathway include the inferior frontal gyrus (opercular and triangular part), the ventral portions of the precentral gyrus, and the anterior portions of the insula (forming together the left frontal operculum (L-FO)). Posteriorly, the main hubs are the posterior sector of the insula, the ventral portions of the supramarginal gyrus, and Sylvian parietal temporal region (Spt), forming, together with the upper parts of the posterior superior temporal gyrus and sulcus, the left temporoparietal junction (L-TPJ). Area Spt is located in the posterior part of the left planum temporale (PT) region, where speech perception and production systems converge.

In contrast to these left dominant structures and networks, ventral pathways are bilaterally distributed into both hemispheres, and the major hubs include the superior temporal gyrus (STG), superior temporal sulcus (STS), middle and inferior temporal gyri (MTG/ITG), and the anterior temporal lobe (ATL). The ventral stream connects the frontal cortices to the occipital, parietal, and temporal lobes, via long white matter (WM) tracts, including the external capsule (EC), the inferior fronto-occipital fascicle (IFOF), the inferior longitudinal fascicle (ILF), and the uncinate fascicle (UF).

Traditionally, neuropsychologists and other neuroscientists concentrated their research on specific small elements of language processing. What is now known is that the human organizes its interactions for communication under in a situationally specific manner involving multifunctional processing of multimodal input from the environment. Different groups of words, forming different groups of meanings, connected with different emotional aspects, involve different parts of our brain, far beyond the strictly defined language networks (Huth, W, Griffiths, Theunissen, & Gallant, 2016). They found that the distribution of semantically selective areas within the semantic system was relatively symmetrical across the two cerebral hemispheres. A finding that is inconsistent with human lesion studies that support the idea that semantic representation is lateralized to the left hemisphere but, however, completely in line with the bilateral distribution of the ventral stream of the dual-stream model.

The point here is that these networks are incredibly complex and disruption in any component may produce a verbal apraxia or related language difficulty. To the extent that these same structures, many of them motoric, are recruited in other cognitive activities, we can reasonably expect that damage to one of them would produce multiple downstream effects in addition to the apraxic condition that is the focus of this book.

White Matter Degeneration Following Injury

If we are going to have a model that speculates on downstream damage, it would be useful to identify mechanisms on just how this might occur. In addition to the "line being broken" with no information being able to be processed below the point of the break, there are physiological effects that follow injury to white matter. For example, following an initial impact after spinal cord injury (SCI), a cascade of downstream events has been identified. These have been term termed "secondary injury," which culminate in progressive degenerative events in the spinal cord. These secondary injury mechanisms include, in part, ischemia, inflammation, free radical-induced cell death, glutamate excitotoxicity, cytoskeletal degradation, and induction of extrinsic and intrinsic apoptotic pathways. There is expanding evidence that glutamate excitotoxicity plays a key role not only in neuronal cell death but also in delayed posttraumatic spinal cord white matter degeneration (Park, Velumian, & Fehlings, 2004). Cortically, immune-inflammatory processes and the response to several trigger factors such as trauma, hemorrhage, or ischemia cause the release of active inflammatory substances such as cytokines, which are the basis of second-level brain damage. Secondary injury mechanisms include processes such as alteration of ionic homeostasis, increase of neurotransmitter levels, neuronal cellular death, lipid degradation, and immune-inflammatory activation Disruption of motor and cognitive functioning has been reported as associated with this secondary damage (Tuttolomondo, Pecoraro, & Pinto, 2014). It is possible to associate specific disfunction with this secondary damage. For example, Wasserman and Mion (2019) identified cortical white matter degeneration attributable to white matter degeneration causing memory loss. Thus, there is every reason to believe that further damage and function loss might be attributable to a lesion that initially causes apraxia. In addition, there is every reason to believe that there might be apraxic events secondary to lesions that initially do not cause apraxia.

In addition, there is evidence, much of it from animal studies, that suggests that the system that experiences the insult can react to the disruption in unpredictable ways. For example, after damage to the cochlear, the acoustic system can, in some cases, respond by recalibrating itself to partially accommodate the sensory input loss (Salvi, Wang, & Ding, 2000). How these compensatory adjustments might contribute to a particular apraxic condition is not entirely clear, but it is possible that such recalibrations might negatively impact fluidity. The same research clearly identifies a multiplicity of follow-on difficulty associated from cochlear damage. Cochlear damage results in neuronal shrinkage, axonal pruning, trans-synaptic degeneration new growth of axons, formation of new synapses, and modifications to the distribution of ascending neural projections. Further, cochlear damage also alters the neurochemistry of the central auditory pathway. Protein synthesis is significantly and rapidly downregulated after cochlear destruction or inactivation and glucose metabolism are modified. Neurotransmission in the central auditory pathway is also altered by cochlear damage. This information is presented to highlight the point that downstream and, in some cases, upstream changes are the rule rather than the exception when disruption of a neural pathway occurs.

Neural Network Damage Models

As might be implied from the above, there are at least two ways to look at possible effects from damage to a neural network component. The first is to look at damage to the major gray matter components of any particular system. The second is to look at damage to the white matter connectivity components of the system (Farah, O'Reilly, & Vecera, 1993). Logically, this leads to a third possibility: situations where both gray and white matter are damaged. These three possibilities do not even address all the possibilities when discussing apraxia. We must consider the situation, such as in developmental apraxia, where there is not observable damage to the system and yet the system does not function as it should.

There is substantial and expanding literature on gray matter and white matter damage after head injury and insult (Fu, et al., 2021). This research indicates that the pathophysiological presentation of white matter damage involves axonal damage, demyelination, and mature oligodendrocyte loss. Studies of a variety of other acute brain insults have indicated that white matter damage is strongly correlated with cognitive deficits, neurological deficits, and depression. (Mutha, Sainburg, & Haaland, 2010). As we have pointed out, white matter damage in the basal ganglia has been associated with apraxic sequelae (Pramstaller & Marsden, 1996). White matter damage has been identified as the major etiological factor in ideomotor(limb) apraxia (Leiguarda.R., 2001).

The extant research provides a clear delineation for the role of the basal ganglia in the presentation of apraxic symptomology. The hypothetical multiple roles of the basal ganglia in object-oriented action and, as a result, praxis would include among others (a) the selection of the kinematic parameters and the direction of arm movements, (b) working as a core element of brain systems involved in the timing and representation of action sequences, (c) encoding behavioral context, and (d) working as a subcortical component of the parieto-frontal circuits dedicated to sensorimotor transformation.

Interestingly, multiple studies suggest that basal ganglia pathology per se may not be the proximal cause of overt apraxia. It is when it is combined with dysfunction of the cortical components of the neural systems involved in sequencing, sensorimotor transformation, and response selection that different types of ideomotor praxis deficits would become clinically manifested.

This makes the point rather clearly. Here a component network of a more complex and integrated network system dedicated to purposeful movement is damaged and the downstream impact is apraxia. That while matter damage could occur at multiple sites in the subcortical complex and, as long as the same cortical areas were involved, the resultant functional behavioral disruption would be the same. When combined with different cortical areas involved in different areas of function, such as speech, these same subcortical white matter deficiencies would result in different forms of praxis.

It should be recalled that as far as a clear understanding of the apraxic elements of these disorders, it should be recalled that one of the definitions of apraxia specifies that the disruption of ability to perform skilled movements cannot be explained by the more fundamental motor disorders typical of patients with movement disorders with clear etiology (i.e., Parkinson's). That is to say, that the same disrupted movement caused by disruption of the same circuitry would be labeled as a praxis if the individual did not have a movement disorder that explained it.

The above is not meant to imply that it is only white matter disconnection in subcortical areas that contributes to praxis. That is not the case. Research demonstrates that pathological white matter alterations in a densely connected fronto-temporo-parietal network of short and long association fibers is associated with limb apraxia deficits. Major disconnection affected temporo-parietal and temporo-temporal connections. Gray matter areas with a high number of disconnections included inferior parietal lobe, middle and superior temporal gyrus, inferior and middle frontal lobe, precentral gyrus, putamen, and caudate nucleus (Rosenzoph, et al., 2020).

References

Barrios, J., Weng, W., England, R., Reifenberg, E., & Douglass, A. (2020). Hypothalamic dopamine neurons control sensorimotor behavior by modulating brainstem premotor nuclei in zebrafish. *Current Biology, 30*(23), 4606–4619. https://doi.org/10.1016/j.cub.2020.09.002

Chvatal, S., & Ting, L. (2012). Voluntary and reactive recruitment of locomotor muscle synergies during perturbed walking. *The Journal of Neuroscience, 32*(35), 12237–12250. https://doi.org/10.1523/JNEUROSCI.6344-11.2012

Conterno, M., Kümmerer, D., Dressing, A., Glauche, V., Urbach, H., Weiler, C., & Rijntjes, R. (2021). Speech apraxia and oral apraxia: Association or dissociation? A multivariate lesion–symptom mapping study in acute stroke patients. *Experimental Brain Research, 240*, 39. https://doi.org/10.1007/s00221-021-06224-3

Cooper, R. (2007). Tool use and related errors in ideational apraxia: The quantitative simulation of patient error profiles. *Cortex, 43*(3), 319–337.

De Renzi, E., & Lucchelli, F. (1988). Ideational apraxia. *Brain, 111*(5), 1173–1185. https://doi.org/10.1093/brain/111.5.1173

Dumont, C., Ska, B., & Joanette, Y. (2000). Conceptual apraxia and semantic memory deficit in Alzheimer's disease: Two sides of the same coin? *Journal of the International Neuropsychological Society, 6*(6), 693–703. https://doi.org/10.1017/S1355617700666079

Farah, M. J., O'Reilly, R. C., & Vecera, S. P. (1993). Dissociated overt and covert recognition as an emergent property of a lesioned neural network. *Psychological Review, 100*(4), 571–588. https://doi.org/10.1037/0033-295X.100.4.571

Foki, T., Vanbellingen, C. T., Pirker, A. L., Bohlhalter, S., Nyffeler, T., Kraemmer, J., et al. (2016). Limb-kinetic apraxia affects activities of daily living in Parkinson's disease: A multi-center study. *European Journal of Neurology, 23*(8), 1301–1307. https://doi.org/10.1111/ene.13021

Frank, M., Loughry, B., O'Reilly, R. (2001). Interactions between frontal cortex and basal ganglia in working memory: A computational model. *Cognitive, Affective, & Behavioral Neuroscience, 1*, 137–160. https://doi.org/10.3758/CABN.1.2.137

Fu, X., Zhou, G., Zhuang, J., Xu, C., Zhou, H., Peng, Y., et al. (2021). White matter injury after intracerebral hemorrhage. *Frontiers in Neurology, 12*, 562090. https://doi.org/10.3389/fneur.2021.562090

Hazy, T. F. (2007). Towards an executive without a homunculus: Computational models of the prefrontal cortex/basal ganglia system. *Philosophical Transactions of the Royal Society of London. Series B, Biological Sciences, 362*, 1601–1613.

Heilman, K., Maher, L., Greenwald, M., & Rothi, L. (1997). Conceptualized apraxia from lateralized esions. *Neurology, 49*(2), 10.1212/WNL.49.2.457.

Hickok, G., Houde, J., & Rong, F. (2011). Sensorimotor integration in speech processing: computational basis and neural organization. *Neuron, 69*(3), 407–422. https://doi.org/10.1016/j.neuron.2011.01.019

Hickok, G. (2012). The cortical organization of speech processing: Feedback control and predictive coding the context of a dual-stream model. *Journal of Communication Disorders, 45*(6), 393–403. https://doi.org/10.1016/j.jcomdis.2012.06.004

Huth, A., de Heer, W. A., Griffiths, W., Theunissen, F., & Gallant, J. (2016). Natural speech reveals the semantic maps that tile human cerebral cortex. *Nature, 532*(7600), 453–459. https://doi.org/10.1038/nature17637

Kelley, A., Shiltz, C., & Landry, C. (2005). Neural systems recruited by drug- and food-related cues: Studies of gene activation in corticolimbic regions. *Physiology & Behavior, 86*(1–2), 11–14. https://doi.org/10.1016/j.physbeh.2005.06.018

Kirrie, B., Granier, J., & Robin, D. (2008). Understanding the nature of apraxia of speech: Theory, analysis, and treatment. *Neuropsychological Trends, 4*, 7–44.

Koziol, L. B. (2009). *Subcortical structures and cognition*. Springer.

Koziol, L., & Budding, D. (2009). *Subcortical structures and cognition*. Springer.

Leiguarda, C. D., & Marsden, C. (2000). Limb apraxias: Higher-order disorders of sensorimotor integration. *Brain, 123*(Pt 5), 650–879. https://doi.org/10.1093/brain/123.5.860

Leiguarda, R. (2001). Limb apraxia: Cortical or subcortical. *NeuroImage, 14*(1), 5137–5141. https://doi.org/10.1006/nimg.2001.0833

Menon, V. (2013). Developmental pathways to functional brain networks: Emerging principles. *Trends in Cognitive Sciences, 17*. https://doi.org/10.1016/j.tics.2013.09.015

Middleton, F., & Strick, P. (2000). Basal ganglia output and cognition: Evidence from anatomical, behavioral, and clinical studies. *Brain and Cognition, 42*(2), 183–200. https://doi.org/10.1006/brcg.1999.1099

Moser, D., Basilakos, A., Fillmore, P., & Fridriksson, J. (2016). Brain damage associated with apraxia of speech: Evidence from case studies. *Neurocase, 22*(4), 346–356. https://doi.org/10.1080/13554794.2016.1172645

Mutha, P., Sainburg, R., & Haaland, K. (2010). Coordination deficits in ideomotor apraxia during visually targeted reaching reflect impaired visuomotor transformations. *Neuropsychologia, 48*(13), 3855–3867. https://doi.org/10.1016/j.neuropsychologia.2010.09.018

Nasios, G., Dardiostis, E., & Messinis, L. (2019). From Broca and Wernicke to the neuromodulation era: Insights of brain language networks for neurorehabilitation. *Behavioural Neurology, 2019*. https://doi.org/10.1155/2019/9894571

Park, E., Velumian, A., & Fehlings, M. (2004). Mechanisms of spinal cord injury: A review with an emphasis on the implications for white matter degeneration. *Journal of Neurotrauma, 21*(6). https://doi.org/10.1089/0897715041269641, on line.

Pramstaller, P., & Marsden, C. (1996). The basal ganglia and apraxia. *Brain, 119*(1), 319–340. https://doi.org/10.1093/brain/119.1.319

Rakison, D. (2010). Perceptual categorization and concepts. In G. Bremner & T. Wachs (Eds.), *The Wiley-Blackwell handbook of infant. Wiley*. https://doi.org/10.1002/9781444327564.ch7

Rosenzopf, H., Wiesen, D., Basilakos, A., Yourganov, G., Bonilha, L., Fridriksson, J., … Sperber, C. (2022). Mapping the human praxis network: an investigation of white matter disconnection in limb apraxia of gesture production. *Brain Communications, 4*(1), 1–14. https://doi.org/10.1093/braincomms/fcac004

Salvi, R., Wang, J., & Ding, D. (2000). Auditory plasticity and hyperactivity following cochlear damage. *Hearing Research, 147*, 261–274.

Seven, Y., Mantilla, C., & Sieck, G. (2014). Recruitment of rat diaphragm motor units across motor behaviors with different levels of diaphragm activation. *Journal of Applied Physiology, 117*(11), 1308–1316. https://doi.org/10.1152/japplphysiol.01395.2013

Sunderland, A., & Shiner, C. (2007). Ideomotor apraxia and functional ability. *Cortex, 43*(3), 359–367. https://doi.org/10.1016/S0010-9452(08)70461-1

Teverovsky, E., Bickel, J., & Feldman, H. (2009). Functional characteristics of children diagnosed with childhood apraxia of speech. *Disability and Rehabilitation, 31*(2), 94–102. https://doi.org/10.1080/09638280701795030

Tuttolomondo, A., Pecoraro, R., & Pinto, A. (2014). Studies of selective TNF inhibitors in the treatment of brain injury from stroke and trauma: A review of the evidence to date. *Drug Design, Development and Therapy, 8*, 2221–2238. https://doi.org/10.2147/DDDT.S67655

Wang, M. L. (2014a). Co-occurring development of early childhood communication and motor skills: Results from a population based longitudinal study. *Child: Care, Health and Development*, 77–84.

Wang, M. L. (2014b). The developmental relationship between language and motor performance from 3 to 5 years of age: A prospective longitudinal population study. *BMC Psychology, 2*, 34. https://doi.org/10.1186/s40359-014-0034-3

Wasserman, T., & Mion, A. (2019). The progression of memory loss secondary to TBI-induced white matter attenuation: A review of the literature and case exemplar. *Journal of Pediatric Neuropsychology, 5*(1–2), 31–40.

Wasserman, T., & Wasserman, L. D. (2020). *Motivation, effort and the neural network model*. Springer.

Wessel, J., & Aron, A. (2017). On the globality of motor suppression: Unexpected events and their influence on behavior and cognition. *Neuron, 93*(2), 259–280. https://doi.org/10.1016/j.neuron.2016.12.013

Chapter 6
Developmental Coordination Disorder

One way of looking at the etiology of apraxia from a developmental perspective is to look at what happens when a functional circuit is disrupted by injury or disease. There is another way to consider. What happens when core motor circuits fail to initiate or develop appropriately? Neural network modeling would suggest that when this occurs, the ongoing, forward development of the individual could be negatively affected in multiple ways, to varying degrees, resulting in numerous disorders arising later in the developmental sequence. Some of these movement disorders may, in fact, be classified as apraxic conditions. In summary, these early motor networks comprise the foundation of more complex motor-based actions in synchrony with other neural pathways. Finally, it should be remembered that these newborn present neural networks are recruited for the numerous complex cognitive and motor skills that develop as we progress toward adulthood. As such, we can expect that if one of these foundational networks is disrupted, its inclusion in the network configuration for more complex behaviors would result in disruptions to the expression of all those subsequent behaviors, as well as impacting other network configurations secondary to their shared pathways. We cannot overstate the importance of considering this perspective. For those of us in the world of pediatric neuropsychology, whether it is in research, clinical practice, or neuropsychological evaluations, we must begin to look at the developing brain of a child differently than we do that of an adult. We must understand that applying a measure, whether in a neuropsychological testing or in research, that is, labeling a deficit rather than attending to areas of weakness, may cause us to miss the effects of a single or more likely multiple areas of impact on the cognitive and daily functioning of a developing child. As motor pathways and behaviors are developing even prenatally, we stress that disruption to this system is not a standalone disruption.

T. Wasserman, L. D. Wasserman, *Apraxia: The Neural Network Model*,
Neural Network Model: Applications and Implications,
https://doi.org/10.1007/978-3-031-24105-5_6

Developmental Coordination Disorder (DCD)

Developmental coordination disorder refers to a neurodevelopmental disorder characterized by deficits in both gross and fine motor skills. DCD is a heterogenous disorder with various phenotypical presentations. DCD is a condition involving limitations in gross motor, postural, and/or fine motor performance that are not attributable to other neurological disorders. Presentation varied across children and depends, in part, on their level of anticipatory motor control, response to specific task demands, and ability to attend to feedback to achieve flexible, adaptive movement. Children with DCD rely primarily on vision for feedback, frequently use "fixing" strategies, and exhibit limited motor repertoires. As a result of their movement problems, they tend to avoid physical activity and are prone to secondary impairments, including decreased strength and power (Missiuna et al., 2003). DCD affects a child's ability to execute voluntary coordinated motor actions. This results in poorly articulated, clumsy, slow, or inaccurate motor expression. Four main hypotheses have been postulated to explain DCD in terms of deficits in visuospatial functions, procedural learning, internal modeling, or executive functions. Neuroimaging studies are limited but have underlined several brain regions, including the parietal, frontal, and cerebellar cortices (Biotteau, 2020).

The History of Developmental Coordination Disorder

A developmental disorder affecting motor movement was initially termed "developmental dyspraxia" (Langford, 1955) and described motor difficulties and gestural and visuospatial dyspraxia. Attempts at describing the same disorder included labels such as developmental apraxia, childhood dyspraxia, and sensory motor integration disorder (Biotteau, 2020). Sensory integration disorder, currently termed Ayres Sensory Integration (ASI), was hypothesized to result from inefficient integration or organization of sensory information within the central nervous system (Ayres, 1972) established well before contemporary neuroimaging techniques were available, and remains a cornerstone treatment for occupational therapy interventions.

The DSM V describes developmental coordination disorder (DCD) as a neurodevelopmental disorder (American Psychiatric Association, 2013) along with other stereotypic and tic disorders. This neurodevelopmental umbrella also includes childhood apraxia of speech, which is highlighted in another chapter in this volume, referred to as speech sound disorders under the subheading of "Associated Features" and described as a disorder for which "other areas of motor coordination may be impaired as in developmental coordination disorder." In short, developmental coordination disorder is seen as the "umbrella" disorder under which other motor disorders fall, including childhood apraxia of speech. While the DSM V refers to overlapping phenotypes, this chapter is designed to highlight shared neural networks as a means of better understanding the often-shared phenotypical features found across these diagnostic categories and to highlight how neural network theory explains the ramifications developmentally, academically, and socially which often accompany this diagnostic category.

As we have highlighted elsewhere, confusion and ambiguity in definitional terms abound for many of the diagnostic categories. In an attempt to address the confusion, the World Health Organization, in 1992, termed the disorder "specific developmental disorder of motor function." In 1987, the term developmental coordination disorder was adopted by the American Psychiatric Association. While we laud the DSM V recognition of the disorders having neurodevelopmental underpinnings, including possible genetic and biomarker risk factors, the DSM V remains largely atheoretical and descriptive. In other words, ultimately, the DSM V lists a "disorder" based upon phenotype. Developmental coordination disorder is no exception.

Estimates of the prevalence of DCD vary according to the population of subjects and the definition utilized and range roughly from 5 to 8 percent, with a predominance of males diagnosed ranging from 2:1 to 3:1 (Biotteau, 2020).

DCD Early Signs and Phenotypical Presentations

Expressed (phenotype) difficulties as a result of DCD vary across ages but are observed early in the developmental course (Biotteau, 2020). Our current bent is to often adapt a "wait and see" attitude with early development and we provide a wide berth for the appearance of developmental milestones. Although we can applaud the acceptance and implementation of early intervention programs, even those are based upon the idea remediation rather than interception. However, there is research to suggest that developmental coordination disorder provides risk factor signs early. A recent study (Hua et al., 2022) looked at the association between onset of crawling and of independent walking with later motor development. The population was a total of 8395 children between the ages of 3 and 6 in China who were assessed at 3–4 and at 5–6 years old via the Movement Assessment Battery for Children, second Edition. The groups were categorized into "significant motor impairment" and "at risk" compared to typically developing children. They found that a 1-month delay in crawling increased the risk of significant overall (total score on MABC-2) motor impairment by 5.3 percent when compared to typically developing children. Compared to typically developing children, a 1-month delay in the onset of independent walking increased the risk of overall motor impairment by 7.7 percent. The risk became more pronounced with a 21.7 percent increase for "significant motor impairment" group and by 11.9 percent for the at risk of motor impairment group. The study confirms an association between delayed gross motor milestone achievement, crawling and walking, and subsequent motor impairment. Hua et al. extrapolate this association with other findings indicating that neurological evidence for the crawling milestone has been shown to be accompanied by neural changes which lead to cortical organization efficiency.

Phenotypical signs include poor postural control as noted by hypertonia or hypotonia, poor distal control and hand coordination, impaired balance, and difficulty in motor-based skills learning. Sensorimotor coordination is noted by poor sequencing of movement, poor use of movement feedback mechanisms, timing, and anticipation (prior to actual movement). As a result, areas of difficulty can include skills in dressing, utilizing tools such as scissors and eating utensils, tools, writing, playing sports, etc. (Gueze, 2001). Children with developmental coordination disorder often have lower academic achievement, reduced participation in social activities, which can lead to a more sedentary lifestyle and social isolation (Rinat, 2020). In addition, there are higher rates of anxiety and depression (Harrowell, 2017). While the predominant feature of DCD is motor learning and expression, difficulties with gross or fine motor, or both. And while the diagnostic category of developmental coordination disorder is a standalone diagnosis, DCD often co-occurs with language impairment and learning disabilities (Zwicker, 2009). In fact, children with DCD often have at least one other diagnosis including attention-deficit hyperactivity disorder, autism spectrum disorder, learning disabilities, and specific language impairment. ADHD is believed to be the most common comorbidly occurring disorder, with a prevalence of over 50 percent of DCD children also presenting with ADHD (Watemberg, 2007). The fact that there is a shared genetic component suggests that developmental coordination disorder is likely sharing etiological components with other developmental disorders as well (Martin, 2006). The shared phenotype presentations suggest shared connectome pathways.

A meta-analysis conducted by Wilson and McKenzie (1998) looked at "perceptual motor" problems in children with DCD, highlighting their difficulties in areas of visualizing movement and visual spatial analysis. In fact, they found that the greatest area of deficit was in visual processing, regardless of whether or not the task included a motor component.

Conversely, a study looking at the relationship between cognitive function and motor skills and their relation to school performance in students ages 8–14 (Fernandes, 2016) found a positive relationship between motor coordination and total score on the academic achievement test as well as on the block design and cancelation tests of the Wechsler Intelligence Scale for Children-IV. The authors conclude that visual motor coordination and visual selective attention, although not agility, are positively associated with academic achievement and cognitive function. This makes a great deal of sense to the current authors as it speaks to the need for visual motor coordination and visual selection in order to be successful in many areas of academic skills including scanning reading pages, scanning mathematical formulas, and writing.

As noted above, phenotyping varies. In an attempt to better define the presenting phenotypes as they present in DCD, Green (2008) looked at intervention for children grouped by level of severity of motor involvement and perceptual skills. They found support for subtyping particularly five subgroups based upon perceptual and motor performance. For example, one subtype was explored based upon the magnitude of movement difficulties and whether or not fine motor problems exceeded that of gross motor problems as well as complex motor skills grouping. They found that groups of children with visual perceptual deficits and with both visual perceptual and motor impairment presented with higher impact of motor impairment. The authors (Green, 2008) point out that there was considerable overlap and confounding secondary to comorbidities, which might be considered a weakness in terms of the particular study. However, for the purposes of this discussion, this speaks to how difficult it is to find a child for whom only a single domain is impacted. That finding a child for whom the impact is restricted to a single domain is the exception rather than the rule.

The concept of executive function as a single domain has been discussed by the current authors elsewhere. However, for the purposes of the current discussion, let us agree to look at executive function as a means of looking at multiple areas of functioning. Toward addressing the long-term trajectory of executive function components, Bernardi et al. (2018) looked at children between the ages of 7 and 11. They were assessed twice, 2 years apart. The authors found that developmental gains were similar between the DCD group and controls. However, the gains still reflected a gap between groups, that is, the children diagnosed with DCD performed more poorly than the control group of children on all nonverbal executive function tasks and the verbal fluency tasks at both times of assessment, 2 years apart. Of course, the obvious point of importance for the purposes of this volume is the notability that these children, diagnosed with observable motor deficits, are presenting with deficits well beyond the realm of motor.

The aforementioned study also included a group of children who presented with poor motor skills but no formal diagnosis. These children showed less pervasive executive function problems than those formally diagnosed. However, they did show difficulties, particularly in the areas of fluency and working memory.

In reality then, can we say that although we utilize a diagnostic category, we may be missing the impact of the identified area on other areas of functioning by labeling an area of deficit without understanding or educating others, such as parents and teachers, as to the extent of impact because of interrelatedness of neural pathways (connectome). In our effort to address this, we often list multiple diagnostic categories to account for the multiple areas of deficit. However, are we truly providing a deep as well as wide picture of a given child we have observed or evaluated if we are, again, not explaining the neural pathway interrelatedness of brain-based behavior and skill sets?

And what about the child who is at risk, but not presenting with weakness of sufficient severity to warrant a diagnosis? If under research paradigms we are looking at whole groups of children with undiagnosed weaknesses, but expressed weaknesses, are we not thereby ignoring the impact of the weaknesses on their academic and social performance? Again, the current authors wish to highlight the importance of recognizing the possibility, or probability, that soft signs, areas of weakness rather than outright deficit, are likely concomitant areas of concern with significant consequences.

Genetics Play a Role in Developmental Coordination Disorder

Genetic research as to etiology is still limited. The available research does point to a genetic role in the etiology of the disorder. A summary of the available data and research is provided: A family cluster (Gaines, 2008) was found in a Canadian family consisting of a (married) mother and eight children, five of whom met the criteria for DCD. These children also presented with speech articulation difficulties. Five of the seven children did not crawl and milestone attainment for independent walking was at the late end of normal. Four of the five children were late in attaining language milestones such as (no) two-word utterances by 2 years of age and presenting with limited vocabulary. The results of psychologist performed intellectual assessment indicated normal intellectual functioning, with a common weakness of processing speed. The authors discuss the likelihood of shared genetic causality across disorders.

There has been some modest attention to a region of chromosome 16. For example, the CNV 16p11.2 deletion, which results in childhood apraxia of speech, is also implicated in motor coordination difficulties (Cunningham, 2019). Another study looked at copy number variations (CNVs) (Mosca, 2016) in 82 children with DCD, with or without ADHD and/or a reading disorder. They found an increased rate of large and rare genic CNVs. Of these, 26 percent were found to have de novo rare CNV. Of the inherited CNVs, 64 percent were inherited from a parent with a neurodevelopmental disorder. In addition, twin studies have revealed genetic contribution estimates from 0.44 (Moruzzi, 2010) to 0.8 (Martin, 2006). Mountford (2021) point out that the effect of any individual CNV is difficult to determine and that individual CNVs may result in highly heterogeneous phenotypes.

Neuroimaging and Brain Studies

Following the course of study outlined for most disorders discussed in this volume, the hunt for the etiology of DCD commenced with assumptions about lesions. As far back as the 1960s, works by neurologists and neuropsychologists were looking at the possible involvement of cortical areas. Work by Geschwind et al., (1975) talked about possible disconnection syndromes. An assessment by Luria (Luria, 1973) talked about the role of the basal ganglia, parietal, and frontal lobes in motor deficits. The underdevelopment of the cerebellum in premature infants led Lesny (Lesny, 1980) to suggest the involvement of the cerebellum.

Children with developmental coordination disorder present with functional difficulties in posture, motor learning, and sensorimotor coordination (Zwicker, 2009). A comprehensive review article by Zwicker (2009) considers the role of neural correlates, including the cerebellum, parietal lobe, basal ganglia, and corpus callosum. Considering the role of the cerebellum in motor coordination, balance, and posture, the cerebellum is a likely choice for cortical involvement (Zwicker, 2009). Further, consideration of the role of the parietal lobe in processing visual spatial information, coupled with research indicating visual spatial dysfunction in children with DCD (Green, 2008), makes the parietal lobe another neural contender for involvement in DCD.

A study by Querne et al. (2008) can be used to highlight an important point when considering the neurophysiological integrity of a child's brain-based behaviors for example, during a neuropsychological evaluation or more cursory, perhaps age-based pediatrician visit. Querne et al. were interested in looking at the impact of DCD on neural connectivity during a go/no-go task. Utilizing fMRI they found that children with DCD scored similarly to controls on a measure of correct inhibition. However, their responses were slower and more variable. Utilizing structural equation modeling, they found an increase in path coefficients from both middle frontal cortex and anterior cingulate cortex to inferior parietal cortex, particularly in the left hemisphere in the DCD children. They found that path coefficients between the striatum and parietal cortex decreased in the right hemisphere. Based upon this data, Querne et al. hypothesize that DCD may reflect developmentally abnormal brain hemispheric specialization. They also hypothesized that the connectivity issue found in the middle frontal cortex-anterior cingulate cortex to inferior parietal cortex network pathway indicates that children with DCD have a greater difficulty in easily or promptly switching between initiation (go) and inhibition (no-go) responses. Perhaps most interestingly, they hypothesize that children with developmental coordination disorder compensate for the poor efficiency of the aforementioned neural network pathway through an increased engagement of the anterior cingulate cortex. This strategy would prevent excessive commission errors. This hypothesis is interesting for two reasons. Firstly, it speaks to neural plasticity in allowing for one cortical region to compensate for another. Secondly, it raises the question of when a child, with risk factors or mild connectivity issues, would present with compensatory behaviors versus when the system would become overwhelmed and pathognomonic signs are expressed. In other words, how many children do we work with who may be experiencing compromised neural pathway integrity but are able to compensate up to a given point, often masking the neural compromise? What happens when this compensatory system is stressed? Are we perhaps looking at the child who in a resting state appears fine, but when asked to sit upright and write classroom notes, or write an essay under timed conditions, that is, to maintain postural control and engage in a task requiring rapid fine motor coordination skills, begins to decompensate? The implications for this with respect to neuropsychological evaluation as well as the question of a child's upward limit in an academic setting should be given strong consideration.

The current state of affairs for very preterm infants reflects drastic increases in survival rates. We are, however, first understanding what the degree of prematurity may have on the developing brain. For example, a recent study looked at motor brain areas in very preterm infants that was defined as infants with a gestational age under 30 weeks and a birthweight under 1250 grams. Volumetric imaging was performed at the infant's term equivalent age. At 7 years of age, volumetric imaging was repeated and diffusion tensor imaging was performed. At the term age equivalent (Dewey, 2019), smaller brain volume was found for total volume, cortical gray matter, cerebellum, caudate accumbens, pallidum, and thalamus in children deemed at risk for DCD. The authors also found similar patterns when the children were reevaluated at 7 years of age, that is, there was no catchup for brain growth in the at-risk population. In fact, the children in the at-risk group presented with altered microstructure in multiple white matter tracts. This was particularly true for the motor areas.

Returning to neuroimaging studies, a later review of MRI such as neuroimaging studies (Biotteau, 2016) indicated that the brains of children with developmental coordination disorder present with atypical neuroanatomy. The findings point to an extensive neural network involving the parietal and frontal regions, the basal ganglia, the cerebellum, the parietal lobe, and parts of the frontal lobe. Biotteau et al. (2016) report on the literature associated with DCD and that which strongly suggests the involvement of the cerebellum and its network connections. Their review includes findings of visual distortions performed during motor tasks, difficulty with touching finger to nose, and rapid alternating hand movements among those finding pointing to the cerebellum or cerebellar loops being involved in DCD. Biotteau (2016) also contend that the cerebellum is not the only neural structure involved. They suggest that the basal ganglia, with associations with regulation of movement, are also correlates of neural involvement. Taken together Biotteau (2016) hypothesizes cortico-striatal and cortico-cerebellar network dysfunction.

Utilizing another major area of child development as an example, let us look at the evidence for neural connection between motor network and language and the implications for disturbances by association. In an interesting study, Jäncke (2007) utilized voxel-based morphometry from high-resolution MRI scans, to search for anomalies outside the typical language-based cortical areas. In this study of 42 children, 21 with developmental language disorder and 21 typical children, the comparison of white to gray matter was assessed. In addition, simple hand motor tests were used to assess for possible motor impairments in the children with developmental language disorder. The results are noteworthy. Jancke et al. found decreased white matter volume in a left hemisphere network which comprises the motor cortex, dorsal premotor cortex, ventral premotor cortex, and planum polare on the superior temporal gyrus. Specifically, these results are strongly indicative of the fact that children with a developmental language disorder have "anomalous anatomy" in a left-sided network which is comprised of both motor and language areas, indicating regionally identical areas for both domains. This provides stronger support to the current authors' contention that the current direction of looking for and identifying individual domains of dysfunction, to correlate with, for example, the DSM diagnostic categories, misses the probable impact of early disruption to any one area of the associated neural pathways and larger connectome regions.

In addition to measures of functional activity, some studies have looked at macrostructure or volume. These studies have been focused on cortical regions. For example, one study (Langevin et al., 2015) looked at cortical thickness in children with co-occurring attention-deficit disorder. As mentioned elsewhere, ADHD co-occurs with DCD in up to 50 percent of cases. Their interest was in assessing whether the effects of the co-occurring neurodevelopmental disorders affected the pattern of cortical development in a manner distinct from having a single disorder. Langevin et al. found greater and more widespread reduced cortical thickness in children with co-occurring DCD and ADHD than found for children with DCD or ADHD alone. The cortical thinning was found to be widespread, with concentrations in the frontal, parietal, and temporal lobes, and was correlated with measures of motor functioning and attentional functioning. This finding is compelling all on its own. We now have to look at the rate of ADHD co-occurring with DCD. And while the current authors do not have the answer, we do wonder about how many of these children have impact on reward and attention circuitry without meeting criteria for a formal diagnosis of ADHD.

(Note: Both the cerebellum and the basal ganglia are discussed in greater detail elsewhere in this volume. The reader is encouraged to review these sections in order to better understand the involvement of these cortical and subcortical regions in the initiation and regulation of voluntary motor movement and coordination. In particular, the reader will be directed to the implications of these regions as mechanisms working in unison in the developing brain and the expression of deficits in associated disabilities such as childhood apraxia of speech.)

DCD and the Impact on Other Neural Substrates

How Embedded in Other Systems Is the Motor System?

Historically, as we have discussed, the brain was considered to be composed of modular systems that were discrete and dissociable from each other. Seminal work by Wernicke and Broca, based upon lesion models, ascribed functional properties to specific area of the brain (i.e., the left hemisphere and language). The motor networks were no exception as they were considered to be an independent domain. Traditionally then, the neural substrates serving language functions and actions were considered dissociable and independent of the motor functional systems (Mirabella, 2017).

That thinking, however, began to change following advances in neuroscience and neuroimaging. An early overview in the work of Koziol et al. (2012) and others outlined how these neural network systems were integrated and that this integration was essential for complex human behavior. For example, Bak's disease model of motor neuron disease symptom presentation (Bak, 2012) proposed that the cognitive and motor symptoms which present in motor neuron disease reflect the same neurodegenerative process spreading along functional connections.

The current authors wish to suggest that just as the neurodegenerative process of motor neuron disease affects the closest functional links to the motor system, including the processing of verbs and action words, this model provides a back-tracing ability to understand how language function and embedded meaning advanced in the developing brain. To date, there is a full body of research to indicate that the motor system is highly associated with constructs and their subserving neural pathways including executive function (Wilson, 2020), attention (Kirst et al., 2017), learning disabilities (Zwicker, 2009), language, and autism spectrum disorder (Fulceri et al., 2019).

Toward this point, using a longitudinal study, Wilson et al. (2020) looked at 186 children who met the DCD criteria based upon the DSM 5. They were screened with McCarron Assessment of Neuromuscular Development at two periods over the course of 2 years. The Groton Maze Learning Test served as the measure of executive function. They found that 41 percent of the children diagnosed with DCD showed significantly lower levels of executive functioning as compared to children with typical motor development. This was true for both time points. This finding suggests that children with persisting DCD (which we know can persist into adulthood) demonstrated poorer executive function development than those with typical motor development or who demonstrated remitting DCD. We use this example because despite differences about the discussion of executive function as a standalone domain, this speaks to how skills associated with executive function, such as attention, motivation, persistence, etc., can theoretically be affected as the effect of motor coordination disorder impacts developing neural connections (Wasserman & Wasserman, 2013).

In a study (Piek, 2008) designed to assess the merits of utilizing measures of motor performance for children between 4 months and 4 years of age to predict motor and cognitive performance at school age, parents were asked to complete the Ages and Stages Questionnaires (ASQ). At school age both motor and cognitive ability were assessed using the McCarron Assessment of Neuromuscular Development for fine and gross motor abilities and the Wechsler Intelligence Scale for Children-IV for cognitive ability assessment. In a sample of 33 children, after controlling for SES, the fine motor trajectory information was not found to account for a significant proportion of variance for fine motor performance or cognitive performance. However, with controlling for SES, the ASQ gross motor trajectory did account for a significant proportion of the variance for cognitive performance. In addition, a significant predictive relationship for the gross motor trajectory information and the subtests on the Wechsler Scales for working memory and processing speed may be considered components of, or impacting the components of, executive function and efficiency on specific tasks. This study adds to the body of research supporting the potential impact of early gross motor development on later developing cognitive skills.

In addition, there is some evidence to indicate that an impacted motor system is associated with action-based language processing. Utilizing a go/no-go task, the processing of action verbs in children with developmental coordination disorder was compared to that of typical children. Two versions of the go/no-go task were utilized in which verbs expressing hand, foot, or abstract action were presented. In the "semantic" task, arm-reaching movement toward a target is required when either hand or foot actions are presented. The subjects are to refrain from reaching when abstract verbs are presented. A second version of the paradigm was also presented wherein the subjects were asked to utilize color discrimination rather than the semantic meaning of the verb to decide on whether to reach or not. That is to say, the decision to move is based upon the color of the verb presented rather than the semantic meaning of the verb presented. The results indicated that children with DCD did not demonstrate any difference between verb categories. Typically developing children, in contrast, showed an increase in reaction time to a verb involved in the same effector used to give the response. That is to say, when the meaning of the verb was the cue for reaching, both reaction time and percentage of error increased for typically developing children. The authors (Mirabella, 2017) conclude that this is a pathognomonic sign of the motor system impacting language processing.

Are there risk factors that don't meet pathognomonic levels? What are the potential implications? Some of these questions were considered in a published doctoral dissertation by Goyen (Goyen, 2005) who noted that infants born under 29 weeks gestation (extremely premature) or extremely low birth weight (under 1000 grams) are at high risk for major and minor sequelae, but the research on these children is often limited to assessing for major deficits. The majority of these children are often termed "apparently normal" with "normal intelligence" and no major sensorineural disabilities. However, Goyen (2005) notes that these children present with "minor motor dysfunction," the impact of which is not investigated. Using an embedded multiple study paradigm, Goyen found the following: in a longitudinal study, children were assessed with the Peabody Developmental Motor Scales at the corrected (for prematurity) age of 18 months and again at 3 and then 5 years of age. Goyen found that 64 percent of the children presented with persistent fine motor problems throughout this time frame. In addition, the proportion of children with gross motor deficits actually increased from 18 months (corrected) to the 5-year mark with 81 percent of the children now showing gross motor impact. The second study looked at the impact of motor function in school-aged children from an "apparently normal" high-risk group. This included children with an IQ < 85 and no identified sensorineural disability. The results indicated a significantly higher presentation of DCD compared to the control group. That is to say, utilizing the Movement Assessment Battery for Children and a battery of sensorimotor tests, the high-risk group presented with 42 percent falling in the DCD category compared to 8 percent in the control group. Of note, it was what are considered "neurological soft signs" that contributed to the diagnosis of developmental coordination disorder in the high-risk group. This included postural praxis and sequencing praxis. These findings speak to often unrecognized weakness children must endure or compensate for but ones which most certainly impact the quality of their everyday efforts. In fact, study 3 did find poorer handwriting legibility and speed in comparison to the children's controls in a classroom setting. These children were the same studied in the prior sub-study allowing for an assessment of comorbidity between DCD and handwriting dysfunction. The finding was that of the high-risk children identified as meeting the criteria for DCD, there was a 43 percent comorbidity level for handwriting dysfunction.

Motor Networks in the Newborn and Their Involvement with Later Skills Development

The question of whether movement is produced by active (motor programs) or reactive (reflex) means is quite literally an age-old question, dating back to Aristotle. More recently, this question was fueled by the studies of Ivan Pavlov. Pavlov developed a theory of inborn and conditioned reflexes, according to which all movement is an extension of inborn or conditioned reflexes. He posited that new movement emerges as a result of the creation of repetitive excitation neurons creating new neural pathways. Also highly influential was the work of a neurophysiologist, Sir Charles Sherrington, who posited that movement is modulated by the parameters of reflexes. For example, he discovered muscle spindles which initiate the stretch reflex, a reflex he maintained was necessary for posture and balance. It was Sherrington who coined the terms "synapse" and "neurons," and his work helped to shape our understanding of the brain and spinal cord, as well as efferent and afferent nerve fibers (Latash, 2008). In contrast was the argument by Bernstein (2003) for motor programs. This theory of generalized motor programs posited that patterns of mechanical variables of muscle and joint torque were encoded in the central nervous system (Latash, 2008). In this paradigm, a motor pattern is associated with a motor program. This brings us to the equilibrium-point hypothesis (Feldman & Levin, 1995) which combines elements of the reflex model and the motor program model. A detailed review of the studies emanating from these models, looking at muscles, enervation, equilibrium and multi joint, whole body movement, is far beyond the scope of this chapter and, can be found in the work of Latash (2008).

From the perspective of child development and neural pathways, we can agree that core systems of the brain are established during the gestational course and are foundational to infants' emerging developmental competencies. Among the earliest to mature are the motor and sensory systems, which support the ability of the infant to interact with and receive input from the world (Thomason et al., 2018). From their formation these neural systems are highly malleable which supports a learned fit between the early environment and the infant brain. The brain is primed at birth to receive inputs from sensory organs, and the signals received play an essential role in advancing neurodevelopmental processes. Experimental disruption to normal occurrence and propagation of activity through sensorimotor systems leads to permanent loss of function in those systems and lasting atypical cortical organization. Thus, sensorimotor systems are present at birth, and receptive to signals from the environment, which instruct further developmental patterning of neural systems. Moreover, these systems can produce behavior, enabling the developing organism, or infant, to build representations of stimulus-response properties through interaction with the environment.

What are the elements of the network? Thanks to advances in neuroimaging and the neurosciences, there is ample data to demonstrate that this robust fetal sensorimotor neural network includes regions of the motor and sensory cortices, cerebellum, thalamus, posterior cingulate cortex, and striatum. Also included are regions of the posterior cingulate cortex, supplementary motor cortex, medial temporal lobe, and superior frontal gyrus (Thomason et al., 2018).

Functional Expression in Later Development

Although once considered to possibly remediate on its own through maturation, there is ample evidence that DCD can persist into adolescence and adulthood. Studies clearly indicate that deficits in motor coordination extend into adulthood with resulting effects on academic functioning, non-academic functioning, with concomitant impact on the emotional state of the affected persons (Tal-Saba, 2012). A study by Cousins and Smyth (2003) recruited individual between the ages of 18 and 65 who had been diagnosed previously with DCD or dyspraxia. The participants were assessed on motor dexterity, handwriting, construction, balance, avoidance of obstacles, reaction time, movement time, and sequencing. The performance of the DCD participants was marked by greater slowness and variability of movement. Many of the participants had difficulties with sequencing. The data indicates that motor difficulties, and its associated complications, do persist into adulthood.

As mentioned previously, there is a high degree of associated features between DCD and ADHD (Watemberg, 2007). Looking at the concept of executive function in young adults with developmental coordination disorder as compared to controls (Tal Saban, 2014), participants with DCD completed the BRIEF-A to assess executive function skills and the WURS questionnaire to assess attention issues. The executive function profiles of persons with DCD and borderline DCD indicated significantly poorer functioning than those of the control group, and no significant differences regarding attention issues were found between the DCD and borderline DCD groups. The results of the study also suggest that executive functions can be affected with or without concomitant attention issues.

Also of interest is a study (Cleaton et al., 2021) specifically intending to look at gender differences in presentation. Cleaton et al. found that in adults (aged 16–25) diagnosed with DCD, women reported more impact in gross and non-motor activities. They also reported a negative impact on participation in activities. In contrast, men reported greater fine motor difficulties. There are so many fascinating questions that can be asked given this kind of information. For example, given the age of the groups, were boys identified because of school-based behavior, specifically the typical need in a classroom to take notes? Are women more easily able to state that they are not good in sports? Did these weaknesses impact social and/or attention areas of functioning? Gender provides one more area of interest for consideration when looking at phenotype presentations.

Child Development: The Result of the Integration of Movement, Language, and Cognitive Processes

Action understanding is a critical foundation for developing social cognitive constructs. The ability to understand actions is at the base of empathy, theory of mind, cooperation, and other skills including language (Salo, 2019). Actions are behavior and motor based. Salo (2019) suggest that activation of the motor system during the observation of actions underlies both action understanding and the larger construct of communication.

When Does the Development of the Motor System Begin?

In a study of fetal movement and development (Einspieler et al., 2021), a point, perhaps central to this chapter, is highlighted. Einspieler et al. state "The term sensory is always used first when we discuss the central nervous system (sensori-motor) as a functional unit" followed by "but the actual ontogeny of behaviour is quite the opposite. The developing nervous system in its early stages ought to be seen as a motor-sensory organ, therefore we should put the term motor first." They cite multiple sources, dating back to 1885, and confirmed by modern technology, which establishes that spontaneous motility occurs in utero, even preceding external (sensory) input. The term "central pattern generator" refers to the underlying neural circuitry of the endogenously generated activity, which, modulated by the periphery, is not triggered by external sensory stimulation. Of great significance is the term "rhythmicity," a term we have stressed the importance of in the chapter on language, stressed here for motor movement. Specifically, rhythmicity, "which is inherent not only in alternating movements for locomotion, sucking and breathing movements, but also in the alternation of short phases of activity followed by longer phases of inactivity," is a typical pattern of fetal behavior. They point out that contrary to popular notions, the fetus is not typically in a fixed, flexed position. Rather, there are a multitude of fetal movement patterns which are spontaneously generated, and these movement patterns are closely associated with development of peripheral and central structures. That is to say, these movement patterns are integral to muscular neural development. Many of these movements already reflect an integrating system. For example, at 8–10 weeks gestation, the entire body movement is observed. Actually, there are two movement patterns observed. There are startles that initiated in the limbs which spread to the neck and trunk. There are also slower, more complex movements called general movements. Their presentation is simultaneous and points to an adaptive pattern since startles often induce a general movement. This is a good example of early modulation, a process necessary for almost every conceivable human behavior.

Some motor movements can be seen in utero and become a function later on. For example, yawning, a behavior occurring across species, is hypothesized to impact arousal and communication as it increases cerebrospinal fluid circulation. Beginning at 14 weeks gestation, rhythmic jaw openings and closings followed by swallowing movements can be observed. The neuronal network is formed and functional by 28 weeks gestation and consists of suck-swallow-breathe patterns reflecting a rhythmic motor sequence (Shandley, 2021), again, complex motor sequences with functional purpose later. Einsplier et al. (2021) point out that fetal sucking changes the composition of the fluid in the nasal and laryngeal pathways which is critical for chemo-sensation development. In addition, there is considerable literature indicating that suck ability serves not only as a marker for oral feeding skills but for its association with neuromotor integrity, neuromodulation, and sensorimotor systems (Poore, 2009) as well as later speech-language disorders.

Pointing has also been observed in utero (Einspieler et al., 2021) and is a motor behavior, sophisticated in that it requires digital isolation, and is later used as a communication strategy.

"Embryonic/fetal movements are an integral part of typical development, as skeletal, muscular, and neural developments in particular are activity-dependent. If embryonic/fetal neuromuscular activity is silenced pharmacologically or by disease, the population of spinal motor neurons, the transmitter specification, the pattern of neuromuscular synaptic contact, and genetically determined cell death develop atypically." The impact of these factors can be observed in the fetus. "In case of brain dysfunction, fetal general movements alter their sequence and gestalt, which suggests a dysfunction of the developing nervous system" (Einspieler et al., 2021). While one might not initially conceive of this as apraxia, it clearly relates to disturbed motor behavior perhaps affected by external factors such as maternal drug use, which in turn can be impacting central nervous system development. The expression is noted by alterations in motor sequences and presentations in utero.

From the perspective of neuropsychology and child development, the implications are huge. First, motor development precedes cognition. Second, motor development "even" in utero is showing patterns of behaviors which are later directed to be functional in the expression and reception of communication as well as the processing of incoming information. Third, modulation of go/no-go behavior begins in utero with motor behavior. We have the beginnings of neural substrates critical for integrating all aspects of human behavior.

By perceiving this period through the early stages of child development as simply "developmental," we are missing critical information necessary for a complete understanding of a child's brain-based behavior.

From a pediatric neuropsychology perspective, we are potentially underestimating the impact of soft signs on a child's academic, social, and physical development. That is to say, the error of waiting for pathognomonic signs to emerge as measured by "standardized" norms. As regards the ability of a neuropsychologist to assess these functions, it is accurate to say that they can be assessed, but perhaps not "tested" as far as normative instruments are concerned. It is the integrity of these motor-sensory systems that can be assessed using procedures such as in the Neonatal Behavioral Assessment Scale (Brazelton, 1973) which provides useful qualitative data on early neural integrity, by assessing response patterns to sensory input, and the results of which can be extrapolated to future cognitive activity. This knowledge can be used to generate intervention plans when necessary, thereby allowing neuropsychologists to meaningfully participate in the care of these at-risk infants.

With regard to neuropsychological assessment at later points in a child's development, many neuropsychologists often make what we would consider to be a mistake, that of under-inquiring about and/or observational testing of early motor development and tying that to other domains and to the presenting reason for referral. Observation is one of our strengths. While we are focusing training on the utilization of tests as measures, we need to also remember to observe. When he was stringing beads, was he successful? But did he have to balance both string and hands on a hard surface or was he able to elevate his hand? Was the stringing smooth or did he drop one or two beads first? How did that child descend the stairs? Was he sure of his movements and talking at the same time or did he run his foot along the edge of the stair and rotate his body toward the banister for more security? Was he able to stand on one foot or did he reach for a surface to lean on first? These indicators may not be on a standardized measure, but they are diagnostic. And if they are on a standardized measure, be careful on how you score it. Is getting the bead on the string the point? Or is the quality of the sequencing and movements the important factor?

From a clinical standpoint, this may mean underestimating the impact of dysfunctional systems such as dyspraxia vs. apraxia. From a societal perspective, it means we may be missing a vital period for intervention services which may, if delivered during early developmental critical periods, afford greater remediation than if delivered later.

References

American Psychiatric Association. (2013). Diagnostic and statistical manual of mental disorders fifth edition.

Ayres, J. (1972). Types of sensory integrative dysfunction among disabled learners. *American Journal of Occupational Therapy, 26*(1), 13–18.

Bak, T. H. (2012). What wires together dies together: Verbs, actions and neurodegeneration in motor neuron disease. *Cortex, 48*(7), 936–944.

Bernardi, M. L. (2018). Executive functions in children with developmental coordination disorder: a 2-year follow-up study. *Developmental Medicine and Child Neurology*, 306–313.

Bernstein, N. (2003). *Contemporary studies on the physiology of the of the neural process*. Smysl.

Biotteau, M. C. (2016). Neural signature of DCD: A critical review of MRI neuroimaging studies. Frontiers in Neurology. https://doi.org/10.3389/fneur.2016.00227

Biotteau, M. A. (2020). Developemental coordination disorder. In A. B. Gallagher (Ed.), Handbook of clinical neurology. Vol 174 *Neurocognitive development: Disorder and disabilities* (pp. 3–20). Elsevier.

Brazelton, T. B. (1973). *Neonatal behavioral assessment scale*.

Cleaton, A. T.-S., Tal-Saban, M., Hill, E. L., & Kirby, A. (2021). Gender and age differences in the presentation of at-risk or probable developmental coordination disorder in adults. *Research in Developmental Disabilities, 115*, 104010. https://doi.org/10.1016/j.ridd.2021.104010

Cousins, M. & Smyth, M. M. (2003). Developmental coordination impairments in adulthood. *Human Movement Science, 22*, 433–459. https://doi.org/10.1016/j.humov.2003.09.003. PMID: 14624827.

Cunningham, A. C. (2019). Coordination difficulties, IQ and psychopathology in children with high-risk copy number variants. *Psychological Medicine, 51*, 290–299. https://doi.org/10.1017/S0033291719003210

Dewey, D. T. (2019). Very preterm children at risk for developmental coordination disorder have brain alterations in motor areas. *Acta Paediatrica, 108*(9), 1649. https://doi.org/10.1111/apa.14786

Einspieler, C. P., Prayer, D., & Marschik, P. B. (2021). Fetal movements; the origin of human behaviour. *Developmental Medicine & Child Neurology, 63*(10), 1142–1148.

Feldman, A. G., & Levin, M. F. (1995). Positional frames of reference in motor control: Their origin and use. *Behavioral and Brain Sciences, 18*, 723–806.

Fernandes, W. S.-P. (2016). Motor coordination correlates with academic achievement and cognitive function in children. *Frontiers in Psychology, 7*. https://doi.org/10.3389/fpsyg.2016.00318

Fulceri, F., Grossi, E., Contaldo, A., Narzisa, A., Apicella, F., Parrini, I., et al. (2019, January 9). Motor skills as moderators of core symptoms in autism spectrum disorders: Preliminary data from an exploratory analysis with artificial neural networks. *Frontiers in Psychology*. https://doi.org/10.3389/fpsyg.2018.02683

Gaines, R. C. (2008). Clinical expression of developmental coordination disorder in a large Canadian family. *Paediatrics and Child Health, 13*, 763–768.

Geshwind, H., Tenaillon, A., Samii, K., Nitenberg, G., & Farah, E. (1975). Evaluation des lesions tricuspidiennes par la cineangiographie. *Coeur, 6*, 687–703.

Goyen, T. (2005). Motor dysfunction in apparently normal high-risk children. *Academia.edu*. https://www.academia.edu/27667038/Motor_dysfunction_in_apparently_normal_high_risk_children

Green, D. C. (2008). Does subtype of developmental coordination disorder count: Is there a differential effect on outcome following intervention? *Human Movement Science, 27*, 363. https://doi.org/10.1016/j.humov.2008.02.009

Gueze, R. J.-E. (2001). Clinical and research diagnostic criteria for developmental coordination disorder: A review and discussion. *Human Movement Science, 20*(1-2), 7–47.

Harrowell, I. H. (2017). Mental health outcomes of developmental coordination disorder in late adolescence. *Developmental Medicine & Child Neurology, 59*(9), 973–979.

Hua, J. W., Williams GJ, Jin H, Chen J, Xu M, Zhou Y, Gu G, Du W (2022). Early motor milestones in infancy and later motor impairments: A population-based data linkage study. *Psychiatry*. https://doi.org/10.3389/fpsyt.2022.809181

Jäncke, L. S. (2007). Decreased white-matter density in a left-sided fronto-temporal network in children with developmental language disorder: Evidence for anatomical anomalies in a motor-language network. *Brain and Language*, 91–98.

Kirst, C., Modes, C., & Magnasco, M. (2017). Shifting attention to dynamics: Self-reconfiguration of neural networks. *Current Opinion in Systems Biology, 3*, 132–140. https://doi.org/10.1016/j.coisb.2017.04.006

Koziol, L., Budding, D., & Chidekel, D. (2012). From movement to thought: Executive function, embodied cognition, and the cerebellum. *Cerebellum, 11*(2), 505–525. https://doi.org/10.1007/s12311-011-0321-y

Langevin, L. M., MacMaster, F. P., & Dewey, D. (2015). Distinct patterns of cortical thinning in concurrent motor and attention disorders. *Developmental Medicine and Child Neurology, 3*, 257–264.

Langford, W. (1955). Developmental dyspraxia – Abnormal clumsiness. *Bulletin of the Orton Society, 5*, 3–7.

Latash, M. (2008). Evolution of motor control: From reflexes and motor programs to the equilibrium-point hypothesis. *Journal of Human Kinetics, 19*, 3–24.

Lesny, I. (1980). Developmental dyspraxia-dysgnosia as a cause of congenital children's clumsiness. *Brain Development, 2*, 69–71. https://doi.org/10.1016/S0387-7604(80)80009-X

Luria, A. (1973). *The working brain*. Basic Books.

Martin, N. P. (2006). DCD and ADHD: A genetic study of their shared aetiology. *Human Movement Science, 25*, 110–124.

Mirabella, G. D. (2017). Developpmental coordination disorder affects the processing of action relate verbs. *Frontiers in Human Neuroscience, 10*. https://doi.org/10.3389/fnhum.2016.00661

Missiuna, C., Rivard, L., & Bartlett, D. (2003). Early identification and risk management of children with developmental coordination disorder. *Pediatric Physical Therapy, 15*(1), 32–38.

Moruzzi, S. P.-G. (2010). Clumsiness and psychopathology: Causation or shared etiology? A twin study with the CBCL 6–18 questionnaire in a general school-age population sample. *Human Movement Science, 29*, 326–338. https://doi.org/10.1016/j.humov.2010.01.005

Mosca, S. L. (2016). Copy-number variations are enriched for neurodevelopmental genes in children with developmental coordination disorder. *Journal of Medical Genetics, 53*(12), 812–819. https://doi.org/10.1136/jmedgenet-2016-103818

Mountford, H. H. (2021). Genome-wide association study of motor coordination. *Frontiers in Human Neuroscience*. https://doi.org/10.3389/fnhum.2021.669902

Piek, J. D. (2008). The role of early fine and gross motor development on later motor and cognitive ability. *Human Movement Science, 5*, 668–681.

Poore, M. B. (2009). Suck predicts neuromotor integrity and developmental outcomes. *Perspective on speech and Orofacial Disorders., 19*, 44. https://doi.org/10.1044/ssod19.1.44

Querne, L., & Berquin, P. (2008, 1244). Dysfunction of the attentional brain network in children with Developmental Coordination Disorder: A fMRI study. *Brain Research*, 89–102.

Rinat, S. I.-N. (2020). Children with developmental coordination disorder show altered functional connectivity compared to peers. *Neuroimage: Clinical, 27*. https://doi.org/10.1016/j.nicl.2020.102309

Salo, V. F. (2019). The role of the motor system in action understanding and communication: Evidence from human infants and non human primates. *Developmental Psychobiology, 61*(3), 390–401.

Shandley, S. C. (2021). Abnormal nutritive sucking as an indicator of neonatal brain injury. *Frontiers in Pediatrics, 8*. https://doi.org/10.3389/fped.2020.599633

Tal Saban, M. O. (2014). Executive function and attention in young adults with and without Developmental Coordination Disorder – A comparative study. *Research in Developmental Disabilities, 35*, 2644–2650.

Tal-Saba, M. Z. (2012). The functional profile of young adults with suspected developmental coordination disorder (DCD). *Research in Developmental Disabilities, 33*, 2193–2202. https://doi.org/10.1016/j.ridd.2012.06.005

Thomason, M., Hect, J., Waller, R., Manning, J., Stacks, A., Beeghly, M., et al. (2018). Prenatal neural origins of infant motor development: Associations between fetal brain and infant motor development. *Developmental Psychopathology, 30*(3), 763–772. https://doi.org/10.1017/S095457941800072X

Wasserman, T., & Wasserman, L. (2013). Towards a unifying model of executive function. *Applied Neuropsychology: Child, 2*(2), 88–96. https://doi.org/10.1080/21622965.2013.748394

Watemberg, N. W.-S. (2007). Developmental coordination disorder in children with attention-deficit–hyperactivity disorder and physical therapy intervention. *Developmental Medicine & Child Neurology, 920-925*(49), 12.

Wilson, P. H., & McKenzie, B. E. (1998). Information processing eficits associated with developmental coordination disorder: A meta-analysis of research findings. *Jornal of Child Psychology, 39*, 829–840.

Wilson, P. R.-G. (2020). Cognitive and motor function in developmental coordination disorder. *Developmental Medicine and Child Neurology*, 1317–1323.

Zwicker, J. M. (2009). Neural correlates of developmental coordination disorder: A review of hypotheses. *Child Neurology, 24*, 1273–1281.

Chapter 7
Childhood Apraxia of Speech

Since, as we have reported, the inspiration for this book was a child with childhood apraxia of speech, we thought it's only fitting to cover this apraxic condition in more detail. We also note that the developmental nature of the disorder and the lack, in most cases, of an identifiable etiology provide fertile ground for a discussion of neural network modeling. Specifically, this chapter will review the current understandings of CAS based upon descriptive diagnostic characteristics, followed by an integration of neuroimaging and genetic information. Following this a second chapter will detail our understanding of neural network development and how brain-based development may be affected by and impact the expression of unfolding developmental skills across language, cognitive, academic, and social venues.

What Is Childhood Apraxia of Speech?

Based on the phenotypical nature of the existing definitions, this seems like a straightforward question. However, just as there is much confusion about the definition of apraxia proper, ambiguity extends into the discussion of what is a childhood apraxia of speech.

According to the American Speech-Language-Hearing Association (ASHA) (American Speech Hearing Association, 2022), childhood apraxia of speech (CAS) is a neurological childhood (pediatric) speech sound disorder in which the precision and consistency of movements underlying speech are impaired in the absence of neuromuscular deficits (e.g., abnormal reflexes, abnormal tone). As stated in this definition, CAS may occur as a result of known neurological impairment, in association with complex neurobehavioral disorders of known and unknown origin, or as an idiopathic neurogenic speech sound disorder. The core impairment in planning

T. Wasserman, L. D. Wasserman, *Apraxia: The Neural Network Model*,
Neural Network Model: Applications and Implications,
https://doi.org/10.1007/978-3-031-24105-5_7

and/or programming spatiotemporal parameters of movement sequences results in errors in speech sound production and prosody (Childhood Apraxia of Speech, 2022).

The term childhood apraxia of speech (CAS), as used by ASHA, covers all forms and presentations of apraxia of speech in childhood whether or not the etiology is congenital or acquired and whether or not it is associated with a specific etiology.

ASHA prefers CAS over other terms used for this disorder, including "developmental apraxia of speech" and "developmental verbal dyspraxia," which typically refer to idiopathic presentations and not to acquired neurological etiologies. The rationale, as described on their website, states that they are concerned that the "inclusion of the term 'developmental' in reference to childhood apraxia might be incorrectly interpreted as indicating that children can 'grow out of' this disorder." Unlike a speech delay, they note that the characteristics of CAS are likely to persist past the developmental period (Lewis et al., 2004). Other expert sources make note of the definition. For example, the Mayo Clinic website (Mayo Clinic, 2022) notes that "CAS is sometimes referred to as Developmental Apraxia. They agree with ASHA when they go on to say that children with CAS don't necessarily grow out of CAS as they develop. They highlight critical differences when they point out that, as compared to children with delayed speech or developmental language disorders where children follow usual patterns in development of speech and sounds, but they develop more slowly than usual." Children with CAS don't make typical developmental sound errors. It is not an issue of delayed development.

A formalized definition of CAS is presented in the Diagnostic and Statistical Manual of Mental Disorders, 5th edition (American Psychiatric Association, 2013) which includes CAS in the category of speech sound disorder. According to the DSM 5 which prefers the term verbal dyspraxia, CAS is defined as:

(A) Persistent difficulty with speech sound production that interferes with speech intelligibility or prevents verbal communication of messages.
(B) The disturbance causes limitations in effective communication that interfere with social participation, academic achievement, or occupational performance, individually or in any combination.
(C) Onset of symptoms is in the early developmental period.
(D) The difficulties are not attributable to congenital or acquired conditions, such as cerebral palsy, cleft palate, deafness or hearing loss, traumatic brain injury, or other medical or neurological conditions.

The DSM 5 goes on to describe how speech production describes the clear articulation of the phonemes that, in combination, make up spoken words. It notes how "speech sound production requires both the phonological knowledge of speech sounds and the ability to coordinate the movements of the articulators (i.e., jaw, tongue, and lips) with breathing and vocalizing for speech." It goes on to clarify that "Children with speech production difficulties may experience difficulty with phonological knowledge of speech sounds or the ability to coordinate movements for speech in varying degrees." Speech sound disorder is thus heterogenous and multidimensional in its underlying mechanisms and includes phonological disorder and articulation disorder.

Under the "associated features supporting diagnosis" section in the DSM 5, it is noted that a language disorder, particularly expressive deficits, may be found to co-occur with speech sound disorder. Thus, it is considered possible that CAS can occur in the absence of disordered language. While this is possible, we believe this occurrence to be rare.

The DSM 5 also suggests that "If the ability to rapidly coordinate the articulators is a particular aspect of difficulty, there may be history of delay or incoordination acquiring skills that also utilize the articulators and related facial musculature; among others, these skills include chewing, maintaining mouth closure, and blowing the nose. Other areas of motor coordination may be impaired. Verbal dyspraxia is described in the DSM 5 as a disorder in which other areas of motor coordination may be impaired, as in Developmental Coordination Disorder." From a neural network perspective, these associated conditions are not surprising. It suggests that a thorough assessment of verbal dyspraxia (CAS) routinely includes assessment of all aspects of motor coordination.

Is There a Difference Between CAS and Verbal Dyspraxia?

If we refer back to the ASHA definition, we see that there are three categories of etiologies of CAS:

(A) CAS can occur as a result of a neurological impairment (i.e., stroke, traumatic brain injury, infection). As this apraxia would be the result of trauma, one could expect there to be positive findings on brain MRI scans.
(B) CAS can occur as a result of a neurobehavioral disorder, that is, genetic, metabolic, and/or mitochondrial disorders. This group assumes that CAS then occurs as a result of conditions such as chromosome disorders or in association with disorders such as autism.
(C) CAS can occur as an idiopathic speech sound disorder. This means that the apraxia is of unknown origin, so there is no evidence of either a neurological impairment or neurobehavioral condition.

ASHA clarifies that they use the term *childhood apraxia of speech* (CAS) as an umbrella term for all presentations of apraxia of speech in childhood, whether the etiology is congenital or acquired. In contrast, The DSM 5 focuses on the present disorder manifestations but recognizes a potential association to the larger issue of motor dysfunction. In both cases, the presentation is the focus irrespective of etiology.

So, What Can We Definitively Say About the Definition of CAS?

Let's start by defining the process of speech. The National Institute on Deafness and Other Communication Disorders (National Institute of Deafness and Other Communication Disorders, 2022) describes speech in the following manner: speech is produced through a series of precisely coordinated muscle movements involving breathing, phonation (voice production), and articulation (movement of the throat, palate, tongue, and lips).

We know that estimations of delays in speech and language acquisition in 5-year-old children are at approximately 10–12 percent for speech and language, 7 percent for language only, and 8 percent for speech delay only (Law, 2000; Norbury, 2016). Of this population the presentation rate for CAS has been estimated to be 2.4 percent for the idiopathic subset and 4.3 percent when associated with complex neurodevelopmental disorder (Shriberg, 2019). We also know that CAS is considered a disorder affecting speech.

The prevalence of CAS has reportedly increased substantially during the past decades. For example, in a study of 12,000 to 15,000 estimated diagnostic outcomes for children referred with speech delay of unknown origin from 1998 to 2004, a staff of 15 speech language pathologists in a large metropolitan hospital diagnosed 516 (3.4–4.3%) of these children as having suspected CAS (Delaney & Kent, 2004). There are several reasons given for this increase. Among them are Birth-to-Three Legislation, increased information and recognition, and reimbursement requirements that are based on diagnostic codes (ASHA, 2007).

The Idea of CAS Has Historically Been Controversial

From a historical perspective, the term CAS has been quite controversial as a clinical diagnosis. In 1981, Guyette and Diedrich (1981) reviewed more than 100 studies. They found inconsistencies with each aspect of the studies, that is, population characteristics and diagnostic inconsistencies. CAS was noted to be reflective of a neurological issue that precedes speech but one wherein specificity of pathognomonic markers was absent, resulting in the authors labeling CAS as a "label in search of a population." Perhaps more eloquently, from a pediatric developmental perspective, Malmenholt (2020) described CAS as "confusing as we were using the term apraxia for a developmental speech problem, indicating the loss of a skill not yet acquired." It is an interesting observation that causes us, or should cause us, as treating or diagnostic clinicians, to pay attention to risk factors which may not yet be pathognomonic signs.

Apraxia of speech was the model, and we believe, quite different from a pediatric one. As we will talk about later, the model for many areas of neuropsychology was damage to adults. This assumes an already developed system with acquired damage to an already developed cerebral connectome. Clinicians with a pediatric bent will immediately recognize the folly of this conceptualization. Children are developing organisms, and as such, difficulties presenting at a particular age would be assumed to impact future development of the neural pathways and subsequent behavioral outcomes. However, the current diagnostic model clusters behavior into a diagnostic label.

This behavioral descriptor model, while understood to be necessary for communication among clinicians, reflects how behaviors can be found in more than one disorder, or not at all for some in a particular disorder. Hence, we end up with the DSM model which points to the association of disorders, or rather, the possible association of disorders because of the possibility of shared behaviors across diagnostic labels. Specifically, the reader is asked to refer back to the DSM description of a verbal apraxia and its possible relationship to phonological disorders, apraxia, and motor coordination disorders. To be very clear, it is the intent of the current authors to highlight that models have been based upon developed or adult systems. A child is not a developed neurophysiological organism. Rather, a child is developing, and there is potential for any disorder, because of its location or etiology, to impact all or some forward-moving systems.

What Are Some Comorbidity Associations?

Children diagnosed with CAS often have concomitant issues. In a review of literature, Iuzzini-Siegel (2017) found that greater than 50% of children with CAS also present with fine and gross motor deficits. There are estimates of children with CAS having comorbid language impairments ranging from 46 to 82 percent (Murray, 2018) with better receptive than expressive skill capabilities. Children with CAS may also have comorbid dysarthria or a phonological disorder which makes analyzing which symptoms belong to which disorder challenging (Iuzzini-Siegel, 2017). Reading and writing impairments often develop (Lewis, 2004). In fact, one study (Miller et al., 2019) found that in a group of young people, aged 7–17 years of age, diagnosed with either CAS or speech sound disorder, 65 percent of the CAS group, compared to 24 percent of the speech sound disorder group, was classified as low-proficiency readers based upon nonsense and single-word decoding. Within the larger group of low-proficiency readers, no difference was found on overall reading or oral language, or phonological awareness.

Is CAS Underdiagnosed?

A question arises as to whether this is a diagnosis which is underdiagnosed. In the current authors' opinion, this largely remains true with many diagnosticians seemingly reluctant to make the diagnosis, preferring speech delay or specific language impairment. Does this speak to the ambiguity of the diagnostic markers; the current mindset to diagnose based upon the modular, behavioral presentation; or a reluctance to be the diagnostician who has to speak to the parents of a young child about the potential breadth and length, that is, the developmental implications, of the impact of the disorder upon future language, academic, and cognitive development based upon the presenting risk factors which can be sensitive, but not necessarily specific? We cannot say. It is, however, a topic worthy of discussion. What we can point out is that the lack of a highly specific, agreed-upon, diagnostic criteria is likely to contribute to the disorder being underdiagnosed. For example, returning to our issue of definition, we see the confusion within the term. Note that ASHA refers to a childhood apraxia and rejects the inclusion of the term "developmental," while developmental verbal dyspraxia is the term preferred in Ireland and the UK, and verbal dyspraxia is the preferred term in the DSM, although it is included in the section for disorders appearing in childhood.

The current authors wish to highlight that, consistent with the overall DSM diagnostic system, apraxia of speech is diagnosed based upon its overt presentation of disordered speech. In addition, the symptoms of CAS can change both over time and in presentation as a result of treatment (Maasen, 2002). The younger child may present with limited phonetic skills, speech inconsistency, and sequencing difficulties, which may later present as residual prosody and resonance issues. The distinctions, or rather the ambiguity of definitions between the different developmental language disorders (speech delay and language disorder), further contribute to the confusion as to which disorder we are seeing and how these disorders are accounted for in research paradigms.

As can be noted from the latter part of this statement, the definition has gone from the ASHA description to a larger conceptualization involving potential Mu speech focused scale coordination issues, hearing, and touch. The question has arisen as to whether this co-occurrence of speech and language disorders, including CAS with motor disorders, was the result of speech motor difficulties affecting language or a co-occurrence of both speech and language disorder (Murray, 2018).

The Results of Definitional Confusion

Part of the difficulty with being able to define CAS with greater precision lies with the fact that CAS is a low prevalence disorder. Due to its ambiguous definition, studies of CAS often include children with similar, but non-CAS-based language deficits. There is an ongoing inability to delineate the disorder with specificity, that is, the inability to identify CAS as one might do on a particular bacterial infection or identify a genetic biomarker associated with the syndrome. As noted by Allison et al. (2020), disordered speech is the hallmark of both childhood apraxia of speech and apraxia of speech. Differential diagnosis of the disorder in adults and children continues to present major clinical and research challenges (Allison et al., 2020). This is because while both disorders are defined by difficulties presumed to be with motor planning and programming of speech movements, there are no biomarkers for apraxia of speech or childhood apraxia of speech.

Confounded phenotyping also impacts genetic research (Mountford et al., 2022). Again, within this domain the lack of a consensus with respect to diagnostic criteria results in comparisons across research studies difficult. In addition, the definitions and criteria impact sample sizes, further impacting genetic studies.

With respect to developmental speech disorders, various systems have been attempted. The Shriberg Speech Disorders Classification System (Shriberg et al., 2012), which attempted to base the classifications upon presumed etiology, consists of eight subcategories which attempted to base the model on the linking of "etiological process." Level I consisted of distal causes, level II consists of proximal causes including presentation and execution of speech mediated by feedforward and feedback processes, level III attempted behavioral phenotypes which consists of the expressed behavioral markers, and level IV consists of the critical signs of the phenotypes. Shriberg's goal was to identify a conclusive diagnostic marker at each step of the way with attention to both sensitivity and specificity. The resulting model, however, is largely symptomatic descriptions (Terband et al., (2019)) at the behavioral level. Terband et al. (2019) note a similar difficulty with the Stackhouse and Wells Psycholinguistic Framework whose categories are based on the proximal cause (processing) rather than at the core etiology and result in subcategories of phonological disorders based, again, on symptomology. Terband et al. (2019) went on to argue that core impairment, while not clearly distinguishable from each other, nonetheless requires an understanding of the complex interactions between causation. By way of an example, they offer substitution errors which can be viewed as a feature component, a speech-motor component, or a sequencing error component.

The absence of diagnostic markers which are both sensitive and specific then requires the diagnosis be made based upon clinical symptomology. However, there is no satisfactory consensus as to a core of speech symptoms which would reflect sensitive diagnostic criteria. Differential diagnosis is subsequently compromised by the overlap of symptoms across various speech disorders. That is, there is a significant overlap in speech disorder phenotypes.

Specifying this disorder in children becomes further compromised over the course of a child's development as "a congenital speech disorder in children presenting as a motor speech disorder influences a child's development of phonological presentation" (Stackhouse, 1997) "further rendering a lack of specificity in linguistic models" (Maassen, 2002).

The ASHA Technical Report of 2007 (page 4) noted that "Whereas some of the definitions of CAS reviewed by the Committee view the core problem as one of planning and programming (cognitive level) the spatiotemporal properties of movement sequences (behavioral level) underlying speech sound production, others propose that the deficit extends to representational level (cognitive) segmental and or suprasegmental units in both input processing and production." Asha goes on to say that "there is no validated list of diagnostic features that differentiates this symptom complex from other types of childhood speech sound disorders." The Technical

Report raised three speech characteristics which were consistent and considered specific to childhood apraxia of speech. They are:

1. Inconsistent error of consonants and vowels in repeated productions of syllables or words
2. Lengthened and disrupted coarticulatory transitions between sounds and syllables
3. Inappropriate prosody, especially in the realization of lexical or phrasal stress, which is "a core impairment in planning and/or programming spatiotemporal parameters of movement sequences"

An attempt to operationally define CAS was undertaken by Iuzzini-Seigel and Murray (2017). They created a 12-feature checklist of CAS symptoms expanding upon ASHA's primary criteria. Iuzzini-Seigel and Murray (2017) attempted to use the International Classification of Functioning framework to provide improved operationally defined criteria to better assess for the presence of CAS. They included the following speech features commonly associated with CAS: with respect to the first primary criteria as established by ASHA (2007):

1. Vowel error (a vowel production error in which the vowel is substituted for another vowel or not produced accurately)
2. Consonant distortion (a consonant production error in which a speech sound is recognizable as a consonant, but not produced accurately)
3. Speech sound inconsistency, and nasal resonance (resonance sounds are either hyponasal, in which there is not enough airflow out the nose, or hypernasal in which there is too much airflow out of the nose for non-nasal phonemes)
4. Expanding upon lengthened and disrupted co-articulatory transitions, the included intrusive schwa (the insertion of a schwa sound between consonants)
5. Difficulty achieving initial articulatory configurations (initiation of utterance or initial speech sound may be difficult for a child to produce and may sound lengthened or uncoordinated)
6. Groping (prevocal articulatory searching prior to onset of phonation or extraneous oral movements during nonspeech oral motor tasks) for sounds
7. Increased difficulty with multi-syllabic words (a disproportionately increased number of errors as the number of syllables increases)
8. With regard to the third ASHA criteria of inappropriate prosody, they included
9. Stress errors (an error in which appropriate stress is not produced correctly at the lexical (word) or sentence levels)
10. Syllable segregation (a brief or lengthy pause between sound syllables or words)
11. Slow rate

Each was operationally defined, for example, nasal resonance was defined as hypo- or hypernasal resonance. In addition to the mandatory presence of the three primary criteria, additional five characteristics were required for the diagnosis. They contend that children who produced 5 or more features out of the possible 11, as well as speech inconsistency, warrant the CAS diagnosis. Therefore, a cutoff of five features was used. However, they found that school-aged children with a diagnosis of CAS actually tended to present with an average of eight features. This was in contrast to children with speech delay who tended to present with three features and with typically developing children who presented with an average of one feature. They go on to remind us that the features are not pathognomonic. This again presents the difficulty of specificity and sensitivity when discussing a valid and reliable diagnosis of CAS (*definitions provided by Iuzzini-Seigel and Murray 2017).

Identifying the Speech Errors that Characterize CAS

In fact, there have been multiple studies which have attempted to standardize which speech characteristics are affected in children with CAS. For example, variable production of a phoneme (phonemic inconsistency) across multiple options both within and across word positions differentiates children with suspected CAS from phonological disorder (Iuzzini, Inconsistency of speech in children with childhood apraxia of speech, phonological disorders and typical speech, 2012). There is also research (Lewis, 2004) which has found that 100 percent of children with CAS evidenced vowel errors compared with 8 percent of children with an isolated speech sound disorder or a combined speech and language disorder. At school age, 90 percent of the children with CAS continued to make vowel sound errors, whereas 0 percent of the other group did.

For example, in a review of neuroimaging studies, Liegeois et al. (2014) noted that traditionally, both language and speech disorders have been defined as idiopathic. Turning to the burgeoning field of neuroimaging, Liegeois, Mayes, and Morgan note that neuroimaging studies "have uncovered functional and sub-macroscopic structural anomalies within brain systems." They reviewed articles published between 2008 and 2013. Of note, 2602 abstracts were initially identified. Following their exclusion criteria, wherein MRI was required for inclusion, only ten articles remained, five for speech disorder and five for language disorder. However, speaking to the aforementioned problem of specificity and how that impacts research, Mayes and Morgan noted how the "recruitment samples in both SD and LD studies were heterogenous with regard to diagnosis." Further, for speech disorder studies, diagnostic criteria ranged across childhood apraxia of speech, phonetic and phonemic level errors, and articulatory deficits. For language disorder the criteria included a history of language delay, syntax errors, receptive, expressive, lexical, and/or mixed disorders. Again, the lack of specificity is confounding an already confounding syndrome.

Speech: Structure Versus Function

Dr. Edythe Strand (Strand, 2018) of the Mayo Clinic notes that CAS is believed to be the result of deficits in planning and programming of movement gestures for speech production, that it often occurs in conjunction with language and phonological impairment, and that the definition relates to the ability to specify the parameters of movement. She the elaborates: "As a speaker gets ready to talk, particular muscle groups are selected to begin to contract at very specific times to cause structures to begin to move at a certain time in a particular direction, at a certain speed with a certain amount of force, using a specified amount of muscle tension" (Strand, 2018). Although most of us take this process for granted, hearing it broken down as such allows us to appreciate the complexities involved in speech production.

CAS is associated with functional rather than structural deficits (Iuzzini-Seigel, 2017). Children with CAS have no structural impairment which would impact their speech systems. However, they present with difficulties in motor planning and programming across speech systems, including phonation, articulation, respiration, resonance, and prosody (Iuzzini-Seigel, 2017). Iuzzini et al. state that evaluation is conducted through assessment of speech production of single words, such as on the Goldman-Fristoe Test of Articulation, as well as repeated words and phrases and connected speech. Murray (2018) note that polysyllable words and diadochokinetic tasks stress the child's motor system. However, children with speech delay and phonological disorders may also present with errors such as poor accuracy and inconsistencies on polysyllabic words.

One study looking at difficulty in the production of complex phonetic sequences in CAS through observation of coordination between the lips and jaw during speech production was undertaken (Moss, 2012) using a single-syllable, two-syllable, and three-syllable "real words." Support for the hypothesis of disordered speech motor control in CAS was implied by the difficulty noted in children with CAS in their attempts at longer or more complex syllable imitation (three syllables in contrast to a single syllable). Another attempt (Iuzzini-Siegel, 2017) was made to determine if speech inconsistency was a core feature of CAS or driven by a comorbid language impairment and whether speech inconsistency is both sensitive and specific as a diagnostic marker. They found that a token-token inconsistency of monosyllabic words and a phrase (buy Bobby a puppy) was both sensitive and specific in differentiating children with CAS and speech delay, whereas inconsistency using other stimuli was less so, leading to the conclusion that speech inconsistency was sensitive but not specific as it depended upon the stimulus presented.

A not too dissimilar question has arisen with respect to dyslexia. Developmental dyslexia is believed to affect approximately 5 percent of children (Ramus, 2003). Was dyslexia caused by a cognitive deficit specific to representations and processing of speech sounds (phonological theory) or a general sensory motor deficit? This latter theory might include a cerebellar/motor component. Ramus (2003) noted the antagonistic nature of the theories and the fluctuations across theories over time, with each supported by empirical evidence. He concludes that "sensory and motor disorders are present in a significant proportion of developmental dyslexics but play only a limited role in the etiology of reading disability." As we shall see as we continue, ignoring the contribution of sensory motor involvement may be a mistake with respect to both assessment practices and intervention strategies.

1. The current authors stress the importance of developmental factors in assessment, whether that be a neuropsychological assessment or a language assessment. Knowing the developmental history of a child's language and motor development offers us valuable information in piecing together the developmental trajectory of the child's skills by being able to look at risk factors.
2. We know that reading also relies upon fluid phonemic processing. Both children with dyslexia and children with CAS appear to have difficulty with single-word decoding.
3. The automaticity, the fluidity arising from overlearned behaviors, has been discussed elsewhere by the current authors and will be given attention further on in this chapter. For now, the importance lies in recognizing automaticity of reading, in part, on automaticity in motor behaviors, such as those required in rapid naming, a deficit often associated with reading difficulties.

Genetics, Language Disorders, and CAS

Genetic involvement in language disorders has been under study for several decades at this point, with multiple genetic loci and possible genes. Language disorders are considered to be highly heritable and represent complex interactions between genetic and environmental factors (Mountford et al., 2022), a synergy termed epigenetics. That language disorders are highly heritable is overwhelmingly accepted (Mountford et al., 2022). Nonetheless, there is an underwhelming understanding of how genetic coding variability and epigenetics affect language disorders. Genetic etiology is difficult to pinpoint secondary to variations between individuals and complex patterns of inheritability (Andres, 2022). While there have been over 30 genes identified which are associated with speech and/or language disorders, there is still a paucity of explanation of the underlying genetic cause of developmental language disorder (Mountford et al., 2022). It is hypothesized (Andres, 2022) that "the genes suggested [previously] explain a portion of the dynamic process of language acquisition or the complexity of skills that represent language ability." An intriguing additional hypothesis (Andres, 2022) is that because of the complexity of using language, a combination of genes with variable effect size may better explain the both the acquisition of language and why skill acquisition may be disordered.

The study of genetic disorders as related to language disorders falls into one of two categories: monogenic disorders reflect a single change in the DNA which is sufficient to cause a disorder. Complex disorders refer to multiple genetic variations which combine to contribute to a disorder which is also impacted by environment. Monogenic disorders have traditionally been studied within families. Complex genetic disorders incorporate genetic association methodologies.

Monogenetic inheritance reflects when a disorder arises from either recessive or dominant inheritance. Monogenetic variants are extremely rare. The monogenetic variants have a negative effect on the protein for which they encode which in turn results in a deficit in the cell, resulting in the disorder (Mountford et al., 2022).

FOXP2 is one such monogenetic example. The impact of FOXP2 and its impact on the KE family have been highly published and cited (Morgan et al., 2016). It is of importance to note that variants in FOXP2 show dominant inheritance (one copy of the variant) are extremely rare and account for approximately 2 percent of children with CAS. Children impacted by reduced levels of the FOXP2 protein display typical to low-average intelligence and both receptive and expressive language deficits. Gross and fine motor domains are not considered to be impacted. At the current time, FOXP2 variants are not believed to be contributing to other language disorders. Nonetheless, FOXP2 controls the expression of a series of regulating genes for language and motor function, thereby affecting speech motor learning. In fact, in its role as a transcription factor, FOXP2 variants have been shown to affect development of the cerebellum, striatum, and motor cortex, thus involved with cortical and subcortical regions. Shriberg et al. (2012) showed associations between FOXP2 and speech, prosody, voice, cognition, and language.

Assessing a single family, followed since 1993, and in this case had childhood apraxia of speech ruled out, Andres (2022) identified co-segregating rare variants in three genes, with variants in BUD13 reaching genome-wide significance for SLI.

Robinson Crusoe Island is home to a population with a high incidence of speech language impairment. Molecular genetic techniques were used to identify eight coding variants of significance. By then comparing to a larger population outside of this area (UK), Villanueva et al. (2015) found the impact of NFXL1 gene in both populations. They conclude that coding variants within the NFLX1 gene are associated with speech language impairment "within a complex genetic model."

A recent evaluation of children with CAS (Hildebrand, 2020) found a causative variant in 11 of 33 participants in 10 genes. The implication is that as many as 33 percent of children with CAS may have a causative genetic variant which has resulted in their CAS.

In addition, there are copy number variants, which are deletions or duplications of regions of genetic code. Copy number variants can be of little consequence, and some can cause disease. Some copy number variants affect global development, and some have been linked to language disorders. Deletions of chromosome 16p11 have been linked to childhood apraxia of speech (Mountford et al., 2022).

Other genes have been implicated in specific language impairment populations. It may be fully reasonable to anticipate the involvement of multiple genes impacting the phenotype of childhood apraxia of speech as well. Genetics may look to a "genetic complex model" (Mountford et al., 2022) with each variant contributing incrementally to the potential development or expression of disease. Through genetic linkage studies to identify regions of genetic code shared by affected individuals, the specific language impairment consortium found regions on 16q24 and 19q13 highly associated with SLI. Using this technique (Newbury, 2009), it was found that C-Mad inducing protein was associated with language and reading and spelling which was interpreted as impacting language on a larger scale. The list goes on and the reader is referred to the review article by Mountford et al. (2022) for a more comprehensive read. For our current purposes, it is important to note that what has been largely a phenotypically identified disorder is being assessed on a genetic coding level and potentially reflects a developmental rather than a lesioned disease model per se.

This more comprehensive view of CAS was meant to emphasize the complex and heterogeneous nature of CAS. Obviously, the neural network system that underlies this disorder is also complex, containing many sub-networks operating in an interconnected fashion to produce speech, and disruption in a large number of places within this system will produce disrupted motor speech. We now turn our attention to those motor speech networks.

References

Allison, K., Cordella, C., Iuzzini-Seigel, J., & Green, J. (2020). Differential diagnosis of apraxia of speech in children and adults: A scoping view. *Journal of Speech, Language, and Hearing Research*, 2952–2994.

American Psychiatric Association. (2013). *Diagnostic and Statistical Manual of Mental Disorders* (5th ed.).

American Speech Hearing Association. (2022). Retrieved from Childhood Apraxia of Speech: http://ASHA.org

Andres, E. E. (2022). Family based whole exome analysis of specific language impairment identifies rare variants in BUD13, a component of the retention and splicing complex. *Brain Sciences, 12*, 47.

Childhood Apraxia of Speech. (2022). Retrieved from American Speech-Language Hearing Association: ASHA.org

Delaney, A. L., & Kent, R. D. (2004). Developmental profiles of children diagnosed with apraxia of speech. The annual convention of the American-Speech-Language-Hearing Association. Poster. Philadelphia: American-Speech-Language-Hearing Association.

Guyette, T. W., & Diedrich, M. (1981). A critical review of developmental apraxia of speech. *Speech and Language*, 1–49.

Hildebrand, M. J. (2020). Severe childhood speech disorder. *Neurology, 94*, 2148–2167. https://doi.org/10.1212/WNL.0000000000009441

Iuzzini-Seigel, J. (2017). Speech assessment in children with childhood apraxia of speech. *Perspectives of the ASHA Special Interest Groups, 2*, 47.

Iuzzini-Seigel, J., & Murray, E. (2017). Speech assessment in children with childhood apraxia of speech. In *Perspectives of the ASHA Special Interest Groups* (pp. 47–60). American Speech Language Hearing Association.

Law, J. B. (2000). Prevalence and natural history. *International Journal of Language & Communication Disorders, 35*(2), 165–188.

Lewis, B., Fairbairn, L., Hanson, A., Ivengar, S., & Taylor, H. (2004). School age follow up of children with childhood apraxia of speech. *Language, Speech, and Hearing Services in Schools*, 122–140.

Liegeois, F., Mayes, A., & Morgan, A. (2014). Neural correlates of developmental speech and language disorders: Evidence from neuroimaging. *Current Developmental Disorders Reports*, 215–227.

Maassen, B. (2002). Issues contrasting adult acquired versus developmental apraxia of speech. *Seminars in Speech and Language*, 257–266.

Malmenholt, A. (2020). *Exploring childhood apraxia of speech: Speech and language profiles in 5 year olds with suspected apraxia of speech or cleft palate*. Karolinska Instituet Department of Clinical Science, Intervention and Technology.

Mayo Clinic. (2022). Childhood apraxia of speech. Retrieved from Mayo Clinic: https://www.mayoclinic.org/diseases-conditions/childhood-apraxia-of-speech/diagnosis-treatment/drc-20352051

Miller, G., Lewis, B., Benchek, P., & Freebaim, L. (2019). Reading outcomes for individuals with histories of suspected childhood apraxia of speech. *American Journal of Speech-Language Pathology*, 1432–1447.

Morgan, A., Fisher, S., Scheffer, I., & Hildebrand, M. (2016). FOXP2-related speech and language disorders. In M. A. Adam (Ed.), *Gene reviews*. University of Washington.

Moss, A. G. (2012). Interarticulatory coordination of the lips and jaw in childhood apraxia of speech. *Journal of Medical Speech-Language Pathology, 20*(4), 127–132.

Mountford, H., Braden, R., Newbury, D., & Morgan, A. (2022). The genetic and molecular basis of developmental language, *9*(5), 586. https://doi.org/10.3390/children9050586

Murray, E. T. (2018). Comorbid morphological disorder apparent in some children aged 4-5 years with childhood apraxia of speech: Findings from standardised testing. *Clinical Linguistics & Phonetics*, 1–18.

Murray, E., & Iuzzini-Seigel, J. (2017). *Efficacious treatment of children with childhood apraxia of speech according to the International Classification of Functioning*. ASHA Speech Pathology and Audiology Faculty Research and Publications.

National Institute of Deafness and Other Communication Disorders. (2022). Home page. Retrieved from National Institute of Deafness and Other Communication Disorders: https://www.nidcd.nih.gov/

Newbury, D. W. (2009). CMIP and ATP2C2 modulate phonological short term memory in language impairment. *American Journal of Human Genetics*, 264–272.

Norbury, C. F. (2016). The impact of nonverbal ability on prevalence and clinical presentation of and clinical presentation of language disorder: Evidence from a population study. *Journal of Child Psychology and Psychiatry*, 1247–1257.

Ramus, F. (2003). Developmental dyslexia: Specific phonological deficit or general sensorimotor dysfunction. *Current Opinion in Neurobiology, 13*, 212–218.

Shriberg, L. D. (2019). Estimates of prevalence of speech and motor speech disorders in persons with complex neurodevelopmental disorders. *Clinical Linguistics & Phonetics, 33*(8), 707–736.

Shriberg, L., Lohmeier, H., Strand, E., & Jakielskic, K. (2012). Encoding, memory, and transcoding deficits in childhood apraxia of speech. *Clinical Linguistics & Phonetics*, 445–482.

Stackhouse, J. W. (1997). *Children's speech and literacy difficulties 1: A psycholinguistic framework*. Wurr.

Strand, E. (2018, January 9). Diagnosis and management of CAS. Retrieved from youTube: https://www.youtube.com/watch?v=T8nPckWfvG0&ab_channel=ChildhoodApraxiaofSpeechInfo

Terband, H. M., Maasen, B., & Maas, E. (2019). A psycholinguistic framework for diagnosis and treatment planning of developmental speech disorders. *Folia Phoniatrica et Logopaedica, 71*, 216–227.

Villanueva, R., Nudel, A., Hoischen, M., Fernandex, M., & Simpson, N. (2015). Exome sequencing in an admixed isolated population indicates NFLX1 variants confer a risk of specific language impairment. *Genetics*. https://doi.org/10.1371/journal.pgen.1004925

Chapter 8
Neural Network Components of Childhood Apraxia of Speech and Associated Comorbidities

Given the focus on childhood apraxia of speech, we will now turn our attention to the various neural networks, particularly, the motor networks that comprise the underpinning of motor speech. We are mindful that the same extensive analysis could be done for any of the other apraxia but chose this area due to the lack of specificity as to the etiology of most childhood apraxia of speech, interrelatedness and complexity of the network interactions involved, and potential neural and functional associations to other clinical conditions.

Hemispheres and History

The history of our knowledge of the relationship between areas of the cortex and speech can unequivocally be traced back to the work of Broca and Wernicke. In 1861, a neurosurgeon, Paul Broca, reported on the brain of a deceased patient who had been able to understand language, but could not express a full sentence verbally or in writing. Upon autopsy Broca identified a lesion in the left inferior frontal cortex, which came to be known as the Broca's area, known to be responsible for speech processing and comprehension. Broca came to announce "We speak with the left hemisphere" which became the basis for the belief that the "language center was housed in the left hemisphere." In 1871 the German neurologist Carl Wernicke identified the superior temporal lobe as responsible for processing speech through hearing. Lesions at this location impacted the quality of speech. That is, the person could speak, but the speech was incoherent. This area became known as the Wernicke's area. These finding essentially cemented the idea of lateralized language. Note that these models are lesion based in adults. They are also cortico-centric. Wernicke's model was updated by Norman Geschwind and has become known as the

T. Wasserman, L. D. Wasserman, *Apraxia: The Neural Network Model*, Neural Network Model: Applications and Implications,
https://doi.org/10.1007/978-3-031-24105-5_8

Wernicke-Geschwind model. The model attempted to explain the process of speech through related areas of cortex. The model held that information travelled from the ear to the auditory cortex, to the Wernicke's area, to the Broca's area, and to the motor cortex. As the field has progressed, we now know that the two areas are connected by a large nerve fiber bundle, the arcuate fasciculus. This loop does present in the left hemisphere for most right-handed persons. In order to pronounce a word, or series of phonemes, the information is transmitted via the arcuate fasciculus to the Broca's area and on to the motor cortex. The model is not without complications revisions and exceptions but provides a rudimentary schema for the reader for the current time.

Nonetheless, the language center does not operate in isolation or produce fully formulated speech on its own. Various brain regions contribute critical elements of speech. For example, the left hemisphere is largely responsible for comprehension of the spoken words. The right hemisphere is largely responsible for the emotional connotation as it interprets the tone, rhythm and inflection, or prosody of the spoken language. The right hemisphere also allows for the manipulation and integration of categorical information, which facilitates divergent novel thinking. The left hemisphere focuses on individual events. So, for example, where the right might see the forest, the left sees the tree. How might this translate into higher cognitive thinking? It is not only these large gray matter structures that contribute to speech. These structures must be connected by white matter pathways so that their various functions can be integrated. Figure 8.1 is provided to give the reader an idea of the complexity of structural organization that must be achieved in order to achieve one aspect of motor speech.

Arcuate Fasciculus

In a landmark diffusion tensor imaging study, conducted by Catani and de Scholten (2008), 12 right-handed subjects were used to perform 3D tractography images of white matter tracts and in vivo dissections of the major tracts of the brain. Their resulting atlas includes vivid images of numerous tracts. Included is the arcuate fasciculus. The arcuate fasciculus is a white matter bundle that contains both long and short fibers. It is a major anterior/posterior tract that connects the frontal, parietal, and temporal lobes. Two pathways have been identified: The medial pathway connects the Wernicke's region in the temporal lobe to the Broca's region in the frontal lobe. The second is the indirect pathway which is comprised of two segments, the anterior and the posterior. The anterior pathway segment provides a link between the Broca's region in the frontal lobe and the Geschwind's region housed in the inferior parietal lobe. The posterior segment is the link between the Geschwind's region and Wernicke's region. Here we have yet another and seemingly very important example of white matter tracts connecting regions highly associated with language, sensorimotor learning, hand movements, and basic math operations among others. We point this out here to highlight the fact that the white

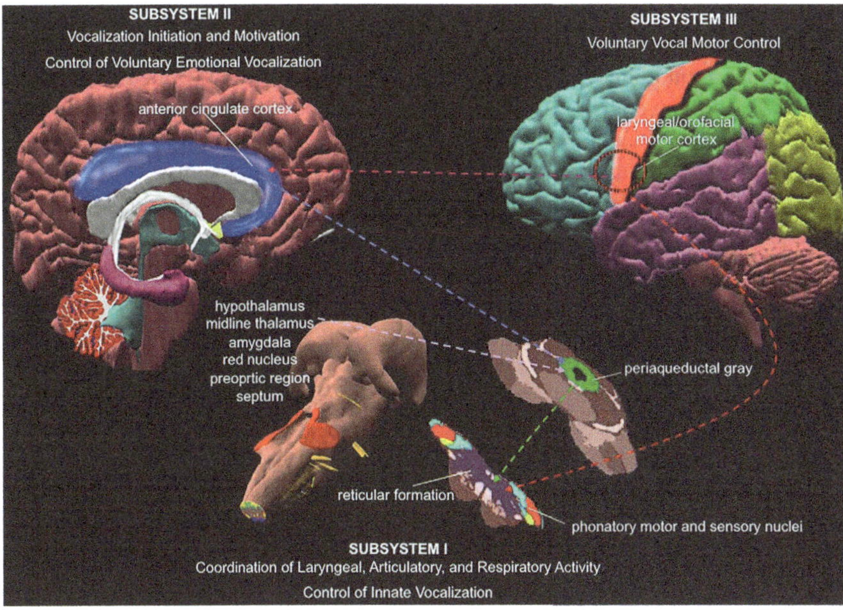

Fig. 8.1 Hierarchical organization of the dual pathway of central voice control
Hierarchical organization of the dual pathway of central voice control. The lowest level (subsystem I) is represented by the sensorimotor phonatory nuclei in the brainstem and spinal cord, which control laryngeal, articulatory, and respiratory muscles during production of innate vocalizations. The higher level within this system (subsystem II) is represented by the periaqueductal gray, cingulate cortex and limbic input structures that control vocalization initiation and motivation as well as voluntary emotional vocalizations. The highest level (subsystem III) is represented by the laryngeal/orofacial motor cortex in the vSMC with its input and output regions that are responsible for voluntary motor control of speech production. Dotted lines indicate direct connections between different regions within the voice-controlling system. (Simonyan et al., 2016)

matter motor structures are recruited for numerous tasks and a disruption of function based in one of these regions would likely have negative impact on a number of output skills in addition to apraxia.

Interconnections of the Arcuate Fasciculus

In fact, the arcuate fasciculus, together with posterior portions of the middle temporal gyrus, presents with differences in humans as compared to other primates and is considered to be a crucial difference in how human language evolved (Sierpowska et al., 2022). They found that connectivity in the posterior temporal lobe, via the arcuate fasciculus, expanded bilaterally to frontal and parietal cortices in humans. In contrast, the ventral tracts show stronger connection to posterior temporal regions in chimpanzees as compared to humans.

They further found that the medial direct pathway, or direct long segment, is larger in the left hemisphere in approximately 80% of the population (Catani et al., 2007). They found interhemispheric differences with greater symmetrical connections were better overall at remembering words (verbal recall) using semantic association. They also found a gender difference, with females tending to be more likely to have this symmetrical pattern of connection.

A longitudinal study by Gao et al. (2022) looked at the vocabulary trajectories of three groups of children ranked as consistently good, catch up, and consistently poor, between the ages of 4 and 10. At age 14, diffusion tensor imaging, using region of interest (ROI)-based tractography, found significantly reduced fractional anisotropy in the left arcuate fasciculus of children in the consistently poor group. The finding was in the posterior and direct segments of the arcuate fasciculus. No differences between groups appeared for the right hemisphere nor in the left anterior segment. Through regression analysis, Yue et al. showed that it was the rate of vocabulary development, rather than initial size of vocabulary, which was a specific predictor of connectivity. The current authors highlight that this may speak to our concern regarding breadth and long-term impact of early developmental disruption.

Hemispheres Do Not Operate in Isolation

As we have pointed out, these neural networks do not operate in isolation, and no one area is responsible for the production of fully functional speech. Neural network modeling posits that these areas, which are responsible for differently and discretely defined functions, are integrated. This integration is made possible by the complex white matter networks that together form the connectome.

Koziol (2014) provided an example of how this might work in practice. He argued that because the right hemisphere can take in the whole scene, so to speak, it becomes possible for this gestalt type processing to set the framework for solving problems that might have similar yet different characteristics. It allows us to take a particular thought or piece of information and use it in a more abstract application to a novel situation. In the process we generate new information. That new information has been acquired through the cross-interactions of both hemispheres. In this way, semantic systems are important not only for language but also for the manipulation of the categories for the divergent thinking often necessary for problem solving. Following this line of thinking, interruption to this process has the potential to disrupt higher-order cognitive thought.

Hemispheres and the Three Rs

A recent study speaks nicely to our discussion of hemispheric function, its interrelatedness, and impact of one area on other cognitive area, in other words possible comorbidities or associations of CAS and comorbid conditions.

We have a good deal of research talking about phonology both for CAS and literacy. We addressed that aspects of language have a strong left hemisphere base. There is research indicating that addition and subtraction are both left lateralized or bilateral (Semenza & Benavides-Varela, 2018) as the visual symbols require interpretation as would a phoneme. The left hemisphere would utilize lexical mechanisms for identifying and producing spoken numerals. Semenza and Benavides-Varela (2018) contend that these lexical mechanisms would be implemented in the "classic" language (Broca's and Wernicke's) areas including the inferior frontal and the superior and middle temporal gyri, as well as basal ganglia and thalamic nuclei." That is, disruption of the pathway at one of several locations may impact math skills as well as reading skills.

While it is not the intent of this chapter to comprehensively address dyslexia, we would note that developmental dyslexia is the most commonly diagnosed learning disorder (Shaywitz, 2005). Although it exists independent of intellectual standing, reading difficulty is often comorbid with dyscalculia (McNorgan, 2021). McNorgan discussed how reading is a process transforming visual or orthographic representations to phonological ones. For those with a reading difficulty, relative to controls, dyslexics show an under activation of the left temporo-parietal cortex and are argued to reflect a failure of audiovisual integration within functionally specialized regions. Interestingly, they also show increased connectivity to posterior right hemisphere areas, specifically the right occipitotemporal cortex and anterior inferior temporal gyrus, possibly a compensatory mechanism (Shaywitz, 2005).

The McNorgan (2021) study also looked at the feedforward neural networks to distinguish between poor and highly skilled readers and between word and pseudoword processing. He mapped multiple functional connectivity networks participating in multiple predictive functional connections. Of interest to our current discussion, McNorgan found three adjacent nodes operating as a functional cluster which spanned the right occipital pole and right calcarine sulcus. They appeared to be terminal points of multiple functional connections within the right hemisphere, which are and are predictive of the poor readers. He also found adjacent nodes belonging to a functional neural cluster in the left occipitotemporal cortex which were terminal points of multiple functional connections with within and across hemispheres predictive of skilled readers. That is, disruption of the pathway may impact reading skills as well.

Why discuss this information in a discussion of CAS? We discuss this for many reasons, firstly, it is because it speaks to a developmental process taking into account the fact that functional networks operate as needed and cross hemispheres. (A comprehensive discussion of connectomes and functional networks may be found in another chapter of this book, and the reader is strongly encouraged to be familiar with the model and current research, largely from neuroimaging, which is currently available). As dyslexia is a more readily defined diagnostic group and is more frequent in presentation than CAS, it allows for larger sample sizes (for that diagnosis) for study and, for our purposes, allows for consideration of a model which highlights bilateral cortical implications. The results of the neuroimaging studies are clear in implicating both hemispheres in processing reading requirements. It ties the process to phonological processing, a process involved in CAS as well, as well as associations to sensorimotor involvement (Ramus, 2003). Associations between reading and math issues are well established. When we look at the aggregate data then, we are afforded a look at how feedforward processes are impacted in a developmental disorder, which, while not CAS, shares components of associated skills and impact. It is then not unreasonable to hypothesize that the impact of a developmental speech apraxia, affecting phonological processing, with known associations to reading and cognitive development, goes well beyond what might be assumed if conceptualizing CAS as "merely" a motor programming problem affecting the production of phonemic sequences.

The Connectome, Development, and CAS

The current authors have discussed elsewhere (Wasserman & Wasserman, 2019) how the regions of the brain are connected by a connectome. This connectome starts out with more localized interconnectivity (small world hubs) and expands across regions as we are exposed to and incorporate information. In fact, neuroimaging studies have revealed structural changes in white matter after learning complex tasks. That is, the neural pathways of the brain are altering in response to stimuli. This is known as a functional network as the network is ever-changing in response to the demands of a particular task. This then, in turn, impacts information processing and performance (Fields, 2010) across cognition, learning, and motor skills development. Fields (2010) states that when new skills are being acquired, the amount of myelin insulating an axon increases, improving the ability of that neuron to fire. This then leads to the potential for more efficient learning and for more efficient learning to lead to the automaticity of the learned behavior. Would it not be reasonable then to assume that if there is a disruption to the process of learning a new skill, this disruption impacts the myelin insulation occurring or that which should be occurring, after the site of impact, thereby impacting the ability to learn higher-order skills more typically associated with that pathway.

Neural pathways also undergo neuronal pruning at various developmental stages. Preston et al. (2014), utilizing voxel-based morphometry, compared gray and white matter volume for children with residual speech sound disorders. The results indicated greater white matter in the corpus callosum for the speech sound error subjects and less white matter in the right occipital gyrus. They speculate that this may reflect an error in developmental pruning.

We know that in adults, apraxia of speech is strongly related to lesions of the left hemisphere; however, in contrast, the majority of children with CAS were found to have normal MRI brain imaging utilizing conventional imaging (Fiori et al., 2016). This suggests that the cerebral anomalies in CAS may be too subtle for detection by standard MRI. More recent research has begun to address this issue. In fact, in children with CAS, using voxel-based morphometry, morphological abnormalities were found in the supramarginal gyrus, Heschel's gyrus, and bilaterally planum temporale (Preston et al., 2014). Kadis et al. (2014) found a thicker left supramarginal gyrus, compared to controls, in the absence of macroscopic lesions in this same population of children with CAS.

In an effort to assess connectome connectivity, Fiori et al. (2016) compared fractional anisotropy as a measure of white matter connectivity in children with CAS. They utilized a whole brain tractography, based on diffusion imaging analysis. The final sample included 13 children with a mean age of 7 years. Fiori et al. found significant differences in fractional anisotropy (FA) in three subnetworks, with FA reduced in children with idiopathic CAS. Two subnetworks were intrahemispheric with one in each hemisphere, and one subnetwork was interhemispheric. Fiori notes that this is consistent with prior hypotheses of altered development of connectivity in CAS (Preston et al., 2014) as well as studies suggesting that it is necessary to have bilateral hemispheric involvement to result in symptomatic apraxia of speech in children (Liegeois & Morgan, 2012).

CAS Is Multifactorial from a Network Perspective

We tend to think in terms of domains. That is, speech and language may be different from each other and different from another domain such as motor development. But we know that there is a very close and undeniable association between early motor development and what the current authors believe are widespread areas of development which transcend our artificially defined constructs or domains. For example, relevant to our current discussion of CAS, it is clear that despite much overlap and lack of specificity, we are discussing neuromotor integrity.

The information provided with respect to cortical involvement, subcortical involvement, and genetic involvement defies our quest for a single agent of causation. It does, however, also point to and highlight the complexity of the human system. Just as there may not be a single genetic variation accounting for speech or language phenotypes, the same can be hypothesized true for a single-entry level of absence or damage. In fact, this position is strongly supported by the current authors; damage from the point of origin impacts all systems moving forward from a vertical brain model perspective.

During the last decade, research has suggested that developmental communication disorders have multifactorial origins at different levels of aggregation (Maassen, 2015). As a developmental disorder, it is unlike adult, acquired disorders (Bishop, 1997). Dysfunction in children will affect the development of other functions, skills, and development which relies on the preceding function being intact from a developmental perspective. Furthermore, Maassen believes the influence of these levels on the resulting behavior is interactive rather than unidirectional. Maassen proposed a developmentally based, perceptual motor model of Childhood Apraxia of Speech. Using a multi-level, multifactorial concept as its foundation, he begins with a discussion of the global outlines of the interactive multi-level model, followed by a discussion of each of the four levels as they relate to CAS, including the interactions between the levels. Acknowledging that little is known about the genetic and neurological background of CAS, Masson's focus is on perceptual-motor level, including to some extent higher cognitive functions such as lexical retrieval. From this developmental perspective, babbling and sensorimotor learning is the foundation for more abstract phonological understanding. Maassen's model begins with phonological encoding in which sensorimotor targets which constitute speech are selected and sequenced in a series. The next stage is motor planning which comprises the selection and sequencing of the articulatory movements necessary to produce these sounds. During the next stage, motor programming is implemented. Maassen (2002) makes the assumption that the core deficit of CAS is a reduced sensorimotor learning capacity. This then leads to poor articulation and poor auditory and somatosensory representation and eventually impacts higher-level processing.

Some have raised the question of whether or not the core problem is with transcoding (planning and programming) or with deficits in auditory perceptual encoding (representational) and/or memory (storage and retrieval). Expanding upon Shriberg's et al. (2019) work, the Syllable Repetition Task (SRT), an 18-item task of non-word repetition (Shriberg et al., 2012), was administered to four groups based upon speech classifications of typical speech, speech delay-typical language, speech delay-language impairment, and CAS. The finding was of lower SRT encoding (the transforming of auditory information into phonemic representation), memory (the storage and retrieval of the representations), and transcoding (the process of planning and programming the representations for expression as a motor gesture such as speech or signing) scores than controls. Velleman (2011), in a review, noted how impact in CAS is cognitive-linguistic in addition to motor planning as noted by the extension of problems with perception and production of vowels, rhymes, and phoneme sequences and further extending into word attack and spelling skills.

In summary, through vastly improved neuroimaging, our more recent knowledge of connectomes allows us to better understand how, although research may need to focus on one aspect of CAS presentations at a time, the impact of disruption at any given point along the network, and/or within given hubs, can be more localized but can absolutely be more pervasive.

The Dual Pathway Model

In fact, the co-occurrence of language and gross and fine motor skills in children with language disorder has been well documented (DiDonato, 2014). One hypothesis for this finding is a dual stream model of speech processing. The dual stream model is based on the fact that the brain has two processes to utilize with speech (Hickok, 2012). On the one hand, speech must be understood, also described as acoustic sound linking to conceptual-semantic representation. On the other hand, speech is spoken and therefore has to be linked to a motor system. The fact that these are separable pathways can be inferred from the fact that one does not preclude the other. We are capable of uttering nonsense words as an example of motor speech without comprehension, and we are sometimes able to comprehend speech without being able to reproduce it.

This dual route model posits that a ventral stream is involved in processing speech for comprehension, i.e., semantic and phonological processing, sound recognition, and the long-term storage of semantic information. The ventral stream involves the superior and middle portions of the temporal lobe.

The dorsal stream is involved in the sensory motor integration which includes articulation of speech sounds. It is an auditory to motor translation. The dorsal stream also is associated with syntactic analysis and phonological memory. The dorsal stream involves the posterior planum temporale and posterior frontal lobe. The dorsal stream is largely left dominant. And while there is a long history of attributing speech to the left hemisphere, the current data indicates that the ventral stream is actually bilaterally organized (Hickok, 2012). In his article (2012) Hickok offers a comprehensive and elucidating review of current neuroimaging findings and contradictions. These will not be repeated here. However, what is largely undisputed is the need for auditory motor integration. The link between auditory and motor interaction dates to Wernicke and remains an important foundational fact for current studies and theory.

The Critical Contribution of the Dorsal Pathway

While both systems are necessary for fully functional speech, Hickok and Poeppel (2007) point to the primacy of the dorsal pathway because "learning to speak is essentially a motor learning task. The primary input to this is sensory, speech in particular. So, there must be a neural mechanism that both codes and maintains instances of speech sounds and can use these sensory traces to guide the tuning of speech gestures so that the sounds are accurately reproduced."

Recent research (Flinker, 2015), rather than using neuroimaging, utilized direct intracranial cortical recordings, through both written and spoken modalities to assess the role of the Broca's area during spoken word operations. They found that by the time actual speech commenced, activation in the Broca's area was quiet, but activity in the motor cortex was apparent. This suggests that the Broca's area contribution is limited to pre-articulatory stages rather than online coordination of the speech articulators.

The beginning of the dorsal pathway is located at the boundary of the temporal and parietal lobes near the Sylvian fissure. The first step of the dorsal pathway begins in the sensory motor interface located in the left Sylvian fissure where the temporal and parietal lobes interface. The Sylvian parietal-temporal area is important for perceiving and reproducing sounds and for phonological short-term memory. Without this area, language acquisition is impaired. The information then moves on to the articulatory network, which is divided into two separate parts. The articulatory network consists of one part which processes motor syllable programs, and the second articulatory network is for motor phoneme programs. In summary, the white matter tracts support different processing with the arcuate fascicle having primary involvement in phonology and articulation and the extreme capsule (EmC) involved in semantics.

In a review of the research, suggested that the dual pathway model adds to our understanding and has valid components; however, the independence of the streams may have been overemphasized. A synergistic relationship between these white matter tracts for language processing and function is more likely. However, research into how cortical and subcortical areas interact is fairly new, and how these systems interact is a current focus. Rolheiser et al. (2011) attempted to assess the contribution of the white matter tracts, with the primary focus on those directly connecting frontal and temporal regions—the arcuate fascicle (AF) and the extreme capsule (EmC). Using a combination of neuropsychological inference, DTI, and comprehensive language testing, Rolheiser et al. (2011) demonstrated that involvement of either the arcuate fascicle, which connects the Wernicke's area and Broca's area, or the extreme capsule is contingent upon the varying demands of different components of language function. This model is very important as it one speaks to the current author's contention (Wasserman & Wasserman, 2020) that neural network recruitment is task specific and provides a portion of the model into understanding how disruption of the development of a neural pathway in developing children can alter the impact or expression of language-based problems in some instances, enough to cause pathognomonic signs and, in others, to cause overlapping behavioral expression. Rolheiser's (2011) results contribute to understanding the interactive nature of neural pathways and, specifically, the contribution of white matter to language by documenting how performance of phonology, morphology, semantics, and syntax makes use of the neural pathways essential for receptive and expressive communication. Rolheiser's work demonstrated a relationship between white matter and behavior which reveals task-specific variability. They conclude that this data, in conjunction with recent studies documenting indirect and secondary white matter pathways relevant to language, demonstrates that it is likely that relevant frontotemporal language connections operate in a collaborative manner. They posit that ultimately behavior emerges as a product of coordinated gray matter activity, as a result of working in conjunction with white matter pathways. And again, that recruitment of pathways is task specific. The current authors would agree.

In fact, the current authors would argue that this is largely the point: that is, childhood development reflects an ever-expanding network of neural pathways. While the mature brain is organized into more functional networks which are altered by being task specific or, put another way, reflect a flexibility in recruitment in order to support various cognitive processes, the developing brain represents an emerging model. The developmental phases represent changes in sensory, motor, and cognitive abilities, and the goal of developmental cognitive neuroscience is to better understand the link between neural substrates and these complex developmental milestones. Fair et al. (2009) documented the now generally accepted fact that brain regions in children communicate with other brain regions on a more local level. That is, regions communicate with closer regions. As the child develops, the cortical communication becomes more distributed (across hubs) ultimately moving from "local" distribution to a highly correlated distributed network, commonly seen in the adult brain.

Cortical and Subcortical Involvement in Motor Speech

The current authors would like to direct the reader to previous work for a moment wherein we have attempted to tie the connectome to motivation (Wasserman & Wasserman, 2020) and the principles of therapy (Wasserman & Wasserman, 2019), as well as the work of Koziol (2014) in tying the vertical brain model to executive functioning. Inherent in all these works is a fundamental understanding of child/human development, learning, and automaticity. While these works literally encompass volumes, there is a core attention to the inclusionary nature of multiple processes which include, but are not limited to, the inclusion of curiosity; directed attention; directed movement and feedback, that is, moving toward; and corrective inhibition of movement, to produce automaticity of learned skills. The analogy to speech and language demands notation. Specifically, consider the process and purpose of movement. Movement requires the arousal of the ventral attention network (Koziol, 2014) for object identification, including arousal of the reward network, and the dorsal attention network for identifying how things work. These two networks interact with the frontoparietal network for goal-directed behavioral control processing, working in unison to create the action control network. The visual system then interacts to sustain attention to a particular object or goal while suppressing attention and movement toward others. The sensory motor network then executes the motor portion of the process. A corresponding process exists for speech. Whereas a shiny red ball may have been the object of curiosity, arousal, and goal-directed behavior for the infant in our prior example, in the speech domain, the object or goal is replaced by an internal representation of the phonological pattern of a word (Hickok, 2012). Hickok posits that the targets are known to be auditory in nature because of work demonstrating that alterations in auditory feedback result in compensatory speech sounds. He points to the work of Guenther et al. (1998) to help demonstrate that a person talking will modify their motor articulations in order to "hit" an auditory target or speech sound, thereby indicating that the target is the sound rather than the motor configuration.

Koziol et al. (2012) note that just as gesturing requires movements to be expressed in a certain order, vocal sound sequences also rely on an organized sequence in order to express a particular meaning. This ties the connection between motor sequencing and verbal sequencing. In fact, this also ties into the subcortical-cortical nature of the process with basal ganglia-cortical loops providing a unique neural architecture for the necessary foundations for sequencing the structure or rules across gestures and vocalizations. From an evolutionary standing, these structures already existed and were specialized over time so that the result is that language is dependent upon the basal ganglia for sequential learning and upon the frontal cortex for the necessary motor programming.

In fact, the current authors wish to remind the reader that intention predates language development. During the sensory motor period, infants begin to demonstrate what appears to be the innate reflex of curiosity (Wasserman & Wasserman, 2020), which results in execution of intent through motor movement. This movement is reinforced and thereby found to be rewarding to the infant-seeking behavior. We also know that categorization precedes language (Rakison & Yermolayeva, 2010) but sets the stage for language development. In this way we can see that language and motor movement are inexorably linked in human development.

Some more recent theoretical work has clarified the underlying auditory motor integration (Hickok et al., 2011) in the dorsal stream. Through recent advances in understanding motor control, speech research has emphasized the role of internal forward models in speech motor control. The basic idea (Hickok et al., 2011) is that the nervous system makes forward predictions about the future state of the motor articulators and the sensory consequences of the predicted actions to control action. The predictions are assumed to be generated by an internal model that receives efference copies of motor commands and then integrates them with information about the current state of the system and past experience of the relation between particular motor commands and their sensory consequences. This internal model allows for a mechanism for detecting and correcting motor errors, that is, motor actions that fail to hit their sensory targets. The ability to suppress errors whether in motor action or speech is very important. It allows us to fine-tune our intent and product. This process of attention to a target and its implementation of behavior, whether behavioral or speech, requires inhibition from attention to or attempts of other behaviors. This inhibition initiates with the basal ganglia, elevating the importance of this subcortical structure to commensurate importance with the cortically based frontal cortices. It is within the cerebellum that this finely tuned computational arithmetic takes place cementing the necessary interplay of the motor areas acting in concert with the cerebellum and basal ganglia loops (Hickok, 2012). The reader will note the expansion of the originally cortical centric model to a cortical subcortical model.

Prediction Errors and Motor Speech

Let us take a moment and review the potential importance of the reference to "detecting and correcting motor errors, that is, motor actions that fail to hit their sensory targets" (Hickok, 2012). Hickok correctly notes that this principle applies to behavior and to speech behavior. In fact, there is a significant body of recent research highlighting the role of prediction errors, the discrepancy between predicted and actual information, and the neural mechanisms engaged as it related to speech in general and CAS in specific. Other researchers also suggest increased prediction error as a factor in CAS.

The current authors refer to the importance of the concept of prediction errors and its role in learning, reward, and motivation (Wasserman & Wasserman, 2020) and the concurrent importance of dopamine in the incorporation and support of brain networks involved in motivation, as well as orienting and cognition. They note that "Models incorporating prediction errors have been invoked to explain complex phenomena such as the transition from goal directed to habitual behavior," a concept which the current authors wish to highlight as applicable to speech production as well. In fact, error prediction is described as "controlling and learning self-directed motor behaviors {as it} involves both an implicit forward model of the effector and explicit model of the task." Also of importance, Popa and Ebner (2019) note that "self-directed motor behavior cannot be cleanly separated from the underlying cognitive context."

Cerebellum and CAS

Much of what was learned about cerebellum function, as with other cerebral areas, originally came from studying the effects of lesions in the area. The cerebellum evolved to allow for the organism to anticipate sensorimotor feedback in order to facilitate rapid execution of behaviors, typically ones which have become automatic. For a long time, the cerebellum's contribution was considered to be limited to proprioception. More recent data indicates that this is a disservice to the cerebellum. The cerebellum is a very old structure evolutionarily speaking. It clearly served a function and was retained. Leiner et al. (1994) noted that during this phylogenic evolution, the growth of the neocortex and cerebral association areas was matched by growth of the lateral cerebellar hemispheres and the dentate nucleus and association connections between these areas. The cerebellum is in fact believed to contain three times as many neurons as the neocortex. Leiner hypothesized that these multiple bilateral cerebro-cortical connections allowed for the engagement of the cerebellum in human cognitive and language functioning.

This was followed by a seminal study by Schmahmann and Sherman (1998) conducted with patients with cerebellar damage, which described symptoms which they termed cerebellar cognitive affective syndrome which included cognitive, visual spatial, emotional impairment, and language impact including agrammatisms and dysprosody. This sparked interest in the cerebellum and its relationship to other subcortical and cortical functions. In addition to other areas such as working memory, executive function, visuospatial function, and affective regulation, research began to look at the role of the cerebellum and language. The cerebellum is characterized by linguistic lateralization, and, from a neuroanatomical perspective, the cerebellum's right hemisphere, which has multiple connections with cerebral cortex language areas, is important for language functions. In fact, there is ample evidence supporting the role of the cerebellum in the production of language, particularly its role in facilitating the serial order of linguistic units or phonemes by regulating the accuracy, speed, and rhythm.

The cerebellum is organized by area. Overlearned or automatic motor behaviors are facilitated within the anterior lobes of the cerebellum. The learning of new sensory motor behaviors, as well as cognitions, is regulated by the posterior and inferior lobes of the cerebellum. The cerebellum assists with behavioral corrections and the predicted outcome of movements. That is, the olivary portion of the cerebellum detects errors and refines its feedback prediction of feedback with each movement. As a coordinated effort, this allows for the organism, or speaking to origination, the brain of the organism, to execute the behavior with increasing precision and accuracy. By informing the neocortex, the cerebro-cerebellar circuit allows for rapid coordination of intention and movement prediction. A sound neurotypical cerebellum then interfaces sensory and motor components, refining the program each time a movement is repeated. In essence, it learns from practice, allowing the behavior or behavioral sequence, to become more precise and automatic. It informs the cerebral cortex about the predicted outcome of movements which can then be stored in the motor and premotor cortex to allow for rapid execution of the behavior (Koziol, 2014). Schmahmann described the cerebellum's role in the regulation of language function as analogous to its role in motor regulation. Likewise, he described the impairment of cerebellar prediction and regulation as a "dysmetria of thought" (1998). The cerebellum has also been implicated in dyslexia, dysgraphia, and aphasia.

Let us consider a possible outcome of cerebellum damage with regard to its role in feedback for movement. The cerebellum's role is modulation of behavior. It does not initiate movement. The cortex is the primary processor of sensory and motor information which the cerebellum modulates. The damage to the cerebellum would result in an inability to compute errors for accuracy. The cerebellum would not be able to perform an online analysis modulating excitatory and inhibitory processes. It would not be able to perform error prediction analysis. For a larger motor movement, the movements would be released through the cortex-basal ganglia loops, e.g., reaching for an object, but without the support from the cerebellum, the movements would be erratic and uncoordinated (Koziol, 2014).

The association of the cerebellum and language regulation is derived from the found neural connections between the cerebellum and neocortex, specifically the Broca's area. Each cerebellar hemisphere both receives and sends information to the contralateral hemisphere. These corticocerebellar tracts connect the lateral parts of the cerebellum with the frontal lobe through ascending and descending pathways. The ascending pathway begins in the dentate nucleus in the cerebellum and goes to the thalamus and to the contralateral areas of the frontal lobe. The motor cortex receives information from the dentate nucleus, and the prefrontal cortex receives information from the ventro-lateral areas. As described elsewhere in this section, the cerebellum is then involved in many aspects of cognition, which are not motor based, including language.

The work of Ackerman et al. (2007) looked at the neural correlates related to the cerebellum with respect to speech, sound perception, and production. The cerebellum also plays a vital role in both gesturing (motor) and speech. The authors note at least two main roles of the cerebellum with respect to language. Ackerman et al. (2007) contend that the cerebellum contributes to the temporal organization of the sound structure of verbal utterances by supporting online sequencing of syllables during overt speech production. They also have evidence for the cerebellum participating in the generation of internal speech through a pre-articulatory verbal code. These changes have been linked to mutations in the FoxP2 gene in particular.

Cerebellar Dysfunction and CAS

Additional studies have specifically assessed the association of cerebellar dysfunction in CAS, attempting to assess cerebellar function in tasks requiring greater complexity and integration. Peter et al. (2020) compared the motor performance of 18 children and adolescents diagnosed with CAS and 11 controls to that of an adult with a likely history of CAS and to an adult with a cerebellar stroke. The first set of conditions included a rapid syllable repetition for repeated same or monosyllables (papapa), disyllables (patapata), and trisyllables (patakapataka). They then included a key tapping task involving tapping the same key with one finger vs tapping two keys with two fingers, alternating the finger taps. A third task assessed fine and gross motor skills and balance. Peter et al. found that the children with CAS have the greatest difficulty, with rapid syllable repetition for the two-syllable condition and less difficulty when switching among three different syllables. They indicated no difficulty when repeating the same syllable. The participant with the cerebella stroke showed deficits in tests of both fine and gross motor ability, as well as in balance. Both repetitive and alternating key tapping was slow in the ipsilateral hand relative to the stroke. Peter concludes that the results are consistent with persisting cerebellar dysfunction that is persisting into adulthood. A similar pattern was found in the key tapping condition with children and adolescents showing difficulty with alternating, but not repetitive key tapping. The subject with CAS performed less well on a test of fine motor ability where the tasks required rapid integration of complex hand movement sequences. Peter et al. (2020) found that the adult with the probable historical diagnosis of CAS obtained motor performance scores similar to those found in the children and adolescents with CAS.

Basal Ganglia and Procedural Memory

There is recognition that a goal of human learning is to make much learning "routinized" or automatic (Koziol, 2009). The repetition of a particular activity and its progressive consolidation of the memory trace of the skills involved in this activity leading to their automaticity are a process known as procedural memory. Procedural memory is involved in daily activities such as driving a car or throwing a ball. There is conflicting data on when the procedural memory system is matured, but it is clearly present early on developmentally speaking. The neural correlates of procedural memory are the subcortical structures, the basal ganglia, and the cerebellum.

Grammar and syntax are rule governed and routinized through the processes of basal ganglia "binding" operations (Koziol, 2014).

The basal ganglia are a group of bilateral subcortical nuclei. The nuclei consist of the striatum, which has a dorsal and ventral component, the globus pallidus, the subthalamic nucleus, and substantia nigra. They do not direct the cortex. Rather, they are a gating mechanism. This cortico-striatal system modulates both behavior and cognition through neural pathways, or loops, by helping in the selection of which behaviors will be executed and which will be suppressed. The basal ganglia gating is not limited to overt behavior. Rather, visual and auditory association areas also project into the striatum.

Ullman and Pierpont (2005) hypothesized a model known as the declarative-procedural model. This model proposes two domains: the mental lexicon and the mental grammar domains. The mental lexicon is comprised of non-rule-based information, our lexicon, or dictionary reserve of words we know as well as words, for example, which need to be memorized such as irregular verbs (buy-buying-bought vs buyed), as well as interpretation of idioms. The mental lexicon is considered to be declarative memory associated and as such temporal lobe (cortical) based. The procedural memory system is associated with rule-based grammar. This domain is associated with cortical-subcortical circuits allowing for us to combine words into complex ideation as well as allowing us to interpret these complex representational strings of words. Rule-based grammar develops early in children and is believed to be based upon procedural learning (Koziol, 2009). Other aspects of language may also be learned in procedural memory, when the knowledge is implicit and involves learning to predict things such as the implicit learning of word boundaries in a stream of speech. There is also a suggestion that procedural memory is impacted in specific language impairment. Children with the diagnosis of specific language impairments have difficulties with the acquisition of grammatical rules. Some have difficulties with motor sequencing. These children have been found to abnormal activation in frontal cortices and specifically the left supplementary motor area as well as in the basal ganglia. The two types of memory are associated within frontal systems, depending on the task. This seems to beg the question of whether impact in the procedural learning system learning will impact declarative memory with implied impact on language comprehension as well as speech production.

Basal ganglia loops are commonly conceptualized to originate and terminate in a given area of cerebral cortex that has direct connectivity with the striatum, which includes the caudate nucleus and the putamen (Bohali et al., 2016). Loops are distinguished based upon cortical origination and termination areas. These areas are usually, but not always, located in the frontal lobe. Recent conceptual work by Bohsali and Crosson (2016) emphasizes three types of basal ganglia loops, each having some common components with others originating from the same cortical area. The direct loop starts in one of several areas of cortex that share direct connectivity with striatal components from the striatum. The direct pathway releases behavior. These loops project to the medial global pallidus and from the medial global pallidus to a thalamic nucleus. The thalamic nucleus projects back to the area of cortex from which the loop originates. Cortico-striatal and thalamic cortical connections are excitatory, and striato-palladal and pallido-thalamic connections are inhibitory. The fourth pathway, the striosomal pathway, projects from the cortical-based paralimbic system to the substantia nigra. This is then providing the basal ganglia with necessary information, information which the basal ganglia uses in the process of learning of new motor behaviors and in lending support for the aforementioned rule-based grammar systems.

Indirect and hyper-direct loops also begin in specific area of cortex. For the indirect loops, the cortex projects to the striatum, similar to direct loops, which are glutamate excitatory connections. However, in this loop, the striatum projects to the lateral global pallidus (gabinergic/inhibitory connections) which in turn projects to the subthalamic nucleus (inhibitory connections). Then the subthalamic nucleus projects back to the medial global pallidus. The medial global pallidus projects to one of the thalamic nuclei mentioned above, and finally the thalamus projects back to the cortical component from which the loop originated.

Like the direct and indirect loops, the hyper-direct loop originates in one of the cortical areas projecting to the basal ganglia, but it differs from these loops by bypassing the striatum. Instead, the cortical component of the loop projects directly to the subthalamic nucleus. In turn, the subthalamic nucleus projects back to the medial global pallidus. The medial global pallidus projects to one of the thalamic nuclei mentioned above and completing the loop. The thalamus projects back to the cortical component from which the loop originated. Basal ganglia models often suggested that loops associated with functionally distinct cortical areas should project to separate and non-overlapping regions within the basal ganglia. Alexander et al. (1986) implied that loops are segregated from one another. Additional studies, however, provide evidence that some basal ganglia loops are integrative, allowing cross-communication between discrete functional networks. Silveri (2021) notes that the cerebellum and the basal ganglia area reciprocally interconnected. It is therefore quite plausible that when damage involves one of these structures, one can likely see the remote effects of abnormal activity in the other. That is, in a functional network, disruption in one area can result in pathology in more remote areas. The current authors would remind the reader that from a developmental perspective, damage to one area would likely impact any neural development in a feedforward program, thus potentially disrupting both neural and behavioral development from that area of disruption forward across integrated networks and subsequently functions.

The neural substrates of the cerebellar, cortex, and association areas represent the cerebellar non-motor functions. The cerebellum and the cerebral cortex, as noted elsewhere, are connected by feedforward cerebellum-thalamus-cortico-ponto-cerebellar pathway. Of importance, segregated functional zones from the cerebellum to heterogenous extra-cerebellar structures are densely connected on a subcortical level. Both the cerebellum and the basal ganglia project to the same primary motor areas; however, most projections are to other areas including the premotor cortex and temporal and parietal areas. This system reflects closed loop architecture with exchanged information between neocortical areas, the basal ganglia, and the cerebellum. The cerebellum, as discussed elsewhere in this section, is believed to compare the current, actual movement with predicted movement it has stored, or learned, through sensory feedback. This model also extends to the cognitive domains. Overall, the recent research indicates that the cerebellum and basal ganglia are indeed part of this highly integrated cortical-subcortical functional network and is involved in motor control as well as associated with cognition and affect.

Broca's Area, Basal Ganglia Loops, and the Supplementary Motor Area (SMA)

As discussed above, research of recent decades has been providing evidence supporting the notion of Broca's area basal ganglia loops (Ullman, 2006). Functional neuroimaging studies measuring regional blood flow effects associated with test performance implicated Broca's area in the basal ganglia to support an overlapping set of language functions. Specifically, both regions are thought to be involved in lexical selection and retrieval, syntax, phonology, as well as higher-order language processing. Functional connectivity studies modeling modulatory relationships between patterns of activation and gray matter regions have shown direct functional connectivity between Broca's area and putamen, pointing to its role of potentially supporting articulatory control and identification of phonological representations of lexical items. Research has, as discussed above, identified pathways connecting Broca's area with the striatum.

The supplementary motor area (SMA) has been shown to be the center for motor planning. This includes motor planning for speech. The supplementary motor area (SMA) occupies the posterior one third of the superior frontal gyrus. Supplementary motor area (SMA) syndrome is defined as temporary paralysis and mutism following damage to the SMA. Although paralysis induced by SMA syndrome is severe during the acute phase, recovery usually occurs within relatively short periods and rarely results in a permanent deficit. There is also a pre-SMA area. The pre-SMA and SMA are differentially involved in the sequencing and initiation of movements, with the pre-SMA acting at a more abstract level than the more motoric SMA (Toga, 2015). One of the first bits of evidence regarding a pre-SMA basal ganglia loop involved in language came from the study of fMRI data to determine frontal, basal ganglia, and thalamic contributions during three facets of language usage: lexical items, semantic vs. phonological information, and rate of generation. The subjects performed four tasks. They had subjects generate lexical/category members for categories. For example, subjects might be asked to generate as many birds as they could, to which they might reply "parakeet, hawk," etc. To determine whether activity was attributable to the semantic nature of this task, subjects also generated words that rhymed with the stimulus word. For example, subjects might be asked to generate as many words as they could that rhymed with rap. Finally, to determine whether activity was unique to the lexical nature of the task, subjects were tasked with generating as many nonsense syllables as they could that began with the beginning and ending consonant blend, for example, "st" at two different rates of generation speed.

They found that a part of the left pre-SMA-dorsal caudate nucleus—ventral anterior thalamic loop—was active during the task for generating words either to a category or to rhyming cues; the loop was not active during the task requiring nonsense syllable generation. They concluded that the loop is associated with the retrieval of words from the lexical library. In addition, diffuse activity in the right basal ganglia (caudate nucleus and putamen) was active during word generation, but not for nonsense syllable generation. The absence of right frontal activity during the word generation task was interpreted to mean that the right basal ganglia activity is used to suppress right frontal activity which in turn prevents right frontal structures from interfering with language production.

With respect to connections between the pre-SMA and Broca's area (Ford et al., 2010), found an anterior-to-posterior gradient with connections between the Broca's area, the Brodmann's area, the supplementary motor area, and the pre-supplementary motor area (SMA). They tied this finding to other findings of the anterior Broca's area being associated with semantics and the posterior Broca's area associated with syntax and phonology. Connectivity between the Broca's area and SMA presents a plausible structural interface for interaction between basal ganglia loops involving these cortical areas. The clear role of the Broca's area in speech production coupled with data indicating SMA involvement in word selection provides support that these basal ganglia loops may interact, providing modulation feedback to ensure the optimal level of speed and accuracy for speech. Broca's area pre-SMA connectivity may be the likely candidate for this mechanism.

Bohasali and Crosson (2016) provide a compelling potential model for Broca's region basal ganglia loop processing. They tie the findings that the Broca's area was modulating activity in the putamen, implicating the putamen to speech initiation and articulation as well as the cortical initiation of phonological representations, a finding supported by prior data. They conclude that the Broca's area is crucially involved in articulatory and phonological processing with a specific emphasis on this circuit, including the putamen, as it supports phonological/articulatory processing. Specifically, phonological representations are likely to be activated within the Broca's area-auditory association area network based on contextual content established by the temporal and inferior parietal cortical networks. They propose that the basal ganglia may be "sharpening the signal to noise ratio of the most contextually appropriate lexical items, There phonological representations, in corresponding articulatory motor programs via the direct loop, while suppressing competing phonological items via the indirect loop" (Bohali et al., 2016). The hyper-direct loop could be resetting the system after the most appropriate phonological representation has been selected, tying this to other pathways within the loops. They propose that Broca's area basal ganglia loops are acting in concert with another basal ganglia loop, specifically the pre-SMA loop to ensure the accuracy of the speech produced so that the actual verbal output both matches the intended expression and addresses processing speed to promote fluidity of the expressed speech.

Citing research from Crosson et al. (2004) and Hagoort (2005), they then suggest that we should be talking about Broca's region rather than Broca's area in particular. This larger region would include the Broca's area, lateral premotor cortex, and pars orbitalis which would be termed the language unification hub of the brain. In fact, Hagoort proposed that the language hub actually consists of three language unification components. The first is syntactic unification. This syntactic unification represents the linking of lexical components into multi-word components utilizing the rules of grammar. The second component is the unification component. This domain unifies our lexical strands into phrases accompanied by appropriate prosody. For example, much social convention is implicated in the phrase "How are you" depending upon the intonation accent on the word "are" vs the word "you." The semantic unification component allows for the understanding of a lexical item within context. These components follow an anterior to posterior functional gradient with subsections of Broca's region supporting various aspects of language, working in unison to support fluid, well-timed speech production. Bohsali and Crosson (2016) suggest that Broca's area and pre-SMA basal ganglia loops work together, combined into the Broca's region, to allow for the transfer of information so that appropriate meaning is assigned (semantic unification) and the items are organized in grammatically correct phrases (syntactic unification) with appropriate intonation applied and with appropriate phonological and articulation initiation.

Language and Motor Cortex in the Interpretation of Speech

The association between motor cortex and spoken speech should be fairly obvious as to the need to move orofacial areas and articulators. Poeppel and Assaneo (2020) wondered whether motor cortex is also involved in interpreting speech. Recognizing that the entrained signals, or the chunking or coupling of oscillating systems, in the auditory cortex are usually hovering at about 4.5 Hz and that this is the average rate of syllables spoken across languages, they attempted to ascertain if there was a neurophysiological basis. They had subjects listen to syllables for nonsense words at rates between 2 and 7 Hz. In fact, they tracked the entrained signal from the auditory cortex to the motor cortex, another example of how various regions of the brain synchronize across tasks, in this case, language perception.

It is interesting to note that the research indicates that, although to a lesser degree, deaf children who sign can also stutter, which seems to concretize the association between language and motor areas, rather than vocalizing areas per se.

Iuzzini-Seigel (2019) looked at whether children with childhood apraxia of speech and other speech disorders and typically developing children would show differences in motor skill attainment in general. Children were classified by language ability and assessed with the Movement Assessment Battery for Children—Second Edition. The results found that children with CAS performed below the normal limit on all components of the motor battery and more poorly than the typical and speech sound disordered children on measures of aiming and catching as well as balance. Iuzzini-Seigel notes how this pattern may impact social, academic, and later on vocational functioning. Iuzzini-Seigel also suggests that what we may be looking at in children with CAS is a "higher order deficit that mediates cognitive-linguistic and motor impairments" in this group. This finding again suggests that the comprised motor system in CAS is also recruited for other motor-driven tasks, and as such this system being compromised will lead to dysfunction in other motor-driven areas. Since, as we have demonstrated, the motor areas are an essential component to most, if not all cognitive activities, this disruption of function should be anticipated to be extensive.

In making our argument that childhood apraxia of speech involves much more than simple disruption of the motor system, we should consider what happens when the semantic/categorical process is disrupted thereby affecting a lack of automaticity for phonemes and sound production. This would result in increasingly disordered cognitive processing utilized to interpret incoming information and to encode it to support developmentally appropriate growth of abstract reasoning. The fact that this system is further impacted, through the process of ongoing development, reflecting increasingly cognitive load, should also be considered.

In Summary

The treatise of both chapters detailing the global nature of CAS is that child development is in effect a bottom-up/feedforward process which potentially impacts multiple areas, and impact in one area potentially impacts other areas depending upon where in the neurophysiological system the problem arises. We have traced potential impact from their genetic etiology in some cases to their behavioral manifestations and then to neural pathway modeling to demonstrate the complexity and the global reach of the potential problems associated with CAS. Where in this course of development the lack of appropriate unfolding of processes occurs will, logically, impact children in somewhat different ways. We may observe the sensitivity and lose the diagnosis because of a lack of specificity.

This addresses both why there is so much confusion as to the pathognomonic signs across disorders and why relying solely on behavioral descriptors is problematic. We need to consider the impact of this diagnostic model on how we end up in a circumlocutious state of diagnosis and behavioral descriptors. That is, we describe descriptors, which sound muddled because of our attempts to put processing issues into a modular diagnostic framework and end up with descriptors of diagnostic categories which do little else than list descriptors. This can be problematic when working with children because we intervene only when pathognomonic signs are fully apparent. And often times we intervene within the domain most notably impacted without an appreciation for the impact in other developmental domains, seeing them as separate and often not targeted if they do not reach the "cutoff" for deficit status. This then impacts intervention with what the current authors believe to be an important fact, the interrelatedness of the identified area with other domains and the need to address the areas presenting with "softer signs." If these two chapters have done their jobs, they will have raised the reader's awareness of an often underdiagnosed disorder, which is not limited to motor planning in the orofacial area, but rather has cortical relatedness to many other areas of child development of skills.

The Implications of Bottom-Up Development for the Functional Implications of CAS

Childhood apraxia of speech represents a developmental disorder. Adult lesion-based studies may have limited applicability in terms of modeling. It is rather important for us to understand the "bottom-up" development of the brain, to truly appreciate the significance of subcortical structures and functions to the higher-level cognitive processes. For example, we know that if a child's behaviors are generated by maturational lags in cerebellar development during the course of early childhood development, a child's presentations may be marked by the manifestation of relatively mild motor difficulty. Actually, motor skill and the quality of motor skills, both gross and fine, can be impacted. For example, the child may have delayed early milestones such as in sitting independently and walking independently. The child may show signs of hypotonia or low muscle tone. This can lead to problems with fine muscular and motor control early on as meeting early developmental milestones and later as impacting how the child sits and writes. Speech production requires fine oral motor control. This is required for articulation of oral motor sequencing in the production of expressing a speech sound and motor associations. Developmental anomalies within these aspects of language system can easily generate phonological processing deficits, and as we know, phonology is a critical foundation for reading and speech production or language. On a pragmatic level, the magnitude of impact would affect the conscious effort required to accomplish reading-related tasks because of "even subtle motor difficulties, reading related tasks would be performed slowly, while in aggregate the diminished allocation of cognitive resources." More effortful cognitive processing would take an additional toll on reading automaticity and comprehension. These observations enable the clinician to understand language and reading development. "They are not pathognomonic signs that indirectly identify a particular disorder. Instead, these are risk factors that serve to predict an increased likelihood of a future diagnosis of dyslexia. This is a critical distinction" (Koziol, 2014). The same can be said for childhood apraxia of speech. That is, childhood apraxia of speech is a developmental disorder with early motor development having a potential association to phonological processing difficulties and subsequent language difficulties with accompanying impact in fine or gross motor behavior or both. Again, these are not pathognomonic signs, but rather risk factors which should alert professionals to the potential benefit of early intervention.

For example, when conducting a neuropsychological evaluation, we should not rely solely on the achieved standard scores. We should be looking at possible risk factors. Other similarly developmental risk factors include difficulty with early identification of letters and letter sound associations, such as asking the child to identify which word in a group has a different starting letter (e.g., bat-ball-doll) or sound blends (br-br-bl). These types of sound word association games require speech, sound awareness, or phonological processing that can be more formally assessed during neuropsychological evaluations. "Performance on these tasks is presumably dependent upon the integrity of frontal parietal networks. However, dependent upon the specific task, numerous other brain regions can be recruited, characterized by changing patterns of functional connectivity in both the left and right cerebral hemispheres."

Treatment of CAS

There are some general principles finding agreement regarding the treatment of CAS. Firstly, it is largely agreed that some activities, although part of the speech pathologist's tool box and of potential face validity, for example, blowing bubbles, are not translating into effective treatment practices for children with CAS. Secondly, CAS is recognized as a "neurological speech sound disorder in which the precision and consistency of movements are impaired" (ASHA, 2022). ASHA emphasizes the need for repetitive planning, programming, and production necessitating the need for intensive and individualized intervention. ASHA highlights a need for both motor programming-based approaches and linguistic approaches. Therefore, there is stress on speech sound movements with the goal of the child developing speech sound skills which are accurate and consistent and which reach a level of automaticity. The linguistic aspect incorporates an emphasis on how to make the speech sounds and how to make sequences of speech sounds and the rules for when sounds and sequences are used. The following is a brief description of motor-based treatment approaches.

The Dynamic Temporal and Tactile Cueing approach uses a cueing hierarchy which is systematically diminished as the child progresses. The system is designed to shape movement gestures. It begins with direct imitation and moves to simultaneous production with provided tactile or gestural cues if direct imitation was not successful. Cues are then faded and the cycle repeats. This approach is recommended for very young children with severe childhood apraxia of speech.

The Nuffield Dyspraxia Program emphasizes the development of phonemes—single speech sounds and simple syllables. The phonological skills are then incorporated into simple word pairs. The goal is a solid "core."

The Rapid Syllable Transition (ReST) program aims to train motor planning flexibility through the repetition of varied sequences of either real or nonsense syllables. This method aims for accurate speech production, rapid and fluent transition across sounds, and accurate syllable stress within words.

The current authors wish to note that other programs exist. For example, the PROMPT program aims to provide Prompts for Restructuring Oral Muscular Phonetic Targets. This program is not limited to children with CAS. Linguistic methods are complementary to motor programs. They emphasize speech function with the aim of helping the child internalize phonological rules. Prosodic facilitation aims to improve intonation. Through rhyming and rhythmic activities, the child is taught to use appropriate intonation to train functional phrases.

As noted elsewhere in this chapter, for some children, difficulties with residual issues including difficulties with unfamiliar multisyllable words, persistent speech sound errors, and struggles with prosody may persist into adulthood. This emphasizes the need for both early identification and intervention.

No doubt many reading this chapter on childhood apraxia of speech will ask since treatment is currently practice-practice-practice, why is this level of understanding important? The authors believe that one of the most important reasons for this level of understanding of the disorder is to debunk the myth that CAS is "simply" a disorder of speech motor dysfunction. It is the hope of the current authors that readers will come a way with a deeper understanding of the need to move away from a behavioral description of CAS as a disorder of phonology to an understanding of how the phonology is intercorrelated with other functions, including motor integration, language comprehension, reading, and arithmetic. There are implications for the trajectory of CAS impacting many other areas of development including social and academic. CAS is not "just" a speech motor disorder.

Secondly, it is hoped that the reader, as a clinician or practitioner, will be more aware of the implications of underdiagnosing this disorder. Treatment for CAS is not a short-term or low-frequency-based intervention. Treatment of CAS requires the overriding of genetic coding, the establishment of neural connections of greater integrity as they traverse from local to larger network integration, and the establishment of greater automaticity for these developmental skills.

Thirdly, it is important for the child and their families to understand that this disorder is not self-limiting. There are implications for all academic areas, and unless the clinician understands the connection between brain-based development and the expression of developmental readiness for academic skill attainment, the family and related teaches will not either.

Fourth is the need to understand the associations of CAS to disordered reading and arithmetic as interpreted by brain-based processes so that the child is supported in areas not typically viewed as directly associated with "a speech problem."

It is important for the clinician to help family and teachers to understand how this "speech" disorder may impact both receptive and expressive language and language communications.

Lastly, there are implications for school-based support services for children with CAS. We currently have a system which affords services to children who show a deficit in a particular academic area. What the current chapter clearly indicates is that supports will potentially be necessary in multiple areas, for although they may not be deficit per se, they are likely impacted. This may mean occupational therapy supports for lingering motor coordination weaknesses to supports for learning to "read" numbers and mathematic signs. Those areas of weakness represent associated processing weaknesses which collectively impact the success of any child.

Owing to the historical professional trajectory of the current authors, we side on the error of caution. We believe strongly in early intervention. We believe strongly that the early years are critical formation years. We believe that it is better to ascertain if there is a presence of risk factor signs coupled with a behavioral expression of multiple signs of CAS and offer intervention services before they become pathognomonic, before they impact a child's social and academic progress and ultimately their self-esteem.

References

Ackermann, H., Mathiak, K., & Riecker, A. (2007). The contribution of the cerebellum to speech production and speech perception: Clinical and functional imaging data. *Cerebellum, 6*(3), 202–213.

Alexander, M. D., DeLong, M. R., & Strick, P. L. (1986). Parallel organization of functionally segregated circuits linking the basal ganglia and cortex. *Annual Review of Neuroscience, 9*, 357–381.

ASHA. (2022). *Childhood Apraxia of Speech*. Retrieved from ASHA: ASHA.ORG

Bishop, D. (1997). *Uncommon understanding: Development and disorders of language comprehension in children*. Taylor & Francis.

Bohali, A., Gullet, J., Mareci, T., Crosson, B., FitzGerald, D., White, K., & Nadeau, S. (2016). Structural connectivity of Broca's region (I7.004). *Neurology, 86*(16 Supplement), I7.004.

Bohsali, A., & Crosson, B. (2016). The basal ganglia and language: A tale of two loops. In J. Soghomonian (Ed.), *Innovations in Cognitive Neuroscience*. Springer. https://doi.org/10.1007/978-3-319-42743-0_10

Catani, M., & de Schotten, M. T. (2008). A diffusion tensor imaging tractography atlas for virtual in vivo dissections. *Cortex, 44*(8), 1105–1132. https://doi.org/10.1016/j.cortex.2008.05.004

Catani, M., Allin, M. P., Husain, M., Pugliese, L., Mesulam, M. M., Murray, R. M., & Jones, D. K. (2007). Symmetries in human brain language pathways correlate with verbal recall. *Proceedings of the Nationall Academy of Sciences U S A, 104*(43), 17163–17168. https://doi.org/10.1073/pnas.0702116104. Epub 2007 Oct 15. PMI.

Crosson, B., et al. (2004). *Left and right basal ganglia and frontal activity during language generation: Contributions to lexical, semantic, and phonological processes* (pp. 1061–1067). Cambridge University Press.

David, D. H., & Rakison, D., Yermolayeva, Y. (2010). Infant categorization. *WIREs Cognitive Science, 1*, 894–905.

DiDonato, A. (2014, May). *New directions in social competence research: Examining developmental trajectories and language minority populations*. Retrieved from ASU.edu: https://keep.lib.asu.edu/_flysystem/fedora/c7/114024/DiDonato_asu_0010E_14024.pdf

Fair, D., Cohen, A., Power, J., Dosenbach, N., Church, J., & Meizen, F., et al. (2009). Functional brain networks develop from a "local to distributed" organization. *PLoS Computational Biology*. https://doi.org/10.1371/journal.pcbi.1000381

Fields, D. (2010). Change in the brain's white matter; the role of the brain's white matter in active learning and memory may be underestimated. *Science, 330*(6005), 768–769.

Fiori, S. G., Guzzetta, A., Mitra, J., Pannek, K., Pasquariello, R., Cipriani, P., Tosetti, M., Cioni, G., Rose, S. E., & Chilosi, A. (2016). Neuroanatomical correlates of childhood apraxia of speech: A connectomic approach. *NeuroImage: Clinical, 12*, 894–901.

Flinker, A. K. (2015). Redefining the role of Broca's area in speech. *Proceedings of the National Academy of Sciences, 112*, 2871–2875. https://doi.org/10.1073/pnas.1414491112

Ford, A., McGregor, K. C., Crosson, B., & White, K. D. (2010). Structural connectivity of Broca's area and medial frontal cortex. *NeuroImage, 52*(4), 1230–1237. https://doi.org/10.1016/j.neuroimage.2010.05.018

Gao, Y., Meng, X., Bai, Z., Liu, X., Zhang, M., Li, H., Ding, G., Liu, L., & Booth, J. R. (2022). Left and right arcuate fasciculi are uniquely related to word reading skills in Chinese-English bilingual children. *Neurobiology of Language, 3*, 109–131. https://doi.org/10.1162/nol_a_00051

Guenther, F., Hanpson, M., & Johnson, D. (1998). A theoretical investigation of reference frames for the planning of speech movements. *Psychological Review, 05*(4), 611–633. https://doi.org/10.1037/0033-295X.105.4.611-633

Hagoort, P. (2005). On Broca, brain, and binding. *Trends in Cognitive Science, 9*(9), 416–423.

Hickok, G. (2012). The cortical organization of speech processing: Feedback control and predictive coding the context of a dual stream model. *Journal of Communication Disorders, 45*(6), 393–402.

Hickok, G., & Poeppel, D. (2007). The cortical organization of speech processing. *Nature Review Neuroscience, 8*(5), 393–402.

Hickok, G., Houde, J., & Rong, F. (2011). Sensorimotor integration in speech processing: Computational basis and neural organization. *Neuron, 69*, 407–422.

Iuzzini-Seigel, J. (2019). Motor performance in children with childhood apraxia of speech and speech sound disorders. *Journal of Speech, Language and Hearing Research, 62*(9), 3220–3233.

Kadis, D. S., Goshulak, D., Namasivayam, A., Pukonen, M., Kroll, R., De Nil, L. F., Pang, E. W., & Lerch, J. P. (2014). Cortical thickness in children receiving intensive therapy for idiopathic apraxia of speech. *Brain Topography, 27*(2), 240–247. https://doi.org/10.1007/s10548-013-0308-8. Published online 2013 Aug 24.

Koziol, L. (2014). *The myth of executive functioning: Missing elements in conceptualization, evaluation, and assessment*. Springer International Publishing.

Koziol, L., Budding, D., & Chidekel, D. (2012). From movement to thought: Executive function, embodied cognition, and the cerebellum. *Cerebellum, 11*(2), 505–525. https://doi.org/10.1007/s12311-011-0321-y

Leiner, H. C., Leiner, A. L., & Dow, R. S. (1994). The underestimated cerebellum. *Human Brain Mapping, 2*(4), 244–254.

Liegeois, F. J., & Morgan, A. T. (2012). Neural bases of childhood speech disorders: Lateralization and plasticity for speech functions during development. *Neuroscience & Biobehavioral Reviews, 36*, 439–458.

Maassen, B. (2002). Issues contrasting adult acquired versus developmental apraxia of speech. *Seminars in Speech and Language, 23*, 257–266.

Maassen, B. (2015). Developmental models of childhood apraxia of speech. In I. R. S. Bahr (Ed.), *Routledge handbook of communication disorders* (pp. 124–133). Routledge/Unesco.

McNorgan, C. (2021). The connectivity fingerprints of highly-skilled and disordered reading persist across cognitive domains. *Frontiers in Computational Neuroscience, 15, 590093*. https://doi.org/10.3389/fncom.2021.590093

Peter, B., Bruce, L., Raaz, C., Williams, E., Pfeiffer, A., & Rogalsky, C. (2020). Comparing global motor characteristics in children and adults with childhood apraxia of speech to a cerebellar stroke patient: Evidence for the cerebellar hypothesis in a developmental motor speech disorder. *Clinical Linguistics and Phonetics, 35*(4), 368–392.

Poeppel, D., & Assaneo, M. F. (2020). Speech rhythms and their neural foundations. *Nature Reviews Neuroscience, 21*(6), 322–334.

Popa, L., & Ebner, T. (2019). Cerebellum, predictions and errors. *Frontiers in Cellular Neuroscience*. https://doi.org/10.3389/fncel.2018.00524

Preston, J. L., Molfese, P. J., Mencl, W. E., Frost, S. J., Hoeft, F., Fulbright, R. K., Landi, N., Grigorenko, E. L., Seki, A., Felsenfeld, S., & Pugh, K. R. (2014). Structural brain differences in school-age children with residual speech sound errors. *Brain and Language, 128*(1), 25–33. https://doi.org/10.1016/j.bandl.2013.11.001

Ramus, F. (2003). Developmental dyslexia: Specific phonological deficit or general sensorimotor dysfunction. *Current Opinion in Neurobiology, 13*(2), 212–218.

Rolheiser, T., Stamatakis, E. A., & Tyler, L. K. (2011). Dynamic processing in the human language system: Synergy between the arcuate fascicle and extreme capsule. *The Journal of Neuroscience, 31*(47), 16949–16957.

Schmahmann, J. D., & Sherman, J. C. (1998). The cerebellar cognitive affective syndrome. *Brain, 121*(4), 561–579.

Semenza, C., & Benavides-Varela, S. (2018). *Reassessing lateralization in calculation*. Royal Society: Biological Sciences.

Shaywitz, S. S. (2005). Dyslexia. *Biological Psychiatry*, 1–13.

Shriberg, L. D., Lohmeier, H. L., Strand, E. A., & Jakielski, K. J. (2012). Encoding, memory, and transcoding deficits in childhood apraxia of speech. *Clinical Linguistics & Phonetics, 26*(5), 445–482.

Shriberg, L. D., Strand, E. A., Jakielski, K. J., & Mabie, H. L. (2019). Estimates of prevalence of speech and motor speech disorders in persons with complex neurodevelopmental disorders. *Clinical Linguistics & Phonetics*, 33(8), 707–736.

Sierpowska, J., Bryant, K., Jannsen, N., & Piai, V. (2022). Comparing human and chimpanzee temporal lobe neuroanatomy reveals modifications to human language hubs beyond the frontotemporal arcuate fasciculus. *Proceedings of the National Academy of Sciences, 119*(28), e2118295119. https://doi.org/10.1073/pnas.2118295119

Silveri, M. (2021). Contribution of the cerebellum and the basal ganglia to language production: Speech, word fluency, and sentence construction - evidence from pathology. *Cerebellum, 20*(2), 282–294.

Simonyan, K., Ackermann, H., Chang, E., & Greenlee, J. (2016). New developments in understanding the complexity of human speech production. *Journal of Neuroscience, 36*(45), 11440–11448. https://doi.org/10.1523/JNEUROSCI.2424-16.2016

Toga, W. (2015). *Brain Mapping*. Elsevier Inc, Academic Press.

Ullman, M. (2006). Is Broca's area part of a basal ganglia thalamocortical circuit? *Cortex, 42*(4), 480–485.

Ullman, M., & Pierpont, E. I. (2005). Specific language impairment is not specific to language: The procedural deficit hypothesis. *Cortex, 41*(3), 399–433.

Velleman, S. (2011). Lexical and phonological development in children with childhood apraxia of speech – A commentary on Stoel-Gammon's 'relationships between lexical and phonological development in young children'. *Journal of Child Language, 38*(1), 82–86.

Wasserman, T., & Wasserman, L. D. (2019). *Therapy and the neural network model*. Springer.

Wasserman, T., & Wasserman, L. D. (2020). *Motivation, effort and the neural network model*. Springer.

Chapter 9
Neuropsychological Assessment of Apraxia: Where Network Reality and Domain Assessment Collide

Neuropsychological assessment is based on the premise that neuropsychological functioning in humans consists of the operation and integration of skill-specific domains. Neuropsychological testing is often cognitively heavy. For example, most neuropsychological assessments will attempt to describe the functioning of language, visuospatial skills, attention, memory, and sensorimotor domains (Koziol, 2014). Each of these domains is responsible for processing (cognitive) information. This processing is broken down into a set of specific activities. Six such activities have been identified:

1. Remembering: Recall or retrieve previous learned information. Example is recite a story that you just read.
2. Understanding: Comprehending the meaning, intention, interpolation, and interpretation of instructions, reading material, and presented problems.
3. Applying: Use a concept/newly learned material in a new situation or unprompted use of an abstraction.
4. Analyzing: Separating material or concepts into component parts so that its organizational structure may be understood. This also includes distinguishing between facts and inferences.
5. Evaluating: Make judgments about the value of ideas or materials.
6. Creating: Builds a structure or pattern from numerous elements. Putting parts together to form a whole, with emphasis on creating a new meaning or structure.

There are other things to consider. Blooms taxonomy, for example (Armstrong, 2010), has areas of psychomotor consideration. These include the following:

1. Perception (awareness): The ability to use sensory cues to guide motor activity. This ranges from sensory stimulation, through cue selection, to translation.
2. Set: Readiness to act. It includes mental, physical, and emotional sets. These three sets are dispositions that predetermine a person's response to different situations. By extension, this can be considered intentionality and therefore potentially related to some forms of apraxia.
3. Guided response: The early stages in learning a complex skill that includes imitation and trial and error. Adequacy of performance is achieved by practicing.

T. Wasserman, L. D. Wasserman, *Apraxia: The Neural Network Model*,
Neural Network Model: Applications and Implications,
https://doi.org/10.1007/978-3-031-24105-5_9

4. Mechanism (basic proficiency): This is the intermediate stage in learning a complex skill. Learned responses have become habitual, and the movements can be performed with some confidence and proficiency.
5. Complex overt response (expert): The skillful performance of motor acts that involve complex movement patterns. Proficiency is indicated by a quick, accurate, and highly coordinated performance, requiring a minimum of energy. This category includes performing without hesitation and automatic performance.
6. Adaptation: Skills are well developed, and the individual can modify movement patterns to fit special requirements.
7. Origination: Creating new movement patterns to fit a particular situation or specific problem. Learning outcomes emphasize creativity based upon highly developed skills.

At first glance, these psychomotor areas would appear to have relevance in identifying treatment approaches that would facilitate the development of the various skills. Neuropsychological assessment would appear to focus on the first set of cognitively based skills and much less on these psychomotor skills. We will be highlighting the value of focusing on the psychomotor skills and suggest ways for neuropsychologists to include them, in a more comprehensive and systematic manner, in their ongoing assessments.

How Many Domains Are There?

As with everything else, there is general agreement as to the concept, but some disagreement as to the exact number of domains. For the purpose of classifying neurocognitive disorders, the Neurocognitive Work Group of the DSM 5 (American Psychiatric Association, 2013) agreed on six principal domains of cognitive function: (1) memory and learning, (2) language, (3) executive functions, (4) complex attention, (5) social cognition, and (6) perceptual and motor functions. Meta-analytic reviews have identified up to seven cognitive domains: attention/working memory, executive functioning, language, verbal memory, visual memory, visuomotor ability, and visuospatial ability (McGinty et al., 2014). Most psychological tests identify four, including verbal skills, visual motor skills, memory, and perceptual motor skills being the most common. As psychological assessment follows the descriptors proffered by the American Psychiatric Association, the six cognitive domains (complex attention, executive function, learning and memory, language, perceptual-motor function, and social cognition) have found themselves an integral part of neuropsychological assessment.

When it comes to the assessment of most apraxic conditions, it seems apparent that the emphasis on cognitive domain assessment that characterizes neuropsychological assessment is not clearly relatable in the assessment of apraxia. Given the fundamental motor nature of apraxic conditions, it behooves us to look at whether neuropsychological tests are designed to assess the conditions that comprise apraxia.

Briefly, this does not seem to be the case. The motor tests that are typically included in a neuropsychological test battery look at how effectively the individual is able to coordinate hand-eye movements, finger dexterity, balance, and motor speed in general (Weintraub, 2000b). For the most part, these assessments are based on behavioral observation, which is fine, or assessments of basic motor speed, which is fine, but do not seem to be geared to assessing white matter dysregulation of motor functioning and conceptualizing how this disruption is functionally important. That is why, with the possible exception of childhood apraxia of speech, most neuropsychologists, if they assess apraxia in the first place, content themselves to a *description* of an observable motor skill dysfunction and leave the treatment to someone else. Given, as we have seen, that based upon network modeling, downstream effects in general, and cognitive effects in particular, of an apraxia producing lesion should be anticipated, perhaps it is wise for neuropsychologists to better develop tools and skills to assess the far-reaching consequences of apraxia in its several forms. Specifically, neuropsychologists have to do better than merely administering tests and reporting standard scores. This is a field based upon the premise that behavior is brain based and it is the purpose of the neuropsychologist to understand and help others understand how this process is unfolding or disrupted in any given individual referred for assessment.

Domains Are Complex and Subsume Multiple Functions

There are issues with domain-based assessment that should be considered. As should be readily apparent, each domain supports a wide variety of activities and knowledge. We can never assess the functioning of an entire domain no matter how many tests we give. We can only sample certain of the many complex skills. What is more concerning from a network perspective is that these domains are considered discrete and largely dissociable from each other. That is, neuropsychologists, for example, believe that there is the ability to assess only visual motor, or receptive language, or memory skills without contamination from other skill areas. As we have demonstrated elsewhere (Wasserman & Wasserman, 2017), there are problems with these ideas. Basically, network modeling is based on the idea, and neuroimaging confirms that networks constantly interact with one another to produce an outcome. Based on that assumption, it would be highly unlikely that we would ever be able to assess only one discrete area of functioning, because the possbility that just one independent network controls the complex functioning assessed by neuropsychological tests is infinitesimally small.

Let's take a look at some of these areas of concern in detail.

Questionable Assumptions Concerning Ability of Neuropsychological Tests

The neuropsychological assessment of apraxia is hampered by certain assumptions that have traditionally characterized neuropsychological test function. Examining these assumptions and challenging them based upon networking principles will point to the way forward for including apraxias into neuropsychological testing considerations.

Assumption: Most Disorders Are Produced by Discrete and Dissociable Neuropsychological Deficits

There is an assumption that once we diagnose a specific clinical condition, ADHD, for example, we somehow understand what has gone wrong with the neural network underpinning that skill. For example, if a person is diagnosed as having ADHD, we often provide feedback detaining the same descriptors presented in the DSM though that is an explanation of brain-based behavior. Child has been referred for inattentiveness and impulsivity, diagnosed with ADHD, and parent receives the explanation that child has ADHD so he is inattentive and impulsive. A more neural-based explanation would allow one to reliably assume fronto-striatal network abnormalities contributing to ADHD (Bush, 2010) or that the deficits are specifically related to dysfunction of the reticular activating system which is a basal ganglia structure that is the major relay system among the many pathways that enter and leave the brain. Only this assumption is not entirely accurate.

Neuropsychological studies of attention-deficit hyperactivity disorder (ADHD) actually identify a broad range of processes that are dysregulated in attention-deficit hyperactivity disorder. These include areas of executive dysfunction including inhibitory and working memory deficits, as well as non-executive deficits (perception; memory timing) (Sonuga-Barke et al., 2010). Alterations in motivational and reward processes have also been identified (Wasserman & Wasserman, 2015).

Moreover, even the most robust neuropsychological effects are only moderate in size and often fall short of the level required for diagnosis. Sonuga-Barke et al. point out that Nigg et al. (2005) found only 30% of patients with deficits on at least three tasks on a large executive function assessment battery. They believed that this pattern of limited associations across distinct domains highlights the neuropsychological heterogeneity in ADHD.

Originally, the dual pathway model of attention-deficit hyperactivity disorder (Sonuga-Barke, 2003) posited that this heterogeneity was the result of two, more or less, independent patterns of deficit each affecting some ADHD patients and not others: one grounded in dorsal fronto-striatal dysregulation mediated by inhibitory-based executive function and the other underpinned by ventral fronto-striatal circuits and linked to altered signaling of delayed rewards, manifest as delay aversion. There were still a group of patients for which neither of these circumstances were identified. They proposed a third dissociable system based on temporal processing deficits in conjunction with basal ganglia. As we have suggested, later research has identified still others. The point here is that there is not one clear dysfunctional system in ADHD or in many other disorders. There are many. If you diagnose ADHD on behavioral criteria, which is how it is done, you have no knowledge which of the many potential causal systems are implicated.

There is research to suggest that the same issue arises when attempting to assess the role of executive function (EF) in psychopathology. Research investigating phenotypic and genetic overlap of three EF latent variables (a common EF factor predicting response inhibition, working memory updating, and mental set shifting tasks and updating- and shifting-specific factors) with five impulsivity dimensions (negative and positive urgency, lack of premeditation and perseverance, and sensation seeking) found common EF and multiple impulsivity dimensions, particularly negative urgency, independently predicted externalizing psychopathology. The research demonstrated that multiple impulsivity dimensions, but not common EF, predicted internalizing psychopathology (Friedman et al., 2020). These results suggested that EFs and self-reported impulsivity tap different aspects of control that are both relevant for psychopathology. EFs and impulsivity appear to "capture somewhat overlapping but phenotypically and genetically separable constructs. Importantly, they are both valid measures of individual differences that are independently relevant for understanding externalizing psychopathology. Thus, EF and impulsivity are not interchangeable" (pg536). Assessing this accurately means that assessment has the ability to discretely and accurately assess each construct. Given the confusion in multiple definitions of both constructs, the answer is at best ambiguous (Bickel, 2012). This research suggested that EF and impulsivity are generally considered conceptually distinct, but, in fact, they may be antipodes (i.e., widely separated on a common continuum, upon which they are related). The authors highlight a quote by Hermann Hesse "Scientific thought often progresses by recognizing heterogeneity in phenomena formally considered homogenous. This evolution sometimes involves identifying small components and conceptualizing how they fit together to produce larger phenomena" (pg361). We concur. If you identify a person as having ADHD using behavioral criteria, then that's what you know. You do not know for sure what the specific neurological underpinning is as it could be several things or a combination of several things.

The same situation pertains to understanding the neuropsychological underpinning of obsessive-compulsive disorder. For example, a multi-parameter MRI study revealed specific white matter abnormalities in OCD suggesting tract disorganization as main feature, reflected by local changes in fiber directionality. This altered anatomical connectivity *might play* a specific role in OCD pathophysiology (Garibotto et al., 2010). Specifically, OCD patients showed significantly lower fractional anisotropy values and altered principal diffusion direction along a wide range of network structures. These included the corpus callosum, cingulum, superior longitudinal fasciculus, and inferior fronto-occipital fasciculus bilaterally. In addition, a track-based analysis of the inferior fronto-occipital fasciculus confirmed a significant bilateral FA reduction. Lower FA values in the inferior fronto-occipital fasciculus, superior longitudinal fasciculus, and corpus callosum correlated with symptom severity and neuropsychological performance. Here we have a suggestion of a rather complex network with many components that is somehow dysfunctional. We do not know how or why, and we do not know if the problem emanates from a specific place or that the entire network is somehow compromised. More recent research confirmed this idea by demonstrating that OCD patients presented widespread microstructural abnormalities in distributed working memory tracts and that heterogeneity of dysfunction characterized their findings (Zang et al., 2021).

Finally, there is research to suggest that the problems associated with OCD are related to white matter myelination as opposed to a structural or neural transmitter-based dysfunction (Maleki et al., 2020). They found no significant group differences in brain structures were observed between OCD and healthy controls. Rather, they found that MTR, an indicator of myelination, was positively associated with OCD symptom severity in numerous regions including the OFC, striatum, CC, insula, and cingulum. Specifically, they found that higher myelination was found in certain brain regions in more severe OCD patients.

In summary, existing functional connectivity studies of obsessive-compulsive disorder (OCD) provide considerable support for a model of network dysfunction. That being said, these group-level observations have failed to yield neuroimaging biomarkers sufficient to serve as a test for the OCD diagnosis, predict current or future symptoms, or predict treatment response, perhaps because these studies failed to account for the substantial intersubject variability in structural and functional brain organization (Brennan et al., 2019).

This situation becomes more problematic when it is recognized that you cannot assess discrete elements of a neural pathway independently of its other component parts or from the task you are using to assess it.

Assumption: We Can Assess Components of a Neural Network Independently of Its Other Components

We have stated that many constructs that are taken for granted in modern neuropsychology, fluid intelligence, and executive function among them can best be explained by conceptionalizing them as a collection of task-specific processes engaged in an integrated recruited network involved in problem solving. However, fractionalizing an organically integrated network in an attempt to describe elements of its function leads to arbitrarily defined segments that may be interesting to discuss abstractly, but never occur independently in the real-world operation of the system itself (Wasserman & Wasserman, 2017). This would suggest that you cannot assess the functioning of just one component of a highly integrated network recruited to solve a particular task. For example, our meta-analytic review of tests of attention deficit disorder concluded that the assessment of executive functioning by neuropsychological tests inevitably leads to assessment of cortical-subcortical circuitry common to many forms of executive function and, by implication, behavioral functioning (Wasserman & Wasserman, 2013).

As a result of the shared nature of network components, any finding you would generate would be "contaminated" by the operation of other network components that were recruited to solve the particular task used in the assessment. You would be confronted by the problem that network recruitment is task specific, and it is highly probable that no two tasks recruit exactly the same network. For example, when attempting to measure attention, you can use paying attention to an image as a measure of sustained attention. Clearly, the nature of the picture is a factor with individual implications to the viewer. Not all pictures evoke the same emotional responses, and some may not evoke any at all. The addition of an emotional component brings onboard networks associated with reward recognition. Thus a similar task might involve the recruitment of dissimilar networks due to the history of the individual being asked to solve the task.

This has wider implications as well. For example, all of the domains of cognition that have been found to relate to motor learning can broadly be classified as fluid cognitive abilities, which are a global cognitive measure reflecting one's abilities for problem solving and learning new things in the absence of prior experience. Thus, it is possible that global fluid cognition, rather than visuospatial working memory specifically, is related to motor learning, and it is impossible to disentangle the two (French et al., 2021).

Assumption: Neuropsychological Tests Were Designed to Assess Brain Function

It is generally accepted that the historical purpose of clinical neuropsychology was to assist in the diagnosis of brain pathology (Chaytor & Schmitter-Edgecombe, 2003). In general, neuropsychological tests were successful in doing so (Long & Kibby, 1995). With the expansion and development of imaging techniques, the role of neuropsychological testing has changed. There are, of course, some disorders, like apraxia, that are not readily diagnosed using imaging techniques or testing. There are also certain disorders, such as cognitive delay, which still require the use of testing to aid in diagnosis. The number of disorders that require testing for identification continues to diminish.

Neuropsychologists have adapted to these changes by broadening the range of neuropsychology practice. Where traditionally physicians have customarily been the primary referral source for neuropsychological assessments, other agencies (schools, employers, lawyers, and insurance companies) now utilize neuropsychology more frequently. As might be expected, this redefinition of scope of practice has brought about a change in the types of questions that neuropsychologists are asked to address. Referrals are moving away from diagnostic questions to questions about cognitive abilities and disabilities, such as the suitability for advanced educational programming, rehabilitation programs, and ability to work, live independently, manage finances, and drive. While the questions have changed, most clinicians continue to utilize test data as the basis of the conclusions they reach regarding the answer to these new questions. The tests themselves have not changed along with the referral questions. That is, the same tests that were developed to answer injury-related diagnostic questions are now used to answer different questions, for which they were not designed. Neuropsychologists have responded by attempting to associate neuropsychological test performance to very specific brain function (Hale et al., 2010). Nevertheless, current neuropsychological tests were not designed to assess neural network functioning and are likely too blunt to do so.

Assumption: Neuropsychological Tests Can Identify Specific, Discrete, and Dissociable Brain-Based Deficits

We are not suggesting that neuropsychological tests do not measure brain function; they clearly do. The question is *what* are we identifying? Firstly, we need to question whether a function has been accurately identified. Most of us are taught that we are testing a particular function. We administer the tests and report on the function using the domain name of the test. There are, however, many examples of tests "with the same domain name" and poor correlation coefficients ostensibly because the task demands are just slightly different (Koziol, 2014).

What we are saying is that our tests tend to measure the operation of a broad set of networks recruited to solve a particular task. Some psychologists write their reports from a domain-based perspective and speak about deficits specific to that domain, for example, visual spatial deficits or verbal memory deficits. We posit that these are neither discrete nor dissociable domains. Two different but related tasks would likely result in the recruitment of two different but related networks. It is questionable whether it is even possible to independently measure a specific subcomponent of a construct such as executive function (Wasserman & Wasserman, 2017).

Pathognomonic Signs in the Assessment of Apraxia

It should be fairly obvious by now that the available neuropsychological assessment instruments possess neither the sensitivity nor specificity to determine the specific functional neuropsychological deficit associated with the apraxic condition we are attempting to assess. Fundamentally, that is because any particular apraxic condition can be due to a disruption of function anywhere in a complex network. The same condition can be produced by lesions to different sites. That is not to say, the neuropsychological assessment data is not useful. It is. Once determined that an individual is experiencing an apraxic condition, test data can provide a thorough look at associated academic and intellectual functioning that reflects large-scale integrated network operation.

How should the practicing neuropsychologist diagnose apraxia? We have long held that neuropsychology is not based on getting the answers from the test. It is using the test data, in conjunction with our body of knowledge, to arrive at a conclusion. This leads us to a discussion of pathognomonic signs.

The term "pathognomonic sign" describes a sign, symptom, or a group of signs or symptoms that is indicative of a specific physical or mental disorder and not associated with other disorders. The sign is a *particular* sign whose presence means that a particular disease is present beyond any doubt. To those of us who are in clinical work, the pathognomonic sign approach is essentially everyday practice. The behavioral symptom clusters associated with the diagnosis of mental health conditions are essentially a list of hypothetically discriminating pathognomonic signs of a particular disorder. The system certainly has its detractors, including the present authors. The fact remains that certain currently used clinical conditions are so broad, vague, and overlapped with other clinical conditions that identifying them by pathognomonic sign is the only available option. Such is also the case for apraxia, especially developmental apraxia. We have argued elsewhere (Wasserman & Wasserman, 2016) that this state of affairs is not conducive to good science and that the system should be replaced with one that classifies dysfunction based upon the underlying neuropsychology. We will argue here for the same thing as regards apraxia. However, as it stands now, the underlying dysfunction of many apraxic conditions is not currently identifiable. There are exceptions of course, such as in the case of adult stroke or brain injury. However, the specific etiology of developmental apraxia and other related language impairments has not been elucidated. That leaves us with pathognomonic sign approach.

If only it was that easy. The following is from the ICD-10-CM (World Health Organization(WHO), 1993), and it highlights the problem. Apraxia is identified as a "group of cognitive disorders characterized by the inability to perform previously learned skills that cannot be attributed to deficits of motor or sensory function. The two major subtypes of this condition are ideomotor (see apraxia, ideomotor) and ideational apraxia, which refers to loss of the ability to mentally formulate the processes involved with performing an action. For example, dressing apraxia may result from an inability to mentally formulate the act of placing clothes on the body." The major point is that apraxia does not describe one specific disorder but rather a group of disorders characterized by the inability to do a motor task. Although the description goes on to say that "aparaxias are generally associated with lesions of the dominant parietal lobe and supramarginal gyrus," that is not always the case. Interestingly, the above definition excludes aparaxias caused by cardiovascular disease, although it does not say why.

Clinical Presentation

So maybe pathognomonic sign approach is not exactly the best idea which leaves the idea of clinical presentation. How does it look to the clinician trying to assess it? What it looks like is a motor disorder wherein a person cannot perform a motor task that they previously could perform. It does get a bit more specific, especially when apraxic disorders of speech are considered. For example, "the most common AOS errors involve place of articulation, with affricates and fricatives most affected (e.g., a word with affricate sounds such as the 'ch' in 'church' will be more difficult to say for apraxic speakers than a word with bilabial phonemes, such as the 'm' in 'mom'). Errors are more common on consonant clusters, rather than singleton consonants (e.g., 'strict' will be more difficult than 'sit') and patients with AOS are more likely to produce errors when asked to repeat nonsense words, as opposed to meaningful words. Patients with AOS often assign equal stress to each word. Pauses between syllables and words are common, as is an overall slowed rate of speech" (Ogar et al., 2005). The problem with this is that these particular abilities are the purview of speech and language pathologists. They are not generally included in a standard neuropsychological assessment and not part of training for most psychologists or neuropsychologists. Perhaps that needs to change.

Developmental Apraxia of Speech and Pathognomonic Sign

There are problems with the pathognomonic sign approach when it comes to developmental apraxia; namely, there do not appear to be a stable set of pathognomonic signs. Research continues to demonstrate, as we have been saying, that developmental communication disorders have multi-factorial origins at different levels of organization (genetic, environmental, neurological, behavioral). Moreover, the influence of these levels of organization on the resulting behavioral output is interactive rather than uni-directional (Maassen, 2015). In addition, relatively little is known about the contribution of two of these factors, the genetic and neurological factors. All of this is further compounded by the possibility that developmental apraxia and acquired apraxia are doubly dissociable disorders and separate entities (Karmiloff-Smith et al., 2003). A thorough review of this issue is in a separate chapter in this volume.

What to Do, What to Do?

As regards apraxia, given the unsatisfactory state of affairs regarding the typical procedures used by neuropsychologists to assess for dysfunction associated with apraxia, what do neuropsychologists have to utilize to accomplish the diagnostic task? The answer is that you assess the functional behavior that manifests as a result of the impairment. Specifically, what does an apraxic individual do that a neurotypical individual does not do. It is not that a practicing neuropsychologist cannot discern behaviors related to a praxis. We are trained observers of behavior. It is that we have been conditioned to think that the observation is not sufficient, norms based, reliable, or valid. We are taught that the only way to validate our work is to have a normed test score. We do not agree. In fact, in a system based on behavioral cluster analysis, the only ecologically valid assessment is assessment of individualized behavior. Group normed tests are not designed to that. This leads to the idea that neuropsychologists should be defined by their knowledge of how the brain works as opposed to obtaining a reliable test score. Tests should be part of our tool kit, but our opinions and diagnoses should, when appropriate, be based on our body of knowledge.

Fortunately, models are available to instruct us in this regard. Speech and language pathologists have identified a cluster of behaviors that characterize acquired apraxia of speech, for example. Apraxia of speech (AOS) has been described as a disorder affecting the ability to translate well-formed and filled phonological frames into accurate movement programs to generate speech. The intra- and inter-articulator timing and spatial errors that characterize the disorder result in core perceptual features used for clinical diagnosis: increased segment and inter-segment durations, distorted phonemes, consistent error type across repeated productions of words, segmentation of syllables, and more equal stress over words and/or sentences (Ballard et al., 2014). This would, of course, imply that the neuropsychologist is, or should be, knowledgeable about these aspects of speech and their assessment. It would also imply that either the current range of neuropsychological tests assesses for these aspects of speech, which they do not, or neuropsychologists expand the range and types of assessment tools they utilize.

We realize that we go into some detail on the speech aparaxias, but the same system is utilized for most other aparaxias as well, for example, limb apraxia. Limb apraxia is a heterogeneous disorder historically defined by exclusion: deficits in skilled movement not caused by weakness, deafferentation, abnormal tone or posture, tremors or chorea, intellectual deterioration, or poor comprehension (Baumard & Le Gall, 2021). Interestingly, research suggests that aparaxias like limb apraxia are not task specific but instead reflect a general inability to move the limb under many and dissociable task conditions (Belanger et al., 1996). This would argue for the disruption of basic motor circuitry.

We realize that this form of assessment sounds distinctly like the type of cluster analysis utilized in the DSM system. This likely represents the current state of the art. We would argue that is somewhat unsatisfactory; however in that there is no identification of the networks involved and no recognition of the fact that the resultant core behaviors could be caused by numerous forms of disruption to the system. The etiology of the various forms of apraxic conditions affecting speech remains unclear. Investigators have speculated about whether the neurological damage in apraxia is affecting the integrity of existing stored speech motor programs, forward modeling, the feedback processes of error detection and/or correction, gradual tuning of motor programs, and/or producing sequences of motor programs. These are clearly components of a complex and integrated network system. It is possible that understanding the exact nature of the apraxic condition will lead to more refined treatment techniques. Of course, it is also possible that what is true for many skills is also true for apraxia; practice repetition and the eventual automaticity of appropriate behavior are the best way to go. At the current time, we just do not have enough information to know.

References

American Speech Hearing Association. (2022). Retrieved from Childhood Apraxia of Speech: http://ASHA.org

American Psychiatric Association. (2013). *Diagnostic and statistical manual of mental disorders* (5th ed.). American Psychiatric Association.

Ahel, I., Rass, U., El-Khamisy, S., Katyal, S., Celements, P., Mckinnon, P., et al. (2006). The neurodegenerative disease protein aprataxin resolves abortive DNA ligation intermediates. *Nature, 443*(12), 713–716. https://doi.org/10.1038/nature05164

Allison, K. C.-S. (2020). Differential diagnosis of apraxia of speech in children and adults: A scoping view. *Journal of Speech, Language, and Hearing Research, 63*, 2952–2994.

American Speech-Language-Hearing Association. (2007). *Childhood apraxia of speech (Position Statement)*. Retrieved from American Speech-Language-Hearing Association: www.Asha.org/policy

Andres, E. E. (2022). Family based whole exome analysis of specific language impairment identifies rare variants in BUD13, a component of the retention and splicing complex. *Brain Sciences, 47*.

Armstrong, P. (2010). *Bloom's taxonomy*. Retrieved from Vanderbilt University Center for Teaching: https://cft.vanderbilt.edu/guides-sub-pages/blooms-taxonomy/

ASHA. (2007). *Childhood apraxia of speech technical report*. American Speech and Language Association.

ASHA. (2021). *Childhood apraxia of speech*. Retrieved from ASHA/Practice Portal/Clinical Topics/: https://www.asha.org/practice-portal/clinical-topics/childhood-apraxia-of-speech/

Ayres, J. (1972). Types of sensory integrative dysfunction among disabled learners. *American Journal of Occupational Therapy, 26*(1), 13–18.

Bak, T. H. (2012). What wires together dies together: Verbs, actions and neurodegeneration in motor neuron disease. *Cortex, 48*(7), 936–944.

Baldassare, A., Lewis, C., Committeri, G., Snyder, A. Z., Romani, G., & Corbetta, M. (2012). Individual variability in functional connectivity predicts performance of a perceptual task. *Proceedings of the National Acadamey Scence U. S. A., 109*, 3516–3521.

Ballard, K., Tourville, J., & Robin, D. (2014). Behavioral, computational, and neuroimaging studies of acquired apraxia of speech. *Frontiers in Human Neuroscience*. https://doi.org/10.3389/fnhum.2014.00892

Bangert, M., Peschel, T., Schlaug, G., Rotte, M., Drescher, D., Hinrichs, H., et al. (2006). Shared networks for auditory and motor processing in professional pianists: Evidence from fMRI conjunction. *NeuroImage, 30*, 917–926.

Barrios, J., Weng, W., England, R., Reifenberg, E., & Douglass, A. (2020). Hypothalamic dopamine neurons control sensorimotor behavior by modulating brainstem premotor nuclei in zebrafish. *Current Biology, 30*(23), 4606–4619. https://doi.org/10.1016/j.cub.2020.09.002

Basso, A., Luzzatti, C., & Spinler, H. (1980). Is ideomotor apraxia the outcome of damage to well-defined regions of the left hemisphere? *Journal of Neurology, Neurosurgery, and Psychiatry, 43*, 118–126.

Batista-García-Ramó, K., & Fernández-Verdecia, C. (2018). What we know about the brain structure–function relationship. *Behavioral Sciences, 8*(39), 1–14. https://doi.org/10.3390/bs8040039

Baumard, J., & Le Gall, D. (2021). The challenge of apraxia: Toward an operational definition? *Cortex, 141*, 55–80. https://doi.org/10.1016/j.cortex.2021.04.001

Belanger, S., Duffy, R., & Coelho, D. (1996). The assessment of limb apraxia: An investigation of task effects and their cause. *Brain and Cognition, 32*(3), 384–404. https://doi.org/10.1006/brcg.1996.0072

Bernstein, N. (2003). *Contemporary studies on the physiology of the of the neural process*. Smysl.

Bickel, W. (2012). Are executive function and impulsivity antipodes? A conceptual reconstruction with special reference to addiction. *Psychopharmacology (Berl).*, *221*(3), 361–387. https://doi.org/10.1007/s00213-012-2689-x

Bieńkiewicz, M., Brandi, M. G., Hughes, C., & Hermsdörfer, J. (2014). The tool in the brain: Apraxia in ADL. Behavioral and neurological correlates of apraxia in daily living. *Frontiers in Psycholology*. https://doi.org/10.3389/fpsyg.2014.00353, on line.

Binkofsky, F., Kunesch, E., Classen, J., Seitz, R., & Freund, H. (2001). Tactile apraxia: Unimodal apractic disorder of tactile object exploration associated with parietal lobe lesions. *Rain, 124*(1), 132–144. https://doi.org/10.1093/brain/124.1.132

Brazelton, T. B. (1973). *Neonatal behavioral assessment scale*.

Brennan, B., Wang, D., Li, M., Perriello, C. R., Elias, J., Van Kirk, N., et al. (2019). Use of an individual-level approach to identify cortical connectivity biomarkers in obsessive-compulsive disorder. *Biological Psychiatry: Cognitive Neuroscience and Neuroimaging, 4*(1), 27–38. https://doi.org/10.1016/j.bpsc.2018.07.014

Bush, G. (2010). Attention-deficit/hyperactivity disorder and attention networks. *Neuropsychopharmacology, 35*(1), 278–300. https://doi.org/10.1038/npp.2009.120

Cabrero, F., & De Jesus, O. (2021, August 30). *Apraxia of lid opening*. Retrieved from National Library of Medicine: https://www.ncbi.nlm.nih.gov/books/NBK560542/

Carrera, E., & Tononi, D. (2014). Diaschisis: Past, present, future. *Brain, 137*(9), 2408–2422. https://doi.org/10.1093/brain/awu101

Cassidy, A. (2016). The clinical assessment of apraxia. *Practical Neurology, 16*, 317–322.

Chaytor, N., & Schmitter-Edgecombe, M. (2003). The ecological validity of neuropsychological tests: A review of the literature on everyday cognitive skills. *Neuropsychology Review, 13*(4), 181–187.

Childhood Apraxia of Speech. (2022). Retrieved from American Speech-Language Hearing Association: ASHA.ORG.

Churchland, M. M., & Shenoy, K. V. (2007). Temporal complexity and heterogeneity of single-neuron activity in premotor and motor cortex. *Journal of Neurophysiology, 97*, 4235–4257.

Chvatal, S., & Ting, L. (2012). Voluntary and reactive recruitment of locomotor muscle synergies during perturbed walking. *The Journal of Neuroscience, 32*(35), 12237–12250. https://doi.org/10.1523/JNEUROSCI.6344-11.2012

Cleaton, A. T.-S. (2021). Gender and age differences in the presentation of at-risk or probable developmental coordination disorder in adults. *Research in Developmental Disabilities, 115*. https://doi.org/10.1016/j.ridd.2021.104010

Coe, B., Witherspoon, K., Rosenfeld, J., et al. (2014). Refining analyses of copy number variation identifies specific genes associated with developmental delay. *Nature Genetics, 46*, 1053–1017.

Cogan, D. (1952). A type of congenital ocular motor apraxia presenting jerky head movements. *Transactions of the American Academy of Ophthalmology and Otolaryngology, 56*, 579–588.

Conterno, M., Kümmerer, D., Dressing, A., Glauche, V., Urbach, H., Weiler, C., & Rijntjes, R. (2021). Speech apraxia and oral apraxia: Association or dissociation? A multivariate lesion–symptom mapping study in acute stroke patients. *Experimental Brain Research, 240*, 39. https://doi.org/10.1007/s00221-021-06224-3

Cooper, R. (2007). Tool use and related errors in ideational apraxia: The quantitative simulation of patient error profiles. *Cortex, 43*(3), 319–337.

Cousins, M. S. (2003). Developmental coordination impairments in adulthood. *Human Movement Science, 22*, 433–459. https://doi.org/10.1016/j.humov.2003.09.003

Cunningham, A. C. (2019). Coordination difficulties, IQ and psychopathology in children with high-risk copy number variants. *Psychological Medicine, 51*, 290–299. https://doi.org/10.1017/S0033291719003210

Darley, F. (1967). Lacunae and research approaches to them. In C. Miliken & F. Darley (Eds.), *Brain mechanisms underlying speech and language*. Grune & Stratton.

Davis, B., Jakielski, K., & Marquardt, T. (1998). Developmental apraxia of speech: Determiners of differential diagnosis. *Clinical Linguistics & Phonetics, 12*, 25–45. https://doi.org/10.3109/02699209808985211
De Renzi, E., & Faglioni, P. (1999). Apraxia. In G. Denes & L. Pizzamiglio (Eds.), *Handbook of clinical and experimental psychiatry*. Psychology Press. https://doi.org/10.4324/9781315791272
De Renzi, E., & Lucchelli, F. (1988). Ideational apraxia. *Brain, 111*(5), 1173–1185. https://doi.org/10.1093/brain/111.5.1173
De Renzi, E., Faglioni, P., & Sorgato, P. (1982). Modality specific and supramodal mechanisms of apraxia. *Brain, 105*, 301–312.
Delaney, A. L., & Kent, R. D. (2004). Developmental profiles of children diagnosed with apraxia of speech. In *The annual convention of the American-Speech-Language-Hearing Association. Poster*. American-Speech-Language-Hearing Association.
Dewey, D. T. (2019). Very preterm children at risk for developmental coordination disorder have brain alterations in motor areas. *Acta Paediatrica, 108*, 9. https://doi.org/10.1111/apa.14786
Donkervoort, M.-S., & Deelman, B. (2000). Prevalence of apraxia among patients with a first left hemisphere stroke in rehabilitation centres and nursing homes. *Clinical Rehabilitation, 14*(2), 130–136.
Duffy, J. (2006). Apraxia of speech in degenerative neurologic disease. *Aphasiology, 20*, 511–527.
Duffy, J. J. (2012). The diagnosis and understanding of apraxia of speech: Why including neurodegenerative etiologies may be important. *Journal of Speech, Language and Hearing Research, 55*(5), S1518–S1522. https://doi.org/10.1044/1092-4388(2012/11-0309)
Duménieu, M., Marquèze-Pouey, B., Russier, M., & Debanne, D. (2021). Mechanisms of plasticity in subcortical visual areas. *Cells, 10*(11), 3162. https://doi.org/10.3390/cells10113162
Dumont, C., Ska, B., & Joanette, Y. (2000). Conceptual apraxia and semantic memory deficit in Alzheimer's disease: Two sides of the same coin? *Journal of the International Neuropsychological Society, 6*(6), 693–703. https://doi.org/10.1017/S1355617700666079
Edelman, G., & Gally, J. (2001). Degeneracy and complexity in biological systems. *Proceedings of the National Academy of Sciences, 98*(24), 13763–13768.
Einspieler, C. P. (2021). Fetal movements; the origin of human behaviour. *Developmental Medicine & Child Neurology, 63*(10), 1142–1148.
Evarts, E. V. (1868). Relation of pyramidal tract activity to force exerted during voluntary movement. *Journal of Neurophysiology, 31*, 14–27.
Farah, M. J., O'Reilly, R. C., & Vecera, S. P. (1993). Dissociated overt and covert recognition as an emergent property of a lesioned neural network. *Psychological Review, 100*(4), 571–588. https://doi.org/10.1037/0033-295X.100.4.571
Feldman, A. G., & Levin, M. F. (1995). Positional frames of reference in motor control: Their origin and use. *Behavioral and Brain Sciences., 18*, 723–806.
Fernandes, W. S.-P. (2016). Motor coordination correlates with academic achievement and cognitive function in children. *Frontiers in Psychology, 7*. https://doi.org/10.3389/fpsyg.2016.00318
Fogassi, L., Ferrari, P., Gesierich, B., Rozzi, S., Chersi, F., & Rizzolatti, G. (2005). Parietal lobe: From action organization to intention understanding. *Science, 308*, 662–667.
Foki, T., Vanbellingen, C. T., Pirker, A. L., Bohlhalter, S., Nyffeler, T., Kraemmer, J., et al. (2016). Limb-kinetic apraxia affects activities of daily living in Parkinson's disease: A multi-center study. *European Journal of Neurology, 23*(8), 1301–1307. https://doi.org/10.1111/ene.13021
Fornito, A., Zalesky, A., & Breakspear, M. (2015). The connectomics of brain disorders. *Nature Reviews|Neuroscience, 16*, 150–172.
French, M., Cohen, M., Pohlig, R., & Reisman, D. (2021). Fluid cognitive abilities are important for learning and retention of a new, explicitly-learned walking pattern in individuals after stroke. *Neurorehabilitation Neural Repair, 35*(5), 419–430. https://doi.org/10.1177/15459683211001025
Friedman, N., Hatoum, A., Gustavson, D., Corley, R., Hewitt, J., & Young, S. (2020). Executive functions and impulsivity are genetically distinct and independently predict psychopathology:

Results from two adult twin studies. *Clinical Psychological Science, 8*(3), 519–536. https://doi.org/10.1177/2167702619898814
Fu, X., Zhou, G., Zhuang, J., Xu, C., Zhou, H., Peng, Y., et al. (2021). White matter injury after intracerebral hemorrhage. *Frontiers in Neurology, 12*, 562090. https://doi.org/10.3389/fneur.2021.562090
Fulceri, F., Grossi, E., Contaldo, A., Narzisa, A., Apicella, F., Parrini, I., et al. (2019). Motor skills as moderators of core symptoms in autism spectrum disorders: Preliminary data from an exploratory analysis with artificial neural networks. *Frontiers in Psychology, 9*. https://doi.org/10.3389/fpsyg.2018.02683
Fuster, J. (1997). Network memory. *Trends in Neuroscience, 20*(10), 451–459. https://doi.org/10.1016/S0166-2236(97)01128-4
Gaines, R. C. (2008). Clinical expression of developmental coordination disorder in a large Canadian family. *Paediatrics and Child Health, 13*, 763–768.
Gainotti, G., & Trojano, L. (2018). Chapter 16 – Constructional apraxia. In G. Vallar & H. Coslett (Eds.), *Handbook of clinical neurology* (Vol. 151, pp. 331–348). Elsevier. https://doi.org/10.1016/B978-0-444-63622-5.00016-4
Gallego, J., Perich, M., Naufel, S., Ethier, C., Solla, S., & Miller, E. (2018). Cortical population activity within a preserved neural manifold underlies multiple motor behaviors. *Nature Communications, 9*, 4233. https://doi.org/10.1038/s41467-018-06560-z
Ganguly, J., & Jog, M. (2020). Tauopathy and movement disorders—Unveiling the chameleons and mimics. *Frontiers in Neurology: Movement Disorders*. https://doi.org/10.3389/fneur.2020.599384
Garibotto, V., Scifo, P., Gorini, A., Alonso, C., Brambati, S., Bellodi, L., & Perani, D. (2010). Disorganization of anatomical connectivity in obsessive compulsive disorder: A multi-parameter diffusion tensor imaging study in a subpopulation of patients. *Neurobiology of Disease, 37*(2), 468–476. https://doi.org/10.1016/j.nbd.2009.11.003
Gerstner, W., Kistler, W., Naud, R., & Paninsk, L. (2014). Neuronal populations. In W. Gerstner, W. Kistler, R. Naud, & L. Paninsk (Eds.), *Neuronal dynamics from single neurons to networks and models of cognition* (pp. 291–322). Cambridge University Press.
Giovannetti, T., Libon, D., Buxbaum, L., & Schwartz, M. (2002). Naturalistic action impairments in dementia. *Neuropsychologia, 40*, 1220–1232.
Gold, L., & Lauritzen, M. N. (2002). Neuronal deactivisation explains decreased cerebellar blood flow in response to focal cerebral ischemia or suppressed neocortical function. *Proceedings of the National Academy Science U. S. A., 99*, 7699–7704.
Gonzales-Rothi, L., & Heilman, K. (1996). Liepmann (1900 and 1905): A definition of apraxia and a model of praxis. In C. Code, Y. Joanette, A. Roch-Lecours, & C. Wallesch (Eds.), *Classic cases in neuropsychology*. Psychology Press.
Goyen, T. (2005). Motor dysfunction in apparently normal high-risk children. *Academia.edu*. https://www.academia.edu/27667038/Motor_dysfunction_in_apparently_normal_high_risk_children
Green, D. C. (2008). Does subtype of developmental coordination disordrere count: Is there a differential effect on outcome following intervention? *Human Movement Science, 27*, 363. https://doi.org/10.1016/j.humov.2008.02.009
Gross, R., & Grossman, M. (2008). Update on apraxia. *Current Neurology and Neuroscince Reports, 8*(6), 490–496. https://doi.org/10.1007/s11910-008-0078-y
Guyette, T. W., & Diedrich, W. M. (1981). A critical review of developmental apraxia of speech. In *Speech and Language* (pp. 1–49).
Hale, J., Alfonso, V., Berninger, V., Bracken, B., Christo, C., Clark, E., et al. (2010). Critical issues in response-to-intervention, comprehensive evaluation, and specific learning disabilities identification and intervention: An expert white paper consensus. *Learning Disability Quarterly, 33*(3), 223–236.
Hamilton, J., Haaland, K., Adair, J., & Brandt, J. (2003). Ideomotor limb apraxia in Huntington's disease: Implications for corticostriate involvement. *Neuropsychologia*, 614–621.

Handiru, V., Alivar, A., Hoxa, A., Saleh, S., Suviseshamuthu, E. S., Yue, G., & Allexandre, D. (2021). Graph-theoretical analysis of EEG functional connectivity during balance perturbation in traumatic brain injury: A pilot study. *Human Brain Mapping, 14*(42), 4427–4447. https://doi.org/10.1002/hbm.25554

Harrowell, I. H. (2017). Mental health outcomes of developmental coordination disorder in late adolescence. *Developmental Medicine & Child Neurology, 59*(9), 973–979.

Hazy, T. F. (2007). Towards an executive without a homunculus: Computational models of the prefrontal cortex/basal ganglia system. *Philosophical Transactions of the Royal Society of London. Series B, Biological Sciences, 362*, 1601–1613.

Heilman, K., Maher, L., Greenwald, M., & Rothi, L. (1997). Conceptualized apraxia from lateralized lesions. *Neurology, 49*(2). https://doi.org/10.1212/WNL.49.2.457

Heilman, K., Rothi, L., & Valenstein, E. (1982). Two forms of ideomotor apraxia. *Neurology, 32*, 342–346.

Hildebrand, M. J. (2020). Severe childhood speech disorder. *Neurology, 94*, 2148–2167.

Holtmaat, A., & Svoboda, K. (2009). Experience-dependent structural synaptic plasticity in the mammalian brain. *National Review Neuroscience, 10*, 647–658.

Honey, C. J., & Sporns, O. (2008). Dynamical consequences of lesions in cortical networks. *Human Brain Mapping, 29*, 802–809.

Honey, C., Sporns, O., Cammoun, G. X., Thiran, J., et al. (2009). Predicting human resting-state functional connectivity from structural connectivity. *Proceedings of the National Academy of Science U. S. A., 106*, 2035–2040.

Hua, J. W. (2022). Early motor milestones in infancy and later motor impairments: A population-based data linkage study. *Psychiatry*. https://doi.org/10.3389/fpsyt.2022.809181

Humphrey, D. R., & Thompson, W. D. (1970). Predicting measures of motor performance from multiple cortical spike trains. *Science, 170*(7), 758–762.

Huth, A., de Heer, W. A., Griffiths, W., Theunissen, F., & Gallant, J. (2016). Natural speech reveals the semantic maps that tile human cerebral cortex. *Nature, 532*(7600), 453–459. https://doi.org/10.1038/nature17637

Iuzzini, J. (2012). *Inconsistency of speech in children with childhood apraxia of speech, phonological disorders, and typical speech*. Indiana University ProQuest Dissertations Publishing.

Iuzzini-Seigel, J. M. (2017). Speech assessment in children with childhood apraxia of speech. In *Perspectives of the ASHA special interest groups* (pp. 47–60). American Speech Langauge Hearing Association.

Iuzzini-Siegel, J. H. (2017). Speech inconsistency in children with childhood apraxia of speech, language impairment and speech delay: Depends on the stimuli. *Journal of Speech Language and Hearing Research*, 1194–1220.

Karmiloff-Smith, A., Scerif, G., & Ansari, D. (2003). Double dissociations in developmental disorders? Theoretically misconceived, empirically dubious. *Cortex, 39*, 161–163.

Kelley, A., Shiltz, C., & Landry, C. (2005). Neural systems recruited by drug- and food-related cues: Studies of gene activation in corticolimbic regions. *Physiology & Behavior, 86*(1–2), 11–14. https://doi.org/10.1016/j.physbeh.2005.06.018

Kertes, A., & Ferro, J. (1984). Lesion size and location in ideomotor apraxia. *Brain, 107*(92), 1–33.

Kirrie, B., Granier, J., & Robin, D. (2008). Understanding the nature of apraxia of speech: Theory, analysis, and treatment. *Neuropsychological Trends, 4*, 7–44.

Kirst, C., Modes, C., & Magnasco, M. (2017). Shifting attention to dynamics: Self-reconfiguration of neural networks. *Current Opinion in Systems Biology, 3*, 132–140. https://doi.org/10.1016/j.coisb.2017.04.006

Koziol, L. (2014). *The myth of executive functioning: Missing elements in conceptualization, evaluation and assessment*. Springer.

Koziol, L. B. (2009). *Subcortical structures and cognition*. Springer.

Koziol, L., Budding, D., & Chidekel, D. (2012). From movement to thought: Executive function, embodied cognition, and the cerebellum. *Cerebellum., 11*(2), 505–525. https://doi.org/10.1007/s12311-011-0321-y

Langevin, L. M. (2015). Distinct patterns of cortical thinning in concurrent motor and attention disorders. *Developmental Medicine and Child Neurology*, (3), 257–264.
Latash, M. (2008). Evolution of motor control: From reflexes and motor programs to the equilibrium-point hypothesis. *Journal of Human Kinetics, 19*(19), 3–24.
Law, J. B. (2000). Prevalence and natural history. *International Journal of Language & Communication Disorders, 35*(2), 165–188.
Leiguarda, C. D., & Marsden, C. (2000). Limb apraxias: Higher-order disorders of sensorimotor integration. *Brain, 123*(Pt 5), 650–879. https://doi.org/10.1093/brain/123.5.860
Leiguarda, R. (2001). Limb apraxia: Cortical or subcortical. *NeuroImage, 14*(1), 5137–5141. https://doi.org/10.1006/nimg.2001.0833
Lesny, I. (1980). Developmental dyspraxia-dysgnosia as a cause of congenital children's clumsiness. *Brain Development, 2*, 69–71. https://doi.org/10.1016/S0387-7604(80)80009-X
Lewis, B. F. (2004). School-age follow up of children with childhood apraxia of speech. *Language, Speech, and Hearing Services in Schools, 35*, 122–140.
Liepmann, S., & Mass, O. (1907). Fall von linksseitiger Agraphie und Apraxie bei rechtsseitiger Lahmung. *Journal of Psychology and Neurology, 10*, 14.
Long, C. J., & Kibby, M. Y. (1995). Ecological validity of neuropsychological tests: A look at neuropsychology's past and the impact. *Advances Medical Psychotherapy, 8*, 59–78.
Luria, A. (1973). *The working brain*. Basic Books.
Luzzi, S., Piccirilli, M., Pessalacia, M., Fabi, K., & Provincialia, L. (2010). Dissociation apraxia secondary to right premotor stroke. *Neuropsychologia, 48*(1), 68–76. https://doi.org/10.1016/j.neuropsychologia.2009.08.010
Maasen, B. (2002). Issues contrasting adult acquired versus developmentla apraxia of speech. *Semin Speech Language*, 257–266.
Maassen, B. (2015). Developmental models of childhood apraxia of speech. In R. Barr & E. Sillimen (Eds.), *Routledge handbook of communication disorder* (pp. 124–133). Routledge.
Maleki, S., Chye, Y., Zhang, X., Parkes, L., Chamberlain, S., Fontenelle, L., et al. (2020). Neural correlates of symptom severity in obsessive-compulsive disorder using magnetization transfer and diffusion tensor imaging. *Psychiatry Research: Neuroimaging, 298*, 111046. https://doi.org/10.1016/j.pscychresns.2020.111046
Malkani, R., & Zadikoff, C. (2011). The apraxias in movement disorders. In N. Galvaez-Jimenez, P. Tuite, & K. Bhatia (Eds.), *Uncommon causes of movement disorders* (pp. 35–45). Cambridge University Press.
Martin, N. P. (2006). DCD and ADHD: A genetic study of their shared aetiology. *Human Movement Science*, 110–124.
Mayo Clinic. (2022). *Childhood apraxia of speech*. Retrieved from Mayo Clinic: https://www.mayoclinic.org/diseases-conditions/childhood-apraxia-of-speech/diagnosis-treatment/drc-20352051
McGinty, H., Phillips, K., Jim, H., Cessna, J., Asvat, Y., Cases, M., et al. (2014). Cognitive functioning in men receiving androgen deprivation therapy for prostate cancer: A systematic review and meta-analysis. *Support Cancer Care, 22*(8), 2271–2280. https://doi.org/10.1007/s00520-014-2285-1
McNeil, M. (2011). *Clinical management of sensorimotor speech disorders*. Thieme.
Menon, V. (2013). Developmental pathways to functional brain networks: Emerging principles. *Trends in Cognitive Sciences, 17*, 627. https://doi.org/10.1016/j.tics.2013.09.015
Meyer, K., & Damasio, A. (2009). Convergence and divergence in a architecture for recognition and memory. *Trends in Neuroscience, 32*(7), 376–382. https://doi.org/10.1016/j.tins.2009.04.002
Middleton, F., & Strick, P. (2000). Basal ganglia output and cognition: Evidence from anatomical, behavioral, and clinical studies. *Brain and Cognition, 42*(2), 183–200. https://doi.org/10.1006/brcg.1999.1099
Miller, G. L.-H. (2019). Reading outcomes for individuals with histories of suspected childhood apraxia of speech. *American Journal of Speech Lanuage Pathology*, 1432–1447.

Mirabella, G. D. (2017). Developmental coordination disorder affects the processing of action relate verbs. *Frontiers in Human Neuroscience, 10*. https://doi.org/10.3389/fnhum.2016.00661
Missiuna, C., Rivard, L., & Bartlett, D. (2003). Early identification and risk management of children with developmental coordination disorder. *Pediatric Physical Therapy, 15*(1), 32–38.
Moncrieff, J. C. (2022). The serotonin theory of depression: A systematic umbrella review of the evidence. *Molecular Psychiatry*, 1. https://doi.org/10.1038/s41380-022-01661-0
Morgan, A., & Webster, R. (2018). Aetiology of childhood apraxia of speech: A clinical practice. *Journal of Paediatrics and Child Health, 54*, 1090–1095. https://doi.org/10.1111/jpc.14150
Morgan, A., Fisher, S., Scheffer, I., & Hildebrand, M. (2016). FOXP2-related speech and language disorders. In M. A. Adam (Ed.), *Gene reviews*. University of Washington.
Moruzzi, S. P.-G. (2010). Clumsiness and psychopathology: Causation or shared etiology? A twin study with the CBCL 6–18 questionnaire in a general school-age population sample. *Human Movement Science*, 326–338. https://doi.org/10.1016/j.humov.2010.01.005
Mosca, S. L. (2016). Copy-number variations are enriched for neurodevelopmental genes in children with developmental coordination disorder. *Journal of Medical Genetics, 12*, 812–819. https://doi.org/10.1136/jmedgenet-2016-103818
Moser, D., Basilakos, A., Fillmore, P., & Fridriksson, J. (2016). Brain damage associated with apraxia of speech: Evidence from case studies. *Neurocase., 22*(4), 346–356. https://doi.org/10.1080/13554794.2016.1172645
Moss, A. G. (2012). Interarticulatory coordination of the lips and jaw in childhood apraxia of speech. *Journal of Medical Speech-Language Pathology., 20*(4), 127–132.
Mountford, H. B. (2022). The genetic and molecular basis of developmental language. *Children, 586*.
Murray, E., McCabe, P., & Ballard, K. J. (2015). A randomized controlled trial for children with childhood apraxia of speech comparing Rapid Syllable Transition treatment and the Nuffield. *Journal of Speech, Language, and Hearing Research, 58*, 669–686. https://doi.org/10.1044/2015_JSLHR-S-13-0179
Mutha, P., Sainburg, R., & Haaland, K. (2010). Coordination deficits in ideomotor apraxia during visually targeted reaching reflect impaired visuomotor transformations. *Neuropsychologia, 48*(13), 3855–3867. https://doi.org/10.1016/j.neuropsychologia.2010.09.018
Nasios, G., Dardiostis, E., & Messinis, L. (2019). From Broca and Wernicke to the neuromodulation era: Insights of brain language networks for neurorehabilitation. *Behavioural Neurology, 2019*. https://doi.org/10.1155/2019/9894571
National Institute of Deafness and Other Communication Disorders. (2022). *Home page*. Retrieved from National Institute of Deafness and Other Communication Disorders: https://www.nidcd.nih.gov/
Newbury, D. W. (2009). CMIP and ATP2C2 modulate phonological short term memory in language impairment. *American Journal of Human Genetics, 85*, 264–272.
Nigg, J., Willcutt, E., Doyle, A., & Sonuga-Barke, E. (2005). Causal heterogeneity in attention-deficit/hyperactivity disorder: Do we need neuropsychologically impaired subtypes? *Biological Psychiatry, 57*, 1224–1230.
Norbury, C. F. (2016). The impact of nonverbal ability on prevalence and clinical presentation of and clinical presentation of language disorder: Evidence from a population study. *Journal of Child Psychology and Psychiatry, 57*, 1247–1257.
NORD. (2021). *Ocular motor apraxia, cogan type*. Retrieved from National Organization of Rare Disorders: https://rarediseases.org/rare-diseases/ocular-motor-apraxia-cogan-type/
Ochipa, C., & Rothi, L. (1992). Conceptual apraxia in alzheimer's disease. *Brain, 115*(Pt 4), 1061–1071.
Ogar, J. M., Dronkers, N. F., Brambati, S. M., Miller, B. L., & Gorno-Tempini, M. L. (2007). Progressive nonfluent aphasia and its characteristic motor speech deficits. *Alzheimer Disease and Associated Disorders*, 523–530.
Ogar, J., Slama, H., Dronkers, N., Amici, S., & Gorno-Tempini, M. (2005). Apraxia of speech: An overview. *Neurocase, 11*, 427–432. https://doi.org/10.1080/13554790500263529

Park, E., Velumian, A., & Fehlings, M. (2004). Mechanisms of spinal cord injury: A review with an emphasis on the implications for white matter degeneration. *Journal of Neurotrauma, 21*(6). https://doi.org/10.1089/0897715041269641, on line.

Park, J. (2017). Apraxia: Review and update. *Journal of Clinical Neurology, 13*(4), 317–324. https://doi.org/10.3988/jcn.2017.13.4.317

Pazzaglia, M., Pizzamiglio, L., Pes, E., & Aglioti, S. (2008). The sound of actions in apraxia. *Current Biology, 18*(22), 1766–1772. https://doi.org/10.1016/j.cub.2008.09.061

Pazzaglia, M., Smania, N., Corato, E., & Aglioti, S. (2008). Neural underpinnings of gesture discrimination in patients with limb apraxia. *The Journal of Neuroscience, 28*(12), 3030–3041. https://doi.org/10.1523/JNEUROSCI.5748-07.2008

Piek, J. D. (2008). The role of early fine and gross motor development on later motor and cognitive ability. *Human Movement Science, 5*, 668–681.

Poore, M. B. (2009). Suck predicts neuromotor integrity and developmental outcomes. *Perspective on Speech and Orofacial Disorders, 19*, 44. https://doi.org/10.1044/ssod19.1.44

Pramstaller, P., & Marsden, C. (1996). The basal ganglia and apraxia. *Brain, 119*(1), 319–340. https://doi.org/10.1093/brain/119.1.319

Ramus, F. (2003). Developmental dyslexia: Specific phonological deficit or general sensorimotor sysfunction. *Current Opinion in Neurobiology, 13*, 212–218.

Rehme, A. K., & Grefkes, C. (2012). Cerebral network disorders after stroke: Evidence from imaging-based connectivity analyses of active and resting brain states in humans. *Journal of Physiology, 591*, 17–51.

Roig, M., Gratacòs, M., Vazquez, E., del Toro, M., Foguet, A., Ferrer, I., & Macaya, A. (2003). Brainstem dysgenesis: Report of five patients with congenital hypotonia, multiple cranial nerve involvement and ocular motor apraxia. *Developmental Medicine & Child Neurology, 45*, 489–493.

Rosenzopf, H., Wiesen, D., Basilakos, A., Yourganov, G., Bonilha, L., Fridriksson, J., et al. (2022). Mapping the human praxis network: An investigation of white matter disconnection in limb apraxia of gesture production. *Brain Communications, 4*(1), 1–14. https://doi.org/10.1093/braincomms/fcac004

Rosenzoph, H., Weisen, D., Basilakos, A., Yourganov, G., Bonilha, L., Rorden, C., et al. (2020, April 17). *Mapping the Human Praxis Network: An investigation of white matter disconnection in limb apraxia*. Retrieved from bioRxiv.org: https://doi.org/10.1101/2020.04.14.041442

Salo, V. F. (2019). The role of the motor stem in action understanding and communication: Evidence from human infants and non human primates. *Developmental Psychobiology, 61*(3), 390–401.

Salvi, R., Wang, J., & Ding, D. (2000). Auditory plasticity and hyperactivity following cochlear damage. *Hearing Research, 147*, 261–274.

Sato, J., Biazoli, C. E., Jr., Zugman, A., Pan, P., Bueno, A., Moura, L., et al. (2021). Long-term stability of the cortical volumetric profile and the functional human connectome throughvout childhood and adolescence. *European Journal of Neuroscience, 54*, 6187–6201. https://doi.org/10.1111/ejn.15435

Saxena, S., & Caroni, P. (2011). Selective neuronal vulnerability in neurodegenerative diseases: From stressor thresholds to degeneration. *Neuron, 71*, 35–48.

Scott, S. H., & Kalaska, J. F. (1997). Reaching movements with similar hand paths but different arm orientations. I. Activity of individual cells in motor cortex. *Journal of Neurophysiology*, 826–852.

Seven, Y., Mantilla, C., & Sieck, G. (2014). Recruitment of rat diaphragm motor units across motor behaviors with different levels of diaphragm activation. *Journal of Applied Physiology, 117*(11), 1308–1316. https://doi.org/10.1152/japplphysiol.01395.2013

Shandley, S. C. (2021). Abnormal nutritive sucking as an indicator of neonatal brain injury. *Frontiers in Pediatrics, 8*. https://doi.org/10.3389/fped.2020.599633

Sharma, V., & Wong, L. (2022). Middle cerebral artery disease. In J. Grotta, G. Albers, J. Broderick, S. Kasner, R. Sacco, A. Day, et al. (Eds.), *Stroke (seventh edition) pathophysiology, diagno-*

sis, and management (pp. 317–346). Elsevier. https://doi.org/10.1016/B978-0-323-69424-7.00024-7

Shriberg, L. D., & Fourakis, M. (2010). Extensions to the speech disorders classification system (SDCS). *Clinical Linguistics & Phonetics, 24*, 795.

Shriberg, L. D. (2019). Estimates of prevalence of speech and motor speech disorders in persons with complex neurodevelopmental disorders. *Clinical Linguistics & Phonetics, 33*(8), 707–736.

Shriberg, L., KwiatkowskiI, J., & Mabie, H. (2019). Estimates of the prevalence of motor speech disorders in children with idiopathic speech delay. *Clinical Linguistics & Phonetics, 33*, 679–706. https://doi.org/10.1080/02699206.2019.1595731

Singer, W. (1993). Synchronization of cortical activity and its putative. *Annual Review of Physiology, 55*, 349–374.

Soliveri, P., Piacentini, S., & Girotti, F. (2005). Limb apraxia in corticobasal degeneration and progressive supranuclear palsy. *Neurology, 64*, 448–453.

Sonuga-Barke, E. (2003). The dual pathway model of AD/HD: An elaboration of neurodevelopmental characteristics. *Neuroscience Biobehavioral Review, 27*, 593–604.

Sonuga-Barke, E., Bitsakou, P., & Thompson, M. (2010). Beyond the dual pathway model: Evidence for the dissociation of timing, inhibitory and delay-related impairments in attention deficit/hyperactivity disorder. *Journal of Child and Adolescent Psychiatry, 345-355*. https://doi.org/10.1016/j.jaac.2009.12.018

Sporns, O., Tononi, G., & Kötter, R. (2005). The human connectome: A structural description of the human brain. *PLoS Computational Biology, 1*, e42. https://doi.org/10.1371/journal.pcbi.0010042

Stackhouse, J. W. (1997). *Children's speech and literacy difficulties 1: A psycholinguistic framework*. Wurr.

Strand, E. (2019, January 9). *Diagnosis and management of CAS*.

Sunderland, A., & Shiner, C. (2007). Ideomotor apraxia and functional ability. *Cortex, 43*(3), 359–367. https://doi.org/10.1016/S0010-9452(08)70461-1

Tal Saban, M. O. (2014). Executive function and attention in young adults with and without developmental coordination disorder – A comparative study. *Research in Developmental Disabilities*, (35), 2644–2650.

Tal-Saba, M. Z. (2012). The functional profile of young adults with suspected developmental coordination disorder (DCD). *Research In Developmental Disabilities*, 2193–2202. https://doi.org/10.1016/j.ridd.2012.06.005

Tarsy, D. (2012). *Movement disorders: A video atlas*. Humana Press.

Terband, H. M. (2019). A psycholinguistic framework for diagnosis and treatment planning of developmental speech disorders. *Folia Phoniatrica et Logopaedica, 5–6*, 216–227.

Tettamanti, M., Buccino, G., Saccuman, M., Gallese, V., Danna, M., Scifo, P., et al. (2005). Listening to action-related sentences activates fronto-parietal motor circuits. *Journal of Cognitive Neuroscience, 17*, 273–281.

Teverovsky, E., Bickel, J., & Feldman, H. (2009). Functional characteristics of children diagnosed with childhood apraxia of speech. *Disability and rehabilitation, 31*(2), 94–102. https://doi.org/10.1080/09638280701795030

The Medical Dictionary. (2021). *Apraxia*. Retrieved from The Medical Dictionary: http://the--medical-dictionary.com/apraxia_article_2.htm

Thomason, M., Hect, J., Waller, R., Manning, J., Stacks, A., Beeghly, M., et al. (2018). Prenatal neural origins of infant motor development: Associations between fetal brain and infant motor development. *Developmental Psychopathology, 30*(3), 763–772. https://doi.org/10.1017/S095457941800072X

Tse, M. (2012). Double duty of tail caudate nucleus neurons. *Nature Reviews Neuroscience, 13*, 11005–11016. https://doi.org/10.1038/nrn3342

Tuttolomondo, A., Pecoraro, R., & Pinto, A. (2014). Studies of selective TNF inhibitors in the treatment of brain injury from stroke and trauma: A review of the evidence to date. *Drug Design, Development and Therapy, 8*, 2221–2238. https://doi.org/10.2147/DDDT.S67655

van den Heuvel, M., & Sporns, O. (2013). Network hubs in the human brain. *Trends in Cognitive Sciences, 17*(12), 683–696. https://doi.org/10.1016/j.tics.2013.09.012

Wang, M. L. (2014a). Co-occurring development of early childhood communication and motor skills: Results from a population based longitudinal study. *Child: Care, Health and Development*, 77–84.

Wang, M. L. (2014b). The developmental relationship between language and motor performance from 3 to 5 years of age: A prospective longitudinal population study. *BMC Psychology, 2*, 34. https://doi.org/10.1186/s40359-014-0034-3

Wasserman, T., & Wasserman, L. (2013). Towards a unifying model of executive function. *Applied Neuropsychology: Child, 2*(2), 88–96. https://doi.org/10.1080/21622965.2013.748394

Wasserman, T., & Wasserman, L. (2015). The misnomer of attention deficit hyperactivity disorder. *Applied Neuropsychology: Child, 4*(2), 116–122. https://doi.org/10.1080/21622965.2015.1005487

Wasserman, T., & Wasserman, L. (2016). *Depathologizing psychopathology*. Springer.

Wasserman, T., & Wasserman, L. (2017). Touching the elephant: The search for fluid intelligence. *Applied Neuropsychology Child., 6*(3), 228–236. https://doi.org/10.1080/21622965.2017.1317489

Watemberg, N. W.-S. (2007). Developmental coordination disorder in children with attention-deficit–hyperactivity disorder and physical therapy intervention. *Developmental Medicine & Child Neurology, 920–925*(49), 12.

Watson, R., & Heilman, K. (1983). Callosal apraxia. *Brain, 106*(2), 391–403. https://doi.org/10.1093/brain/106.2.391

Weintraub, S. (2000a). Neuropsychological assessment of mental state. In M. Mesulam (Ed.), *Principles of behavioral and cognitive neurology* (pp. 135–136). Oxford University Press.

Weintraub, S. (2000b). Neuropsychological assessment of mental state. In I. M. Mesulam (Ed.), *Principles of behavioral and cognitive neurology* (p. 121). Oxford University Press.

Wessel, J., & Aron, A. (2017). On the globality of motor suppression: Unexpected events and their influence on behavior and cognition. *Neuron, 93*(2), 259–280. https://doi.org/10.1016/j.neuron.2016.12.013

Wheaton, L., & Hallet, M. (2007). Ideomotor apraxia: A review. *Journal of the Neurological Sciences, 260*, 1–8. https://doi.org/10.1016/j.jns.2007.04.014

Whiteside, S., Dyson, L., Cowell, P., & Varley, R. (2015). The rlationship between apraxia of speech and oral apraxia: Association or dissociation? *Archives of Clinical Neuropsychology, 30*(7), 670–682. https://doi.org/10.1093/arclin/acv051

Wilson, P. M. (1998). Information processing deficits associated with developmental coordination disorder: A meta-analysis of research findings. *Joornal of Child Psychology*, 829–840.

World Health Organization (WHO). (1993). *The ICD-10 classification of mental and behavioural disorders*. World Health Organization (WHO).

Yadegari, F., Azimian, M., Rahgozar, M., & Shekarchi, B. (2014). Brain areas impaired in oral and verbal apraxic patients. *Iranian Journal of Neurology, 13*(2), 77–82.

Yun, J., Shin, S., & Son, S. (2021). Clinical utility of repeated urimal test of articulation and phonation for patients with childhood apraxia of speech. *Children, 8*(12), 1–7. https://doi.org/10.3390/children8121106

Yuste, R. (2015). From the neuron doctrine to neural networks. *Nature Reviews. Neuroscience, 16*, 487–497. https://doi.org/10.1038/nrn3962

Zadikoff, C., & Lang, A. (2005). Apraxia in movement disorders. *Brain, 128*(7), 1480–1497. https://doi.org/10.1093/brain/awh560

Zang, Z., Ping, L., Zhai, A., & Zhou, Z. (2021). Microstructural white matter abnormalities in obsessive-compulsive disorder: A coordinate-based meta-analysis of diffusion tensor imaging studies. *Asian Journal of Psychiatry, 55*, 102467. https://doi.org/10.1016/j.ajp.2020.102467

Zohary, E., Shadlen, M., & Newsome, W. (1994). Correlated neuronal discharge rate and its implications for psychophysical performance. *Nature, 370*, 140–143.

Zwicker, J. M. (2009). Neural correlates of developmental coordination disorder: A review of hypotheses. *Child Neurology*, 1–9.

Chapter 10
Treatment for Apraxia: Plasticity and Regeneration

Treatment for many apraxia conditions has remained remarkably the same for quite some time. Essentially, the apraxic individual, usually under the guidance of a skilled professional, practices the desired motor sequence until automaticity of the desired sequence is achieved. Treatment relies on neural plasticity to achieve the desired outcome.

Treatment for apraxia conditions of all types represents a significant effort in most rehabilitation facilities. Studies evaluating the level of autonomy in brain-damaged patients have shown how apraxia significantly reduces their levels of autonomy in carrying out everyday activities. Caregivers have reported the need for more assistance with apraxia patients engaged in these activities than with those suffering from other neuropsychological deficits. Apraxic deficit slows down motor rehabilitation in patients with hemiparesis and reduces the ability of patients with severe aphasia to communicate by gesturing (Cantagallo et al., 2013).

Treatment efficacy research is limited. Given the association of apraxia to long-term disability, the evidence base for effective treatment is also surprisingly limited. There are several reasons for this being the case. Perhaps one of the most significant is that apraxia is not a single disorder and successful intervention requires an understanding of what is to be rehabilitated (Worthington, 2016). In addition, for many intervention studies, there is also the lack of a clear theoretical rationale. Although all start with an assessment of apraxia to identify specific cases, these assessments often lack a theoretical basis and lack reliability across studies. Even more significantly, the assessments are rarely used to inform the intervention. In part this is because there is no standard diagnostic process, universal taxonomy of apraxia subtypes, or theoretical consensus regarding potential subtypes (Molloy & Jagoe, 2019). That is not to say that attempts are not being made. For example, there is the Apraxia Battery for Adults, a measure of apraxia in which participants perform various tasks and are assessed on diadochokinetic rate, increasing word length, limb and oral apraxia, latency and utterance time for polysyllabic words, repeated trials test,

T. Wasserman, L. D. Wasserman, *Apraxia: The Neural Network Model*,
Neural Network Model: Applications and Implications,
https://doi.org/10.1007/978-3-031-24105-5_10

and inventory of articulation characteristics. The test was however normed using a sample of 40 persons with apraxia and 49 persons for normative speech, ranging in age from 33 to 93. This limits the instrument in applicability to younger persons, although the test recommends use for persons 9 years and above, and reports noted difficulties in identifying less than severe apraxia, which is interpreted as typical aphasia ("due to language difficulties") (Dabul, 2000).

Additionally, treatment efficacy studies are compromised by the heterogeneous grouping of apraxia within an identified subtype. For example, children diagnosed with speech sound disorders comprise a heterogeneous group who differ in terms of the severity of their condition, underlying cause, speech errors, involvement of other aspects of the linguistic system, and treatment response. Even now, there is no universal and agreed upon classification system for the subtype. Instead, several theoretically differing classification systems have been proposed based on either an etiological (medical) approach, a descriptive-linguistic approach, or a processing approach (Waring & Knight, 2013).

Lack of Consensus for the Selection of Treatments for Apraxia

Perhaps as a result of the issues identified, there is a lack of consensus among treating professionals. For example, in a recent survey of professional speech and language pathologists in the USA and Canada who treat apraxia of speech, respondents reported frequently using an eclectic approach to treat CAS (USA 85%; Canada 89%). That implies that these professionals select multiple and various techniques they deemed effective. From the perspective of hypothesis testing, this means numerous treatment approaches that would complicate any analysis. In the survey no intervention emerged as the most preferred primary treatment for CAS. There were a couple of treatment models that served as core components of many treatment packages. US-based clinicians more commonly reported using the Kaufman Speech to Language Protocol (K-SLP) (33%) and Dynamic, Temporal, and Tactile Cueing (DTTC) (28%), while clinicians in Canada used PROMPT ® (31%) (Gomez et al., 2022). These approaches share common elements.

Classes of Treatment for Apraxia

There are several classes of treatment for apraxia conditions summarized below:

Restorative (Restitutive) Treatments

These interventions attempt to restore impaired processing back to normal function. This has been attempted by trying to improve sensory integration, perceptuo-motor performance, and selective attention. The sensory approach is somewhat unique, as it emanated from perspectives on developmental dyspraxia and was underpinned by the idea that apraxia is due to failure to attend to or integrate functionally appropriate sensory information.

Compensatory (Substitutive) Treatments

Compensatory methods focus on the disability associated with the apraxia and do not attempt to address the underlying impairment. They attempt to teach work arounds or ways of compensating for the disability. One such approach is strategy training (Cantagallo et al., 2013). Strategy training relies on teaching internal strategies and therefore is informatively characterized as a form of metacognitive intervention.

Assistive Technology

Assistive technology is designed to reduce the need for expensive and hard to find professional treatment provided at an intensity that would be effective in the treatment of apraxia conditions. An example of such technology is the coach system (Mihailidis et al., 2006). Coach is a computerized device which attempts to address difficulties with sequencing action subtasks, that is, everyday activities such as handwashing or cutting using a knife via camera, and provides audio and video cues. In between is a complex process of determining the intentions (belief states) of the user on a probabilistic basis to deliver cues effectively.

Treatment Examples

Multiple disciplines including speech therapy, physical therapy, and occupational therapy offer treatment for apraxia conditions. In the area of apraxia of speech, including childhood apraxia of speech, there is a myriad of techniques employed to help an individual recover or develop function. The interesting point about treatment for speech-related apraxic conditions is while there are many specific types of treatment that target different aspects of speech production, the core of these treatments remains the same. For example, "for both children and adults, the treatment for AOS involves speech-language therapy. The specific approach is customized to the individual and considers the severity of their condition and the specific difficulties they have with speech. All of the approaches share core elements. Amongst these elements are:

- Asking for the same word or phrase to be repeated multiple times
- Practicing saying specific syllables or words to the individual learn to move from one sound to another

- Having the individual carefully observe how the therapist's mouth moves when they say words or phrases
- Using visual cues, such as practicing speech in front of a mirror, to remind the individual how to move their mouth to say specific words or phrases" (HealthLine, 2022)

These are the general principles to be sure, but they can be observed in most treatment approaches, including those with research support. For example, the PROMPT Program (Hayden et al., 2010) is a tactile kinesthetic -based treatment method that has been effective in treating motor speech disorders in adults and in children (Dale & Hayden, 2014). Although the PROMPT program is known for its use of tactile information, and its use of the core approaches identified above, there are several other core elements that collectively distinguish it from other treatment programs. These include the following (shared techniques are bolded for emphasis):

- Determination of a communication focus for treatment, that is, an aspect of development in which to embed and focus communication intervention, such as prelinguistic skills, speech subsystem development or rebalancing, activities of daily living, self-help skills, interactive communication routines, play skills, or preacademic or academic learning
- Determination of the uses of PROMPT, such as to develop an interactive focus for oral communication; to map in cognitive-linguistic concepts; or to develop, balance, or restructure speech subsystems and determine sensory modalities most needed in treatment (TKP, visual-auditory)
- Development of goals and objectives that embody the communication focus and work toward motor, language, cognitive, and social function. This entails the use of reciprocal turn taking, including cognitively appropriate words, objects, actions, interactions, and social interaction and/or choice making in almost every interaction between the child and therapist
- Ensuring within each session a high degree of motorphoneme *rehearsal (mass practice using prompts for accuracy of production)* organized so that (a) these motor-phonemes are generalized across various vowel contexts and transitions (distributed practice) and are embedded into novel syllables and words within naturalistic activities and (b) immediate use and transfer of the newly learned PROMPT lexicon are embedded in activities and the natural environment for use with parents, caregivers, or peers.

It is clear that the PROMPT program is highly organized and planned and just as clear that it relies on systematic practice to produce a result. The current authors applaud the emphasis on the development of cognitive linguistic function, thereby recognizing the association of language production with other cognitive domains.

A review of treatments for motor apraxic conditions (West et al., 2008) yielded the same pattern of treatment intervention, one that relied heavily on motor practice (common elements are bolded):

- *Strategy training in daily living activities*: this technique teaches internal (e.g., the patient is taught to verbalize and implement the task steps at the same time) or external (e.g., when aids are used to overcome a functional barrier) compensatory strategies that enable a functional task to be completed. These strategies will not have been used prior to the stroke.

- Sensory stimulation: stimulations including deep pressure, sharp, and soft touch are applied to the patients' limbs.
- Proprioceptive stimulation: the patient leans on and puts weight through their upper and lower limbs.
- *Cueing, verbal, or physical prompts given to enable each stage of the task to be completed.*
- *Chaining (forward or backward): the task is broken down into its component parts.* Using backward chaining the task is completed with facilitation from the therapist apart from the final component, which the patient carries out unaided. If successful next time, further steps are introduced. Forward chaining is the reverse of backward chaining.
- *Normal movement approaches: the therapist facilitates the body through normal movement patterns.*

As indicated, what these techniques all have in common is that they rely on practice of the target behavior until that practice encourages the development of a proficient target behavior. To get that development, they rely on the principles involved with neural plasticity and neural regeneration as the basis for the development of the desired skill.

Neural Plasticity

A central premise of network modeling is that behavior is a result of underlying activity in an individual's nervous system. The primary functional unit of the nervous system is the neuron, although there are numerous other cells. A person's behavioral repertoire is a manifestation of activity in their neural circuits. Following on, changes in a person's behavior is caused by changes to the process of the operation of the neural circuitry. This is true in relation to function loss that the system experiences as a result of damage or disrupted development or, on a more positive note, what occurs with learning. All of this change must be significantly subserved by an underlying change in neuronal connectivity.

Much of the communication between neurons in the nervous system occurs at synapses, and, as a result, changes in behavior are ultimately followed by alterations in the nature, strength, or number of interneuronal synaptic contacts. Repetitive stimulation of synapses can cause long-term potentiation or long-term depression of neurotransmission (Galvan, 2010). The capacity for modifications of synaptic connections between neurons is referred to as synaptic plasticity. Synaptic plasticity therefore subserves learning and memory in its positive forms and apraxia and other disorders when something goes awry. In the case of apraxia, therefore, synaptic plasticity is a likely candidate for a mechanism underlying behavior-modifying changes in neuronal connectivity that mediates treatment and repair of function. There are non-synaptic forms of alterations in neural function. This refers to neuronal plasticity and accounts for phenomena such as intrinsic excitability, cell-wide changes in synaptic composition, and homeostatic plasticity (Sweatt, 2016).

Neural plasticity is defined as the ability to alter a neuronal response to environmental stimuli and is the foundation of learning and memory (Kozubski et al., 2021). Neuronal plasticity is a basic property of the central nervous system. It ensures both the brain's normal functioning and its capacity for partial regeneration. Plasticity encompasses both synaptogenesis during early development and compensatory and corrective plasticity in the adult brain. One way to understand neural plasticity is the ability of the central nervous system (CNS) to adjust in response to changes in the environment (learning), lesions (damage), or acquired dysfunction. This capability of the CNS can involve modifications in overall cognitive strategies to successfully cope with new challenges (i.e., attention, behavioral compensation), recruitment of new/different neural networks, or changes in strength of such connections or specific brain areas in charge of carrying out a particular task such as movement, language, vision, or hearing (Sharma et al., 2013). At the neuronal level, this implies reorienting of the connections between various neurons that create new pathways or networks. At a cellular level, neuronal circuits consist of synaptic connections between axons and dendrites. As these circuits extend over the brain, there is the potential for many possible interactive combinations allowing for great flexibility. Modification of sensory input may induce rapid changes in cortical representations through various mechanisms including unmasking of connections that exist, but are not utilized in the premorbid (pre-rehabilitation) state. At the cellular level, plasticity involves changes in membrane excitability, synaptic plasticity, as well as structural changes in dendritic and axonal anatomy. Plasticity within and across different brain regions is thought to represent the neural basis underlying sensory substitution, in cases of blindness and deafness as well as in the recovery of motor function after cortical lesions like stroke (Nudo et al., 1996). The plastic nature of the human brain lends itself to experience and training-based structural changes leading to functional recovery (Chatterjeea et al., 2021).

Neural plasticity is notable for its adaptive value. It allows the compensatory changes induced by experience to occur in the CNS continuously. It is these experiences that form the basis of treatment which target specific skills or subcomponents of different skills.

The mechanisms of neural plasticity are quite varied. They can vary from extensive morphological modifications, such as those observed in the regeneration of axons and new synapse formation, to subtle molecular changes that alter the cellular response to neurotransmitters (Merceron-Martinez et al., 2021). Functional plasticity can include neurogenesis, regeneration, axonal collateral formation, and reactive synaptogenesis. There is also research that suggests that plasticity takes on different forms as we age. For example, as opposed to new synaptic connections, research suggests that recruitment of wider brain networks in the elderly and after stroke may play a beneficial role in maintaining the ability of individuals to carry out specific tasks or even in facilitating re-learning (Hummel et al., 2010).

Mechanisms of Neural Plasticity

If neural plasticity is the underlying mechanism for functional recovery from apraxia, then it stands to reason that treatment techniques purposefully target activities that would support plasticity. Neuroplasticity can be broken down into two major mechanisms:

- Neuronal regeneration/collateral sprouting: This includes concepts such as synaptic plasticity and neurogenesis.
- Functional reorganization: This includes concepts such as diaschisis, equipotentiality, and vicariation.

We have covered some of these terms already. Of those that we haven't yet mentioned is equipotentiality. Equipotentiality is the theory that the brain has the capacity (in the case of injury) to transfer functional memory from the damaged portion of the brain to other undamaged portions of the brain. Essentially, large areas of cerebral cortex have similar potential to perform particular functions, including learning and other complex processes, so that intact cortical areas may take over functions of damaged or destroyed areas. Vicariation, on the other hand, is the idea that the brain can reorganize and recruit other portions of the brain to accommodate functions that they were not intended to. Diaschisis refers to the concept that damage to one part of the brain could cause a loss of function in another area due to some connected pathway.

As a side note, perhaps a portent of things to come, a very recent finding from the world of anthropology and genetics suggests that what differentiated the modern human brain from that of archaic hominids is a genetic mutation (Pinson, 2022). The finding is that modern human transketolase (TKTL1) mutated from a lysine to arginine amino acid substitution. Thus, while the brain size of the neanderthal and modern human is similar, this modern human variant results in an increase in the abundance of basal radial glia, resulting in the generation of more neocortical neurons than the original variant. Can this genetic information be harnessed for regeneration? There is a considerable amount of inquiry into this potential rehabilitation source. For example, research into using adult neural progenitor cells as a source of cell replacement is being looked at for their clinical application as autologous cell replacement for neurologic diseases such as Parkinson's, trauma such as stroke, and cell-based gene therapy for neurometabolic diseases (Xenia Lojewski, 2014).

Treatment That Supports Neural Plasticity

Although not directly related to existing treatments for apraxia, there are treatments that support neural plasticity. We review them here to show overlap of these treatment approaches with existing treatments for apraxia.

Clinically, several treatment options have been used to facilitate neuroplasticity in restoring function and eliminating unwanted symptoms. For example, mirror therapy is a technique used in phantom limb pain. The individual uses a mirror to cover their amputation and focuses on watching their intact limb perform activities while imaging that both limbs are performing the same activity. The idea is that a patient with phantom limb pain can feel the same sense or emotion of their corresponding normal body part by observing the mirror image. This has been shown to have increased activation and functional connectivity in the frontoparietal network.

One of the most researched rehabilitation techniques is constraint-induced movement therapy (CIMT). This technique is commonly used in patients recovering from stroke. The core technique is to constrain the functional limb and engage the affected limb in repetitive task practice and behavioral shaping. Using functional magnetic resonance imaging (fMRI) technology, patients who engage in this therapy have been shown to have increased activity in their contralateral premotor and secondary somatosensory cortex in association with improved function (Johansen-Berg et al., 2002).

Research has also been focused on influencing neuroplasticity through the modification of environmental factors. Music therapy has been shown to influence neuroplasticity positively. It has been shown to improve cognition and other executive functions. Exercise has been shown to improve episodic memory and processing speed in addition to decrease age-related atrophy of the hippocampus. A healthy diet has also been shown to be helpful for this (The Health Jade Team, 2022).

Brain Injury, Plasticity, and Functional Recovery

It is known that brain insults, such as those that produce apraxic conditions, cause rapid cell death and a disruption of functional circuits, in the affected neural networks including white matter. During and immediately after stroke, neurological functions associated with the infracted (see glossary) area are lost. As the damaged system attempts to recover loss of function associated with cell death, regenerative processes are activated that lead to a varying degree of functional recovery. Factors produced by new neurons and glia, axonal sprouting of surviving neurons, and new synapse formation help to re-establish some of the lost functions. The timing and location of such events are crucial in the success of the regenerative process (Wielock & Nikolich, 2006).

Recovery of function involves three distinct phases: first, reversal of diaschisis and activation of cell repair; second, functional cell plasticity, that is, changing the properties of existing neuronal pathways; and third, neuroanatomical plasticity leading to the formation of new connections. Steps two and three are the basis of normal learning as well as recovery. In humans, recovery processes primarily engage ipsilateral brain regions, although if the damage is severe, contralateral brain areas are also involved.

What Enhances Neural Plasticity?

Environmental Enrichment and Neural Plasticity

Since recovery is, at least in part, based on neural plasticity, treatment approaches should incorporate factors that encourage its development.

Functional recovery is encouraged by experience-driven re-learning. This re-learning can be facilitated by professionals in a systematic way. An experience-rich environment has numerous biological effects that account for plasticity and its positive effect on recovery of function. For example. it enhances dendritic arborization and spine density on the contralateral pyramidal neurons, supporting the notion that the contralateral hemisphere is particularly involved in the recovery process when stimulated by an enriched environment (Johansson, 2004). Research suggests that the recovery-enhancing effect on sensorimotor function after stroke by an enriched environment is not due to generation and recruitment of new neurons to the periinfarct or remote cortical areas. Rather, the increased proliferation of glial cells and neuroblasts might enhance recovery by releasing regenerative factors or by providing cellular constituents, in particular lipids, for axonal growth (Wielock & Nikolich, 2006).

As indicated most forms of intervention for apraxia can be considered a form of environment enrichment, education, or re-education. These interventions consist of targeted practice of the requisite skill until the individual learns to do the skill in a highly automatic efficient manner. Research has demonstrated that many forms of environmental enrichment produce significant changes to components of the network systems. These include improvement in cortical weight and thickness and an increase of dendritic branching and length, the number of dendritic spines, and the size of synapses of some neuronal populations. Additionally, at the molecular level, environmental enrichment induces the expression of brain-derived neurotrophic factor (BDNF) and nerve growth factor (NGF), synaptic proteins (SP), and NMDA (N-methyld-aspartate) and AMPA (-amino-3-hydroxy-5- methyl-4-isoxazole propionic acid) receptor subunits. More importantly, environmental enrichment improves learning and memory at the behavioral level. Environmental enrichment enhances learning and memory in models of neurodegenerative diseases (Merceron-Martinez et al., 2021). These environmental enrichment activities and treatments have the benefit of inducing task-specific change. In sum, there is substantive research evidence that training and practice encourage neural plasticity with the likely outcome of regaining (in the case of brain damage) or acquiring (in the case of childhood apraxia of speech) appropriate function (Bootsma et al., 2021).

There are other factors that can contribute to plasticity. These include the administration of stem cells and the administration of growth factors such as erythropoetin which stimulates the development of new blood vessels and neurons and increases the levels of other growth factors. These, however, are non-targeted improvements, and the research is not yet clear whether merely adding new neurons and blood vessels will improve a specific function impaired by damage. So for the moment, for the practitioner only enriched environments offer the possibility of targeted recovery of function.

Regeneration

Thus far, we have spoken about synaptic and neuronal plasticity. That is the modification or recruitment of new pathways to reclaim function after injury to the original functional pathway, as in the case with many apraxias. There is another, less common, mechanism for the reacquisition of functioning. That is neuronal regeneration. Regeneration of the nervous system requires either the repair or replacement of nerve cells that have been damaged by injury or disease (Steward et al., 2013). There is evidence that neurons can regrow, albeit, slowly and in some cases assist in recovery of function (Stoll & Muller, 1998).

Injuries or damage secondary to illness, to neural network nerves, can result in partial or total loss of motor, sensory, and autonomic functions as in the case of apraxia. This can occur due to the interruption of axons, degeneration of distal nerve fibers, and eventual death of axotomized neurons. Research has demonstrated that functional deficits caused by nerve injuries can be compensated by reinnervation of denervated targets by regenerating injured axons or by collateral branching of undamaged axons, and, as we have discussed, remodeling of nervous system circuitry related to the lost functions. We have hypothesized that plasticity, in the form of rerouting or recruiting, functionally underpins most treatment for apraxia. Regeneration is potentially another way that functional recovery might theoretically be obtained. That promise has not yet been realized.

Limitations of Plasticity

We have seen how plasticity of central connections may compensate functionally for the lack of adequate target reinnervation. There are, however, some limitations. Plasticity has limited effects on disturbed sensory localization or fine motor control after injuries and may even result in maladaptive changes, such as neuropathic pain and hyperreflexia. This is because after being damaged, neurons shift from a transmitter to a regenerative phenotype, activating molecular pathways that support neuronal survival and axonal regeneration. Nerve injuries also induce a cascade of events, at the molecular, cellular, and system levels, initiated by the injury and progressing throughout plastic changes at the spinal cord, brainstem nuclei, thalamus, and brain cortex. Mechanisms involved in these changes include neurochemical changes, functional alterations of excitatory and inhibitory synaptic connections, sprouting of new connections, and reorganization of sensory and motor central maps. At the current time, it is unclear how therapeutic strategies that enhance axonal regeneration promote selective target reinnervation (Naxarro, 2009).

Treatment Going Forward: Neurorehabilitation

Until now, language representation in the brain was considered as being modular, and under this concept, speech treatment was limited to linguistic tasks and conducted separately for each module (i.e., naming or syntax). Given that we now know that language functions stream widely throughout our brain and are interconnected with many other brain functions, we can also recognize the brain's multifunctionality and the mechanisms for its functional reorganization. This new knowledge, coupled with technological progress, with new sophisticated and widely available and affordable tools for neuroimaging and neuromodulation, as well as telerehabilitation, has the potential to shift clinical neuroscience to an era of improved therapeutic strategies for people living with language and communication disorders including apraxia. Approaching poststroke apraxia or aphasia in terms of disrupted networks coupled with understanding how mechanisms of ischemic brain injury may be influenced by therapeutic interventions can offer better treatment strategies of poststroke language disruption such as apraxia in the future. We now know that recovery from many forms of language disruption including apraxia relies upon supportive, ancillary networks, serving in a role supporting the brain's cognitive reserve. The brain must therefore be functionally reorganized, and when these supportive brain regions involved in recovery remain intact, the outcome is more favorable. As we have seen, neuroplasticity is the driving force for this functional reorganization, and neurorehabilitation is the science of enhancing it (Nasios et al., 2019).

References

Ahel, I., Rass, U., El-Khamisy, S., Katyal, S., Celements, P., Mckinnon, P., et al. (2006). The neurodegenerative disease protein aprataxin resolves abortive DNA ligation intermediates. *Nature, 443*(12), 713–716. https://doi.org/10.1038/nature05164

Allison, K. C.-S. (2020). Differential diagnosis of apraxia of speech in children and adults: A scoping view. *Journal of Speech, Language, and Hearing Research, 63*, 2952–2994.

American Speech Hearing Association (ASHA). (2007). *Childhood apraxia of speech technical report*. American Speech and Language Association.

American Speech Hearing Association (ASHA). (2022). Retrieved from Childhood Apraxia of Speech. http://ASHA.org

American Speech-Language-Hearing Association. (2007). *Childhood apraxia of speech (Position Statement)*. Retrieved from American Speech-Language-Hearing Association. www.Asha.org/policy

Andres, E. E. (2022). Family based shole exome analysis of specific language impairment identifies rare variants in BUD13, a component of the retention and splicing complex. *Brain Sciences, 12*, 47.

Armstrong, P. (2010). *Bloom's Taxonomy*. Retrieved from Vanderbilt University Center for Teaching. https://cft.vanderbilt.edu/guides-sub-pages/blooms-taxonomy/

Ayres, J. (1972). Types of sensory integrative dysfunction among disabled learners. *American Journal of Occupational Therapy, 26*(1), 13–18.

Bak, T. H. (2012). What wires together dies together: Verbs, actions and neurodegeneration in motor neuron disease. *Cortex, 48*(7), 936–944.

Baldassarre, A., Lewis, C. M., Committeri, G., Snyder, A. Z., Romani, G. L., & Corbetta, M. (2012). Individual variability in functional connectivity predicts performance of a perceptual task. *Proceedings of the National Acadamey Science U. S. A., 109*, 3516–3521.

Ballard, K., Tourville, J., & Robin, D. (2014, November 3). Behavioral, computational, and neuroimaging studies of acquired apraxia of speech. *Frontiers in Human Neuroscience*. https://doi.org/10.3389/fnhum.2014.00892

Bangert, M., Peschel, T., Schlaug, G., Rotte, M., Drescher, D., Hinrichs, H., et al. (2006). Shared networks for auditory and motor processing in professional pianists: Evidence from fMRI conjunction. *Neuroimage, 30*, 917–926.

Barrios, J., Weng, W., England, R., Reifenberg, E., & Douglass, A. (2020). Hypothalamic dopamine neurons control sensorimotor behavior by modulating brainstem premotor nuclei in zebrafish. *Current Biology, 30*(23), 4606–4619. https://doi.org/10.1016/j.cub.2020.09.002

Basso, A., Luzzatti, C., & Spinler, H. (1980). Is ideomotor apraxia the outcome of damage to well-defined regions of the left hemisphere? *Journal of Neurology, Neurosurgery, and Psychiatry, 43*, 118–126.

Batista-García-Ramó, K., & Fernández-Verdecia, C. (2018). What we know about the brain structure–Function relationship. *Behavioral Sciences, 8*(39), 1–14. https://doi.org/10.3390/bs8040039

Baumard, J., & Le Gall, D. (2021). The challenge of apraxia: Toward an operational definition? *Cortex, 141*, 55–80. https://doi.org/10.1016/j.cortex.2021.04.001

Belanger, S., Duffy, R., & Coelho, D. (1996). The assessment of limb apraxia: An investigation of task effects and their cause. *Brain and Cognition, 32*(3), 384–404. https://doi.org/10.1006/brcg.1996.0072

Bernstein, N. (2003). *Contemporary studies on the physiology of the of the neural process*. Smysl.

Bickel, W. (2012). Are executive function and impulsivity antipodes? A conceptual reconstruction with special reference to addiction. *Psychopharmacology (Berl), 221*(3), 361–387. https://doi.org/10.1007/s00213-012-2689-x

Bieńkiewicz, M., Brandi, M. G., Hughes, C., & Hermsdörfer, J. (2014, April 23). The tool in the brain: Apraxia in ADL. Behavioral and neurological correlates of apraxia in daily living. *Frontiers in Psycholology*. https://doi.org/10.3389/fpsyg.2014.00353, online.

Binkofsky, F., Kunesch, E., Classen, J., Seitz, R., & Freund, H. (2001). Tactile apraxia: Unimodal apractic disorder of tactile object exploration associated with parietal lobe lesions. *Rain, 124*(1), 132–144. https://doi.org/10.1093/brain/124.1.132

Bootsma, J., Caljouw, S., Veldman, M., Maurits, N., Rothwell, J., & Hortobágyi, T. (2021). Neural correlates of motor skill learning are dependent on both age and task difficulty. *Frontiers in Aging Neuroscience, 22*. https://doi.org/10.3389/fnagi.2021.643132

Brazelton, T. B. (1973). Neonatal behavioral assessment scale.

Brennan, B., Wang, D., Li, M., Perriello, C. R., Elias, J., Van Kirk, N., et al. (2019). Use of an individual-level approach to identify cortical connectivity biomarkers in obsessive-compulsive disorder. *Biological Psychiatry: Cognitive Neuroscience and Neuroimaging, 4*(1), 27–38. https://doi.org/10.1016/j.bpsc.2018.07.014

Bush, G. (2010). Attention-deficit/hyperactivity disorder and attention networks. *Neuropsychopharmacology, 35*(1), 278–300. https://doi.org/10.1038/npp.2009.120

Cabrero, F., & De Jesus, O. (2021, August 30). *Apraxia of lid opening*. Retrieved from National Library of Medicine. https://www.ncbi.nlm.nih.gov/books/NBK560542/

Cantagallo, A., Maini, M., & Rumiati, R. (2013). The cognitive rehabilitation of limb apraxia in patients with stroke. *Neuropsychological Rehabilitation, 22*(3), 473–488.

Carrera, E., & Tononi, D. (2014). Diaschisis: Past, present, future. *Brain, 137*(9), 2408–2422. https://doi.org/10.1093/brain/awu101

Cassidy, A. (2016). The clinical assessment of apraxia. *Practical Neurology, 16*, 317–322.

Chatterjeea, D., Hegdeb, S., & Thaut, M. (2021). Neural plasticity: The substratum of music-based interventions in neurorehabilitation. *Neurorehabilitation, 48*, 155–166. https://doi.org/10.3233/NRE-208011

Chaytor, N., & Schmitter-Edgecombe, M. (2003). The ecological validity of neuropsychological tests: A review of the literature on everyday cognitive skills. *Neuropsychology Review, 13*(4), 181–187.

Childhood Apraxia of Speech. (2022). Retrieved from American Speech-Language Hearing Association: ASHA.ORG

Churchland, M. M., & Shenoy, K. V. (2007). Temporal complexity and heterogeneity of single-neuron activity in premotor and motor cortex. *Journal of Neurophysiology, 97*, 4235–4257.

Chvatal, S., & Ting, L. (2012). Voluntary and reactive recruitment of locomotor muscle synergies during perturbed walking. *The Journal of Neuroscience, 32*(35), 12237–12250. https://doi.org/10.1523/JNEUROSCI.6344-11.2012

Cleaton, A. T.-S., Tal-Saban, M., Hill, E. L., & Kirby, A. (2021). Gender and age differences in the presentation of at-risk or probable Developmental Coordination Disorder in adults. *Research in Developmental Disabilities, 115*. https://doi.org/10.1016/j.ridd.2021.104010

Coe, B., Witherspoon, K., Rosenfeld, J., et al. (2014). Refining analyses of copy number variation identifies specific genes associated with developmental delay. *Nature Genetics, 46*, 1053–1017.

Cogan, D. (1952). A type of congenital ocular motor apraxia presenting jerky head movements. *Transactions - American Academy of Ophthalmology and Otolaryngology, 56*, 579–588.

Conterno, M., Kümmerer, D., Dressing, A., Glauche, V., Urbach, H., Weiler, C., & Rijntjes, R. (2021). Speech apraxia and oral apraxia: Association or dissociation? A multivariate lesion–symptom mapping study in acute stroke patients. *Experimental Brain Research*. https://doi.org/10.1007/s00221-021-06224-3

Cooper, R. (2007). Tool use and related errors in ideational apraxia: The quantitative simulation of patient error profiles. *Cortex, 43*(3), 319–337.

Cousins, M. Smyth, M. M (2003). Developmental coordination impairments in adulthood. *Human Movement Science, 22*, 433–459. https://doi.org/10.1016/j.humov.2003.09.003. PMID: 14624827.

Cunningham, A. C. (2019). Coordination difficulties, IQ and psychopathology in children with high-risk copy number variants. *Psychological Medicine, 51*, 290–299. https://doi.org/10.1017/S0033291719003210

Dabul, B. (2000). *Apraxia battery for adults - Second Edition*. Pro-ed.

Dale, P., & Hayden, D. (2014). Treating speech subsystems in childhood apraxia of speech with tactual input: The PROMPT approach. *American Journal of Speech-Language Pathology*, 644–661. https://doi.org/10.1044/1058-0360(2013/12-0055)

Darley, F. (1967). Lacunae and research approaches to them. In C. Miliken & F. Darley (Eds.), *Brain mechanisms underlying speech and language*. Grune & Stratton.

Davis, B., Jakielski, K., & Marquardt, T. (1998). Developmental apraxia of speech: Determiners of differential diagnosis. *Clinical Linguistics & Phonetics, 12*, 25–45. https://doi.org/10.3109/02699209808985211

De Renzi, E., & Faglioni, P. (1999). Apraxia. In G. Denes & L. Pizzamiglio (Eds.), *Handbook of clinical and experimental psychiatry*. Psychology Press. https://doi.org/10.4324/9781315791272

De Renzi, E., & Lucchelli, F. (1988). Ideational apraxia. *Brain, 111*(5), 1173–1185. https://doi.org/10.1093/brain/111.5.1173

De Renzi, E., Faglioni, P., & Sorgato, P. (1982). Modality specific and supramodal mechanisms of Apraxia. *Brain, 105*, 301–312.

Delaney, A. L., & Kent, R. D. (2004). Developmental profiles of children diagnosed with apraxia of speech. *The annual convention of the American-Speech-Language-Hearing Association. Poster*. American-Speech-Language-Hearing Association.

Dewey, D. T. (2019). Very preterm children at risk for developmental coordination disorder have brain alterations in motor areas. *Acta Paediatrica, 108*(9). https://doi.org/10.1111/apa.14786

Donkervoort, M.-S., & Deelman, B. (2000). Prevalence of apraxia among patients with a first left hemisphere stroke in rehabilitation centres and nursing homes. *Clinical Rehabilitation, 14*(2), 130–136.

Duffy, J. (2006). Apraxia of speech in degenerative neurologic disease. *Aphasiology, 20*, 511–527.

Duffy, J. J. (2012). The diagnosis and understanding of apraxia of speech: Why including neurodegenerative etiologies may be important. *Journal of Speech, Language and Hearing Research, 55*(5), S1518–S1522. https://doi.org/10.1044/1092-4388(2012/11-0309)

Duménieu, M., Marquèze-Pouey, B., Russier, M., & Debanne, D. (2021). Mechanisms of plasticity in subcortical visual areas. *Cells, 10*(11), 3162. https://doi.org/10.3390/cells10113162

Dumont, C., Ska, B., & Joanette, Y. (2000). Conceptual apraxia and semantic memory deficit in Alzheimer's disease: Two sides of the same coin? *Journal of the International Neuropsychological Society, 6*(6), 693–703. https://doi.org/10.1017/S1355617700666079

Edelman, G., & Gally, J. (2001). Degeneracy and Complexity in Biological Systems. *Proceedings of the National Academy of Sciences, 98*(24), 13763–13768.

Einspieler, C. P., Prayer, D., & Marschik, P. B. (2021). Fetal movements; The origin of human behaviour. *Developmental Medicine & Child Neurology, 63*(10), 1142–1148.

Evarts, E. V. (1868). Relation of pyramidal tract activity to force exerted during voluntary movement. *Journal of Neurophysiology, 31*, 14–27.

Farah, M. J., O'Reilly, R. C., & Vecera, S. P. (1993). Dissociated overt and covert recognition as an emergent property of a lesioned neural network. *Psychological Review, 100*(4), 571–588. https://doi.org/10.1037/0033-295X.100.4.571

Feldman, A. G., & Levin, M. F. (1995). Positional frames of reference in motor control: Their origin and use. *Behavioral and Brain Sciences, 18*, 723–806.

Fernandes, W. S.-P. (2016). Motor coordination correlates with academic achievement and cognitive function in children. *Frontiers in Psychology*. https://doi.org/10.3389/fpsyg.2016.00318

Fogassi, L., Ferrari, P., Gesierich, B., Rozzi, S., Chersi, F., & Rizzolatti, G. (2005). Parietal lobe: From action organization to intention understanding. *Science, 308*, 662–667.

Foki, T., Vanbellingen, C. T., Pirker, A. L., Bohlhalter, S., Nyffeler, T., Kraemmer, J., et al. (2016). Limb-kinetic apraxia affects activities of daily living in Parkinson's disease: A multi-center study. *European Journal of Neurology, 23*(8), 1301–1307. https://doi.org/10.1111/ene.13021

Fornito, A., Zalesky, A., & Breakspear, M. (2015). The connectomics of brain disorders. *Nature Reviews | Neuroscience, 16*, 150–172.

French, M., Cohen, M., Pohlig, R., & Reisman, D. (2021). Fluid cognitive abilities are important for learning and retention of a new, explicitly-learned walking pattern in individuals after stroke. *Neurorehabilitation Neural Repair, 35*(5), 419–430. https://doi.org/10.1177/15459683211001025

Friedman, N., Hatoum, A., Gustavson, D., Corley, R., Hewitt, J., & Young, S. (2020). Executive functions and impulsivity are genetically distinct and independently predict psychopathology: Results from two adult twin studies. *Clinical Psychological Science, 8*(3), 519–536. https://doi.org/10.1177/2167702619898814

Fu, X., Zhou, G., Zhuang, J., Xu, C., Zhou, H., Peng, Y., et al. (2021). White matter injury after intracerebral hemorrhage. *Frontiers in Neurology, 12*, 562090. https://doi.org/10.3389/fneur.2021.562090

Fulceri, F., Grossi, E., Contaldo, A., Narzisa, A., Apicella, F., Parrini, I., et al. (2019, January 9). Motor skills as moderators of core symptoms in autism spectrum disorders: Preliminary data from an exploratory analysis with artificial neural networks. *Frontiers in Psychology*. https://doi.org/10.3389/fpsyg.2018.02683

Fuster, J. (1997). Network memory. *Trends in Neuroscience, 20*(10), 451–459. https://doi.org/10.1016/S0166-2236(97)01128-4

Gaines, R. C. (2008). Clinical expression of developmental coordination disorder in a large Canadian family. *Paediatrics and Child Health, 13*, 763–768.

Gainotti, G., & Trojano, L. (2018). Chapter 16 - Constructional apraxia. In G. Vallar & H. Coslett (Eds.), *Handbook of clinical neurology* (Vol. 151, pp. 331–348). Elsevier. https://doi.org/10.1016/B978-0-444-63622-5.00016-4

Gallego, J., Perich, M., Naufel, S., Ethier, C., Solla, S., & Miller, E. (2018). Cortical population activity within a preserved neural manifold underlies multiple motor behaviors. *Nature Communication, 9*, 4233. https://doi.org/10.1038/s41467-018-06560-z

Galvan, A. (2010). Neural plasticity of development and learning. *Human Brain Mapping, 31*(6), 879–890. https://doi.org/10.1002/hbm.21029

Ganguly, J., & Jog, M. (2020). Tauopathy and movement disorders—Unveiling the chameleons and mimics. *Frontiers in Neurology: Movement Disorders*. https://doi.org/10.3389/fneur.2020.599384

Garibotto, V., Scifo, P., Gorini, A., Alonso, C., Brambati, S., Bellodi, L., & Perani, D. (2010). Disorganization of anatomical connectivity in obsessive compulsive disorder: A multi-parameter diffusion tensor imaging study in a subpopulation of patients. *Neurobiology of Disease, 37*(2), 468–476. https://doi.org/10.1016/j.nbd.2009.11.003

Gerstner, W., Kistler, W., Naud, R., & Paninsk, L. (2014). Neuronal populations. In W. Gerstner, W. Kistler, R. Naud, & L. Paninsk (Eds.), *Neuronal dynamics from single neurons to networks and models of cognition* (pp. 291–322). Cambridge University Press.

Giovannetti, T., Libon, D., Buxbaum, L., & Schwartz, M. (2002). Naturalistic action impairments in dementia. *Neuropsychologia, 40*, 1220–1232.

Gold, L., & Lauritzen, M. N. (2002). Neuronal deactivisation explains decreased cerebellar blood flow in response to focal cerebral ischemia or suppressed neocortical function. *Proceedings of the. Natlonal Academy. Sciience USA, 99*, 7699–7704.

Gomez, M., McCabe, P., & Purcell, A. (2022). A survey of the clinical management of childhood apraxia of speech in the United States and Canada. *Journal of Communication Disorders, 96*, 106193. https://doi.org/10.1016/j.jcomdis.2022.106193

Gonzales-Rothi, L., & Heilman, K. (1996). Liepmann (1900 and 1905): A definition of apraxia and a model of praxis. In C. Code, Y. Joanette, A. Roch-Lecours, & C. Wallesch (Eds.), *Classic cases in neuropsychology*. Psychology Press.

Goyen, T. (2005). Motor dysfunction in apparently normal high-risk children. *Academia.edu*. https://www.academia.edu/27667038/Motor_dysfunction_in_apparently_normal_high_risk_children

Green, D. C. (2008). Does subtype of developmental coordination disorder Count: Is there a differential effect on outcome following intervention? *Human Movement Science*. https://doi.org/10.1016/j.humov.2008.02.009

Gross, R., & Grossman, M. (2008). Update on apraxia. *Current Neurology and Neuroscience Reports, 8*(6), 490–496. https://doi.org/10.1007/s11910-008-0078-y

Guyette, T. W., & Diedrich, W. M. (1981). A critical review of developmental apraxia of speech. *Speech and Language*, 1–49.

Hale, J., Alfonso, V., Berninger, V., Bracken, B., Christo, C., Clark, E., et al. (2010). Critical issues in response-to-intervention, comprehensive evaluation, and specific learning disabilities identification and intervention: An expert white paper consensus. *Learning Disability Quarterly, 33*(3), 223–238.

Hamilton, J., Haaland, K., Adair, J., & Brandt, J. (2003). Ideomotor limb apraxia in Huntington's disease: Implications for corticostriate involvement. *Neuropsychologia, 41*, 614–621.

Handiru, S. V., Alivar, A., Hoxha, A., Saleh, S., Suviseshamuthu, E. S., Yue, G. H., & Allexandre, D. (2021). Graph-theoretical analysis of EEG functional connectivity during balance perturbation in traumatic brain injury: A pilot study. *Human Brain Mapping, 14*(42), 4427–4447. https://doi.org/10.1002/hbm.25554

Harrowell, I. H. (2017). Mental health outcomes of developmental coordination disorder in late adolescence. *Developmental Medicine & Child Neurology, 59*(9), 973–979.

Hayden, D., Eigen, J., Walker, A., & Olsen, L. (2010). Prompt: A tactually grounded model for the treatment of childhood in speech production disorders. In L. Williams, S. McCleod, & R. McCauley (Eds.), *Treatment for speech sound disorders in children* (pp. 453–474). Brooks.

Hazy, T. F. (2007). Towards an executive without a homunculus: Computational models of the prefrontal cortex/basal ganglia system. *Philosophical Transactions of the Royal Society B: Biological Sciences, 362*, 1601–1613.

HealthLine. (2022). *What's the treatment for apraxia of speech?* Retrieved from Healthline. https://www.healthline.com/health/apraxia-of-speech#treatment

Heilman, K., Rothi, L., & Valenstein, E. (1982). Two forms of ideomotor Apraxia. *Neurology, 32*, 342–346.

Heilman, K., Maher, L., Greenwald, M., & Rothi, L. (1997). Conceptual apraxia from lateralized lesions. *Neurology, 49*(2). https://doi.org/10.1212/WNL.49.2.457

Hildebrand, M. J. (2020). Severe childhood speech disorder. *Neurology, 94*, 2148–2167.

Holtmaat, A., & Svoboda, K. (2009). Experience-dependent structural synaptic plasticity in the mammalian brain. *National Review Neuroscience, 10*, 647–658.

Honey, C. J., & Sporns, O. (2008). Dynamical consequences of lesions in cortical networks. *Human Brain Mapping, 29*, 802–809.

Honey, C., Sporns, O., Cammoun, G. X., Thiran, J., et al. (2009). Predicting human resting-state functional connectivity from structural connectivity. *Proceedings of the National Academy of Science USA, 106*, 2035–2040.

Hua, J. W. Williams GJ, Jin H, Chen J, Xu M, Zhou Y, Gu G, Du W (2022). Early motor milestones in Infancy and later motor impairments: A population based data linkage study. *Psychiatry*. https://doi.org/10.3389/fpsyt.2022.809181

Hummel, F., Heise, K., Celnik, P., et al. (2010). Facilitating skilled right hand motor function in older subjects by anodal polarization over the left primary motor cortex. *Neurociological Aging, 31*, 2160–2168.

Humphrey, D. R., & Thompson, W. D. (1970). Predicting measures of motor performance from multiple cortical spike trains. *Science, 170(7)*, 758–762.

Huth, A. G., De Heer, W. A., Griffiths, T. L., Theunissen, F. E., & Gallant, J. L. (2016). Natural speech reveals the semantic maps that tile human cerebral cortex. *Nature, 532*(7600), 453–459. https://doi.org/10.1038/nature17637

Iuzzini, J. (2012). *Inconsistency of speech in children with childhood apraxia of speech, phonological disorders, and typical speech.* Indiana University ProQuest Dissertations Publishing.

Iuzzini-Seigel, J. M. (2017a). Speech assessment in children with childhood apraxia of speech. In *Perspectives of the ASHA Special Interest Groups* (pp. 47–60). American Speech Language Hearing Association.

Iuzzini-Seigel, J. H. (2017b). Speech inconsistency in children with childhood apraxia of speech. In *Language impairment and Speech Delay: Depends on the Stimuli. J Speech Lang Hear Res*, 1194–1220.

Johansen-Berg, H., Dawes, H., Guy, C., Smith, S. M., Wade, D. T., & Matthews, P. M. (2002). Correlation between motor improvements and altered fMRI activity after rehabilitative therapy. *Brain, 125*, 2731–2742. https://doi.org/10.1093/brain/awf282

Johansson, B. (2004). Functional and cellular effects of environmental enrichment after experimental brain infarcts. *Restorative Neuroscience, 22*, 163–174.

Karmiloff-Smith, A., Scerif, G., & Ansari, D. (2003). Double dissociations in developmental disorders? Theoretically misconceived, empirically dubious. *Cortex, 39*, 161–163.

Kelley, A., Shiltz, C., & Landry, C. (2005). Neural systems recruited by drug- and food-related cues: Studies of gene activation in corticolimbic regions. *Physiology & Behavior, 86*(1–2), 11–14. https://doi.org/10.1016/j.physbeh.2005.06.018

Kertes, A., & Ferro, J. (1984). Lesion size and location in ideomotor apraxia. *Brain, 107*(92), 1–33.

Kirrie, B., Granier, J., & Robin, D. (2008). Understanding the nature of apraxia of speech: Theory, analysis, and treatment. *Neuropsychological Trends, 4*, 7–44.

Kirst, C., Modes, C., & Magnasco, M. (2017). Shifting attention to dynamics: Self-reconfiguration of neural networks. *Current Opinion in Systems Biology, 3*, 132–140. https://doi.org/10.1016/j.coisb.2017.04.006

Koziol, L. B. (2009). *Subcortical structures and cognition*. Springe.

Koziol, L. (2014). *The myth of executive functioning: Missing elements in conceptualization, evalaution and assessment*. Springer.

Koziol, L., Budding, D., & Chidekel, D. (2012). From movement to thought: Executive function, embodied cognition, and the cerebellum. *Cerebellum, 11*(2), 505–525. https://doi.org/10.1007/s12311-011-0321-y

Kozubski, W., Ong, K., Waleszczyk, W., Zabel, M., & Dorszewska, J. (2021). Molecular factors mediating neural cell plasticity changes in dementia brain diseases. *Neural Plasticity, 2021*, 8834645. https://doi.org/10.1155/2021/8834645

Langevin, L. M., MacMaster, F. P., & Dewey, D. (2015). Distinct patterns of cortical thinning in concurrent motor and attention disorders. *Developmental Medicine and Child Neurology, 3*, 257–264.

Latash, M. (2008). Evolution of motor control: From reflexes and motor programs to the equilibrium-point hypothesis. *Journal of Human Kinetics, 19*, 3–24.

Law, J. B. (2000). Prevalence and natural history. *International Journal of Language & Communication Disorders, 35*(2), 165–188.

Leiguarda, R. (2001). Limb apraxia: Cortical or subcortical. *NeuroImage, 14*(1), 5137–5141. https://doi.org/10.1006/nimg.2001.0833

Leiguarda, C. D., & Marsden, C. (2000). Limb apraxias: Higher-order disorders of sensorimotor integration. *Brain, 123*(Pt 5), 650–879. https://doi.org/10.1093/brain/123.5.860

Lesny, I. (1980). Developmental dyspraxia-dysgnosia as a cause of congenital children's clumsiness. *Brain Development*, 69–71. https://doi.org/10.1016/S0387-7604(80)80009-X

Lewis, B. A., Freebairn, L., Hansen, A., Iyengar, S., & Taylor, H. (2004). School-age follow-up of children with childhood apraxia of speech. *Language, Speech, and Hearing in Schools, 35*, 122–140.

Liepmann, S., & Mass, O. (1907). Fall von linksseitiger Agraphie und Apraxie bei rechtsseitiger Lahmung. *Journal of Psychology and Neurology, 10*, 14.

Long, C. J., & Kibby, M. Y. (1995). Ecological validity of neuropsychological tests: A look at neuropsychology's past and the impact. *Advances in Medical Psychotherapy, 8*, 59–78.

Luria, A. (1973). *The working brain*. Basic Books.

Luzzi, S., Piccirilli, M., Pessalacia, M., Fabi, K., & Provincialia, L. (2010). Dissociation apraxia secondary to right premotor stroke. *Neuropsychologia, 48*(1), 68–76. https://doi.org/10.1016/j.neuropsychologia.2009.08.010

Maasen, B. (2002). Issues contrasting adult acquired versus developmentla apraxia of speech. *Seminars in Speech Language, 35*, 257–266.

Maasen, B. (2015). Developmental models of childhood apraxia of speech. In I. R. Barr & E. Sillimen (Eds.), *Routledge handbook of communication disorder* (pp. 124–133). Routledge.

Maleki, S., Chye, Y., Zhang, X., Parkes, L., Chamberlain, S., Fontenelle, L. F., et al. (2020). Neural correlates of symptom severity in obsessive-compulsive disorder using magnetization transfer and diffusion tensor imaging. *Psychiatry Research: Neuroimaging, 298*, 111046. https://doi.org/10.1016/j.pscychresns.2020.111046

Malkani, R., & Zadikoff, C. (2011). The apraxias in movement disorders. In N. Galvaez-Jimenez, P. Tuite, & K. Bhatia (Eds.), *Uncommon causes of movement disorders* (pp. 35–45). Cambridge University Press.

Martin, N. P. (2006). DCD and ADHD: A genetic study of their shared aetiology. *Human Movement Science, 25*, 110–124.

Mayo Clinic. (2022). *Childhood apraxia of speech*. Retrieved from Mayo Clinic. https://www.mayoclinic.org/diseases-conditions/childhood-apraxia-of-speech/diagnosis-treatment/drc-20352051

McGinty, H., Phillips, K., Jim, H., Cessna, J., Asvat, Y., Cases, M., et al. (2014). Cognitive functioning in men receiving androgen deprivation therapy for prostate cancer: A systematic review and meta-analysis. *Supportive Care in Cancer, 22*(8), 2271–2280. https://doi.org/10.1007/s00520-014-2285-1

McNeil, M. (2011). *Clinical management of sensorimotor speech disorders*. Thieme.

Menon, V. (2013). Developmental pathways to functional brain networks: Emerging principles. *Trends in Cognitive Sciences, 17*. https://doi.org/10.1016/j.tics.2013.09.015

Merceron-Martinez, D., Ibaceta-Gonzalez, C., Salazr, C., Almaguer-Melian, W., Bergado-Rosado, J., & Palacios, A. (2021). Alzheimer's disease, neural plasticity, and functional recovery. *Journal of Alzheimer's Disease*. https://doi.org/10.3233/JAD-201178, In press.

Meyer, K., & Damasio, A. (2009). Convergence and divergence in a architecture for recognition and memory. *Trends in Neuroscience, 32*(7), 376–382. https://doi.org/10.1016/j.tins.2009.04.002

Middleton, F., & Strick, P. (2000). Basal ganglia output and cognition: Evidence from anatomical, behavioral, and clinical studies. *Brain and Cognition, 42*(2), 183–200. https://doi.org/10.1006/brcg.1999.1099

Mihailidis, A., Boger, J. N., Craig, T., & Hoey, J. (2006). The COACH prompting systems to assist older adults with dementia through handwashing: An efficacy study. *BMC Geriatrics, 8*, 28. http://www.biomedcentral.com1471-2318/8/28

Miller, G. L.-H. (2019). Reading outcomes for individuals with histories of suspected childhood apraxia of speech. *American Journal of Speech Language Pathology, 28*, 1432–1447.

Mirabella, G. D. (2017). Developmental coordination disorder affects the processing of action relate verbs. *Frontiers in Human Neuroscience*. https://doi.org/10.3389/fnhum.2016.00661

Missiuna, C., Rivard, L., & Bartlett, D. (2003). Early identification and risk management of children with developmental coordination disorder. *Pediatric Physical Therapy, 15*(1), 32–38.

Molloy, J., & Jagoe, C. (2019). Use of diverse diagnostic criteria for acquired apraxia of speech: A scoping review. *International Journal of Language and Communication Disorders, 54*(6), 875–893. https://doi.org/10.1111/1460-6984.12494

Moncrieff, J. C. (2022). The serotonin theory of depression: A systematic umbrella review of the evidence. *Molecular Psychiatry*. https://doi.org/10.1038/s41380-022-01661-0

Morgan, A., & Webster, R. (2018). Aetiology of childhood apraxia of speech: A clinical practice update for paediatricians. *Journal of Paediatrics and Child Health, 54*, 1090–1095. https://doi.org/10.1111/jpc.14150

Morgan, A., Fisher, S., Scheffer, I., & Hildebrand, M. (2016). FOXP2-related speech and language disorders. In M. A. Adam (Ed.), *Gene reviews*. University of Washington.

Moruzzi, S. P.-G. (2010). Clumsiness and psychopathology: Causation or shared etiology? A twin study with the CBCL 6–18 questionnaire in a general school-age population sample. *Human Movement Science, 29*, 326–338. https://doi.org/10.1016/j.humov.2010.01.005

Mosca, S. L. (2016). Copy-number variations are enriched for neurodevelopmental genes in children with developmental coordination disorder. *Journal of Medical Genetics, 53*(12), 812–819. https://doi.org/10.1136/jmedgenet-2016-103818

Moser, D., Basilakos, A., Fillmore, P., & Fridriksson, J. (2016). Brain damage associated with apraxia of speech: Evidence from case studies. *Neurocase, 22*(4), 346–356. https://doi.org/10.1080/13554794.2016.1172645

Moss, A. G. (2012). Interarticulatory coordination of the lips and jaw in childhood apraxia of speech. *Journal of Medical Speech-Language Pathology, 20*(4), 127–132.

Mountford, H. B. (2022). The genetic and molecular basis of developmental language disorder: A review. *Children, 9*, 586.

Murray, E., McCabe, P., & Ballard, K. J. (2015). A randomized controlled trial for children with childhood apraxia of speech comparing Rapid Syllable Transition treatment and the Nuffield. *Journal of Speech, Language, and Hearing Research, 58*, 669–686. https://doi.org/10.1044/2015_JSLHR-S-13-0179

Mutha, P., Sainburg, R., & Haaland, K. (2010). Coordination deficits in ideomotor apraxia during visually targeted reaching reflect impaired visuomotor transformations. *Neuropsychologia, 48*(13), 3855–3867. https://doi.org/10.1016/j.neuropsychologia.2010.09.018

Nasios, G., Dardiostis, E., & Messinis, L. (2019). From Broca and Wernicke to the neuromodulation era: Insights of brain language networks for neurorehabilitation. *Behavioural Neurology, 2019*. https://doi.org/10.1155/2019/9894571

National Institute of Deafness and Other Communication Disorders. (2022). *Home page*. Retrieved from National Institute of Deafness and Other Communication Disorders. https://www.nidcd.nih.gov/

Naxarro, X. (2009). Chapter 27 Neural plasticity after nerve injury and regeneration. *International Review of Neurobiology, 87*, 483–505. https://doi.org/10.1016/S0074-7742(09)87027-X

Newbury, D. W. (2009). CMIP and ATP2C2 Modulate phonological short term memory in language impairment. *The American Journal of Human Genetics, 85*, 264–272.

Norbury, C. F. (2016). The impact of nonverbal ability on prevalence and clinical presentation of and clinical presentation of language disorder: Evidence from a population study. *Journal of Child Psychology and Psychiatry, 57*, 1247–1257.

NORD. (2021). *Ocular Motor Apraxia, Cogan Type*. Retrieved from National Organization of Rare Disorders. https://rarediseases.org/rare-diseases/ocular-motor-apraxia-cogan-type/

Nudo, R., Wise, B., SiFuentes, F., et al. (1996). Neural substrates for the effects of rehabilitative training on motor recovery after ischemic infarct. *Science, 272*, 1791–1794.

Ochipa, C., Rothi, L. J., & Heilman, K. M. (1992). Conceptual apraxia in Alzheimer's disease. *Brain, 115*(Pt 4), 1061–1071.

Ogar, J., Slama, H., Dronkers, N., Amici, S., & Gorno-Tempini, M. (2005). Apraxia of speech: An overview. *Neurocase, 11*, 427–432. https://doi.org/10.1080/13554790500263529

Ogar, J. M., Dronkers, N. F., Brambati, S. M., Miller, B. L., & Gorno-Tempini, M. L. (2007). Progressive nonfluent aphasia and its characteristic motor speech deficits. *Alzheimer Disease and Associated Disorders*, 523–530.

Park, J. (2017). Apraxia: Review and update. *Journal of Clinical Neurology, 13*(4), 317–324. https://doi.org/10.3988/jcn.2017.13.4.317

Park, E., Velumian, A., & Fehlings, M. (2004). Mechanisms of spinal cord injury: A review with an emphasis on the implications for white matter degeneration. *Journal of Neurotrauma, 21*(6), Reviews https://doi.org/10.1089/0897715041269641, online.

Pazzaglia, M., Pizzamiglio, L., Pes, E., & Aglioti, S. (2008a). The sound of actions in apraxia. *Current Biology, 18*(22), 1766–1772. https://doi.org/10.1016/j.cub.2008.09.061

Pazzaglia, M., Smania, N., Corato, E., & Aglioti, S. (2008b). Neural underpinnings of gesture discrimination in patients with limb apraxia. *The Journal of Neuroscience, 28*(12), 3030–3041. https://doi.org/10.1523/JNEUROSCI.5748-07.2008

Piek, J. D. (2008). The role of early fine and gross motor development on later motor and cognitive ability. *Human Movement Science, 27*(5), 668–681.

Pinson, A. X. (2022). Human TKTL1 implies greater neurogenesis in frontal neocortex of modern humans than Neanderthals. *Science, 377*. https://doi.org/10.1126/science.abl6422

Poore, M. B. (2009). Suck predicts neuromotor integrity and developmental outcomes. *Perspective on speech and Orofacial Disorders*. https://doi.org/10.1044/ssod19.1.44.

Pramstaller, P., & Marsden, C. (1996). The basal ganglia and apraxia. *Brain, 119*(1), 319–340. https://doi.org/10.1093/brain/119.1.319

Ramus, F. (2003). Developmental Dyslexia: Specific phonological deficit or general sensorimotor sysfunction. *Current Opinion in Neurobiology, 13*, 212–218.

Rehme, A. K., & Grefkes, C. (2012). Cerebral network disorders after stroke: Evidence from imaging-based connectivity analyses of active and resting brain states in humans. *Journal of Physiology, 591*, 17–51.

Roig, M., Gratacòs, M., Vazquez, E., del Toro, M., Foguet, A., Ferrer, I., & Macaya, A. (2003). Brainstem dysgenesis: Report of five patients with congenital hypotonia, multiple cranial nerve involvement and ocular motor apraxia. *Developmental Medicine & Child Neurology, 45*, 489–493.

Rosenzoph, H., Weisen, D., Basilakos, A., Yourganov, G., Bonilha, L., Rorden, C., … Sperber, C. (2020, April 17). *Mapping the Human Praxis Network: An investigation of white matter disconnection in limb apraxia*. Retrieved from bioRxiv.org. https://doi.org/10.1101/2020.04.14.041442

Rosenzoph, H., Wiesen, D., Basilakos, A., Yourganov, G., Bonilha, L., Fridriksson, J., et al. (2022). Mapping the human praxis network: An investigation of white matter disconnection in limb apraxia of gesture production. *Brain Communications, 4*(1), 1–14. https://doi.org/10.1093/braincomms/fcac004

Salo, V. F. (2019). The role of the motor system in action understanding and communication: Evidence from human infants and non human primates. *Developmental Psychobiology, 61(3)*, 390–401.

Salvi, R., Wang, J., & Ding, D. (2000). Auditory plasticity and hyperactivity following cochlear damage. *Hearing Research, 147*, 261–274.

Sato, J. R., Biazoli Jr., C. E., Zugman, A., Pan, P. M., Bueno, A. P. A., Moura, L. M., … & Jackowski, A. P. (2021). Long-term stability of the cortical volumetric profile and the functional human connectome throughout childhood and adolescence. *European Journal of Neuroscience*, 6187–6201. https://doi.org/10.1111/ejn.15435

Saxena, S., & Caroni, P. (2011). Selective neuronal vulnerability in neurodegenerative diseases: From stressor thresholds to degeneration. *Neuron, 71*, 35–48.

Scott, S. H., & Kalaska, J. F. (1997). Reaching movements with similar hand paths but different arm orientations. I. Activity of individual cells in motor cortex. *Journal of Neurophysiology, 77*, 826–852.

Seven, Y., Mantilla, C., & Sieck, G. (2014). Recruitment of rat diaphragm motor units across motor behaviors with different levels of diaphragm activation. *Journal of Applied Physiology, 117*(11), 1308–1316. https://doi.org/10.1152/japplphysiol.01395.2013

Shandley, S. C. (2021). Abnormal nutritive sucking as an indicator of neonatal brain injury. *Frontiers in Pediatrics*. https://doi.org/10.3389/fped.2020.599633

Sharma, V., & Wong, L. (2022). Middle cerebral artery disease. In J. Grotta, G. Albers, J. Broderick, S. Kasner, R. Sacco, A. Day, et al. (Eds.), *Stroke (Seventh edition) pathophysiology, diagnosis, and management* (pp. 317–346). Elsevier. https://doi.org/10.1016/B978-0-323-69424-7.00024-7

Sharma, N., Classen, J., & Cohen, L. (2013). Neural plasticity and its contribution to functional recovery. *Handbook of Clinical Neurology, 110*, 3–12. https://doi.org/10.1016/B978-0-444-52901-5.00001-0

Shriberg, L. D. (2019). Estimates of prevalence of speech and motor speech disorders in persons with complex neurodevelopmental disorders. *Clinical Linguistics & Phonetics, 33*(8), 707–736.

Shriberg, L. D., Fourakis, M., Hall, S. D., Karlsson, H. B., Lohmeier, H. L., McSweeny, J. L., Potter, N. L., Scheer-Cohen, A. R., Strand, E. A., Tilkens, C. M., & Wilson, D. L. (2010). Extensions to the speech disorders classification system (SDCS). *Clinical Linguistics & Phonetics, 24*, 795–824.

Shriberg, L., KwiatkowskiI, J., & Mabie, H. (2019). Estimates of the prevalence of motor speech disorders in children with idiopathic speech delay. *Clinical Linguistics & Phonetics, 33*, 679–706. https://doi.org/10.1080/02699206.2019.1595731

Singer, W. (1993). Synchronization of cortical activity and its putative. *Annual Review of Physiology, 55*, 349–374.

Soliveri, P., Piacentini, S., & Girotti, F. (2005). Limb apraxia in corticobasal degeneration and progressive supranuclear palsy. *Neurology, 64*, 448–453.

Sonuga-Barke, E. (2003). The dual pathway model of AD/HD: An elaboration of neuro-developmental characteristics. *Neuroscience Biobehavioral Review, 27*, 593–604.

Sonuga-Barke, E., Bitsakou, P., & Thompson, M. (2010). Beyond the dual pathway model: Evidence for the dissociation of timing,inhibitory and delay-related impairments in Attention Deficit/Hyperactivity disorder. *Journal of Child and Adolescent Psychiatry*, 345–355. https://doi.org/10.1016/j.jaac.2009.12.018

Sporns, O., Tononi, G., & Kötter, R. (2005). The human connectome: A structural description of the human brain. *PLOS Computational Biology*. https://doi.org/10.1371/journal.pcbi.0010042

Stackhouse, J. W. (1997). *Children's speech and literacy difficulties 1: A psycholinguistic framework*. Wurr.

Steward, M., Sridhar, A., & Meyer, J. (2013). Neural regeneration. *Current Topics in Microbiology and Immunology, 367*, 153–191. https://doi.org/10.1007/82_2012_302

Stoll, G., & Muller, H. (1998). Nerve injury, axonal degeneration and neural regeneration: Basic insights. *Brain Pathology, 9*, 313–325. https://doi.org/10.1111/j.1750-3639.1999.tb00229.x

Strand, E. (2019, January 9). *Diagnosis and management of CAS*.

Sunderland, A., & Shiner, C. (2007). Ideomotor apraxia and functional ability. *Cortex, 43*(3), 359–367. https://doi.org/10.1016/S0010-9452(08)70461-1

Sweatt, D. (2016). Neural plasticity and behavior- Sixty years of conceptual advances. *Journal of Neuroshemistry, 139*(2), 179–199. https://doi.org/10.1111/jnc.13580

Tal Saban, M. Z. (2012). The functional profile of young adults with suspected developmental coordination disorder (DCD). *Research in Developmental Disabilities, 33*, 2193–2202. https://doi.org/10.1016/j.ridd.2012.06.005

Tal Saban, M. O. (2014). Executive function and attention in young adults with and without Developmental Coordination Disorder – A comparative study. *Research in Developmental Disabilities, 35*, 2644–2650.

Tarsy, D. (2012). *Movement disorders: A video atlas*. Humana Press.

Terband, H. M. (2019). A psycholinguistic framework for diagnosis and treatment planning of developmental speech disorders. *Folia Phoniatrica et Logopaedica, 71*(5–6), 216–227.

Tettamanti, M., Buccino, G., Saccuman, M., Gallese, V., Danna, M., Scifo, P., et al. (2005). Listening to action-related sentences activates fronto-parietal motor circuits. *Journal of Cognitive Neuroscience, 17*, 273–281.

Teverovsky, E., Bickel, J., & Feldman, H. (2009). Functional characteristics of children diagnosed with Childhood Apraxia of Speech. *Disability and Rehabilitation, 31*(2), 94–102. https://doi.org/10.1080/09638280701795030

The Health Jade Team. (2022). *Brain plasticity*. Retrieved from Health Jade. https://healthjade.net/brain-plasticity/

The Medical Dictionary. (2021). *Apraxia*. Retrieved from The Medical Dictionary. http://the-medical-dictionary.com/apraxia_article_2.htm

Thomason, M., Hect, J., Waller, R., Manning, J., Stacks, A., Beeghly, M., et al. (2018). Prenatal neural origins of infant motor development: Associations between fetal brain and infant motor development. *Developmental Psychopathology, 30*(3), 763–772. https://doi.org/10.1017/S095457941800072X

Tse, M. (2012). Double duty of tail caudate nucleus neurons. *Nature Reviews Neuroscience, 13*, 11005–11016. https://doi.org/10.1038/nrn3342

Tuttolomondo, A., Pecoraro, R., & Pinto, A. (2014). Studies of selective TNF inhibitors in the treatment of brain injury from stroke and trauma: A review of the evidence to date. *Drug Design, Development and Therapy, 8*, 2221–2238. https://doi.org/10.2147/DDDT.S67655

van den Heuvel, M., & Sporns, O. (2013). Network hubs in the human brain. *Trends in Cognitive Sciences, 17*(12), 683–696. https://doi.org/10.1016/j.tics.2013.09.012

Wang, M. L. (2014a). Co-occurring development of early childhood communication and motor skills: Results from a population based longitudinal study. *Child: Care, Health and Development, 40*, 77–84.

Wang, M. L. (2014b). The developmental relationship between language and motor performance from 3 to 5 years of age: A prospective longitudinal population study. *BMC Psychology, 2*, 34. https://doi.org/10.1186/s40359-014-0034-3

Waring, R., & Knight, R. (2013). How should children with speech sound disorders be classified? A review and critical evaluation of current classification systems. *Journal of Language & Communication Disorders, 48*(1), 25–40. https://doi.org/10.1111/j.1460-6984.2012.00195.x

Wasserman, T., & Wasserman, L. (2013). Towards a unifying model of executive function. *Applied Neuropsychology: Child, 2*(2), 88–96. https://doi.org/10.1080/21622965.2013.748394

Wasserman, T., & Wasserman, L. (2017). Touching the elephant: The search for fluid intelligence. *Applied Neuropsychology Child, 6*(3), 228–236. https://doi.org/10.1080/21622965.2017.1317489

Watemberg, N. W.-S. (2007). Developmental coordination disorder in children with attention-deficit–hyperactivity disorder and physical therapy intervention. *Developmental Medicine & Child Neurology, 49*(12), 920–925.

Watson, R., & Heilman, K. (1983). Callosal apraxia. *Brain, 106*(2), 391–403. https://doi.org/10.1093/brain/106.2.391

Weintraub, S. (2000a). Neuropsychological assessment of mental state. In M. Mesulam (Ed.), *Principles of behavioral and cognitive neurology* (pp. 135–136). Oxford University Press.
Weintraub, S. (2000b). Neuropsychological assessment of mental state. In M. Mesulam (Ed.), *Principles of behavioral and cognitive neurology* (p. 121). Oxford University Press.
Wessel, J., & Aron, A. (2017). On the globality of motor suppression: Unexpected events and their influence on behavior and cognition. *Neuron, 93*(2), 259–280. https://doi.org/10.1016/j.neuron.2016.12.013
West, C., Bowen, A., Hesketh, A., & Vail, A. (2008). Interventions for motor apraxia following stroke. *Cochrane Database of Systematic Reviews*. https://doi.org/10.1002/14651858.CD004132.pub2
Whiteside, S., Dyson, L., Cowell, P., & Varley, R. (2015). The relationship between apraxia of speech and oral apraxia: Association or dissociation? *Archives of Clinical Neuropsychology, 30*(7), 670–682. https://doi.org/10.1093/arclin/acv051
Wieloch, T., & Nikolich, K. (2006). Mechanisms of neural plasticity following brain injury *Current Opinion in Neurobiology, 16*(3), 258–264.
Wilson, P. M. (1998). information processing deficits associated with developmental coordination disorder: A meta-analysis of research findings. *Journal of Child Psychology, 39*, 829–840.
World Health Organization (WHO). (1993). *The ICD-10 classification of mental and behavioural disorders*. World Health Organization (WHO).
Worthington, A. (2016). Treatments and technologies in the rehabilitation of apraxia and action disorganisation syndrome: A review. *Neurorehabilitation, 39*(1), 163–174. https://doi.org/10.3233/NRE-161348
Xenia Lojewski, L. X.-B.-E. (2014). Human adult white matter progenitor cells are multipotent neuroprogenitors similar to adult hippocampal progenitors. *Stem Cells Translational Medicine, 3*(4), 458–469.
Yadegari, F., Azimian, M., Rahgozar, M., & Shekarchi, B. (2014). Brain areas impaired in oral and verbal apraxic patients. *Iranian Journal of Neurology, 13*(2), 77–82.
Yun, J., Shin, S., & Son, S. (2021). Clinical utility of repeated urimal test of articulation and phonation for patients with childhood apraxia of speech. *Children, 8*(12), 1–7. https://doi.org/10.3390/children8121106
Yuste, R. (2015). From the neuron doctrine to neural networks. *Nature Reviews Neuroscience, 16*, 487–497. https://doi.org/10.1038/nrn3962
Zadikoff, C. L., & Lang, A. (2005). Apraxia in movement disorders. *Brain, 128*(7), 1480–1497. https://doi.org/10.1093/brain/awh560
Zang, Z., Ping, L., Zhai, A., & Zhou, Z. (2021). Microstructural white matter abnormalities in obsessive-compulsive disorder: A coordinate-based meta-analysis of diffusion tensor imaging studies. *Asian Journal of Psychiatry, 55*, 102467. https://doi.org/10.1016/j.ajp.2020.102467
Zohary, E., Shadlen, M., & Newsome, W. (1994). Correlated neuronal discharge rate and its implications for psychophysical performance. *Nature, 370*, 140–143.
Zwicker, J. M. (2009). Neural correlates of developmental coordination disorder: A review of hypotheses. *Child Neurology, 24*, 1273–1281.

Chapter 11
Understanding Apraxia Going Forward

Perhaps the clearest thing that we can conclude is that currently the science surrounding apraxia remains largely behaviorally defined. However, as we have emphasized, this state of affairs limits the development of new clinical applications. In addition, defining things behaviorally means that we conduct research based upon their behavioral definitions, and as we have seen, these definitions lack both specificity and sensitivity when considered from a neural network perspective. Some of this rests with inconsistencies in many of the behavioral definitions for all but the most isolated apraxia (i.e., eye blink apraxia), such as apraxia and childhood apraxia of speech. The current labels merely describe the behavioral manifestation of a particular type of behavioral dysfunction.

From a neural network perspective, the current diagnostic label of apraxia is bereft of meaning past the idea that a certain complex motor function is not taking place as it should. There are presumptions related to these diagnostic labels to be sure. The presumption is that there is underlying neurological damage and, as we have seen, there is research that identifies certain areas of the brain in relation to certain types of apraxic conditions. However, despite significant gains in research and neuroimaging studies, this is insufficient to clarify the situation, that is, the specificity of the etiology of the disorder, as multiple areas of insult can result in similar behavioral disorders and, the inverse, many of these brain networks overlap several apraxic conditions. In sum, we have difficulties in the area of sensitivity of diagnostic labels for some apraxia and specificity for most.

From a mental health perspective, this should not be surprising as the totality of our current nosology is based on behaviorally classified manifestations of a disorder. We recognize that this has value in that the system provides a common language with which to discuss these issues and facilitates discussion between professionals. There is also a potential benefit emanating from the fact that these behaviorally defined clusters may represent an underlying commonality that might be identified in the future.

T. Wasserman, L. D. Wasserman, *Apraxia: The Neural Network Model*, Neural Network Model: Applications and Implications,
https://doi.org/10.1007/978-3-031-24105-5_11

From a neurological perspective, the current state of affairs reflects a great deal of informative research as compared to the original hypotheses concerning neocortex-based lesions. Nonetheless, much work remains to be done, specifically, improving specificity and sensitivity in identifying specific network dysfunction associated with specific behavioral outcomes. Despite this research, etiology remains unclear.

While it is true to say that a person with verbal apraxia has certain specific dysfunctional behaviors, it is also true to say that those behaviors could be produced by a variety of lesions to locations among the constituent networks involved in this very complex behavior. A review of the etiology of patients identified with apraxia of speech (AOS) can provide an illustration: while patients identified as having apraxia of speech (AOS), defined as an articulatory disorder, were found to have damage to the left superior precentral gyrus of the insula (Ogar et al., 2006), additional involvement of neighboring brain areas was associated with more severe forms of both AOS and related language deficits, such as aphasia. In other words, while the core of apraxia of speech might be one area, the actual variety of clinical manifestations and dysfunction is associated with other areas that are somewhat more diffusely distributed. This would make understanding the underlying network dysfunction in verbal apraxia somewhat identifiable if it were not for the fact that there have been suggestions that apraxia can be due to deep subcortical lesions, which raises the question as to whether damage to the basal ganglia or thalamus can cause apraxia as well (Pramstaller & Marsden, 1996). This, of course, makes sense given the motor components that are central to apraxic conditions.

A similar situation exists in other forms of apraxia. For example, research demonstrates that although conceptual praxis representations are stored in the left hemisphere, analysis of lesion sites does not reveal where in the left hemisphere they may be stored (Heilman et al., 1997). Thus, disruption anywhere in this complex system could produce the same output dysfunction.

The Problem of Diagnosis

We have written about what we perceive is the multiplicity of problems associated with the currently used behaviorally based diagnostic nosologies (Wasserman & Wasserman, 2016). Among our concerns is the issue of the inability of the current nosology's ability to contribute to the advance of brain behavior science, particularly neural network science. Perhaps the science surrounding the etiology of apraxia in general and developmental apraxia in specific provides one of the clearest examples of our ongoing concerns. The diagnosis and understanding of apraxia conditions have not changed much at all in the last 50 years and not enough from when it was described 100 years ago. The diagnosis of apraxia is made based upon the inability to functionally coordinate the movement or intentionality of a specific muscle group to produce a desired outcome. The gold standard for diagnosing things such as childhood apraxia of speech (CAS) remains expert judgment of perceptual features (Murray et al., 2015a). Treatment in the form of practice or muscle strengthening follows. There is no need to understand the underlying neurological/neuropsychological dysfunction although it is assumed that there is damage somewhere in the networks contributing to the final target movement.

Given what we know about apraxia, perhaps this is as good as it gets, and we do not require anything fancier. Diagnosis, after all, should inform treatment. As far as apraxia conditions are concerned, treatment is based on behavioral practice designed to encourage the automation of the desired behavior. As it stands, at the current time, from a treatment perspective, it may not be necessary to know where in a neural network the dysfunction arises, as that knowledge may not contribute to treatment. After all, if there was damage to a particular white matter network component, for example, the solution would be to foster neural plasticity by practicing functional movement anyway. The exact location or general type of insult, apart from a malignant tumor, would make little or no difference as far as treatment goes. We cannot target a specific area. We know, however, that repeated practice will, in some instances, lead to functional recovery. Perhaps this is a satisfactory circumstance as it is all that is needed for treatment. For us, this is not the case.

Our most far-reaching concern regards the failure of a behavioral system to generate research that would identify and expand our knowledge concerning how damage of dysfunction of the white matter networks that subserve function causes the problems that identify themselves for treatment. In fact, we have argued and stand by our concerns that these behavioral descriptors, which may have clinical utility, actually impede research. This concern is evident in both treatment of and research concerning ADHD. The melding of dozens of potential combinations of behavioral clusters confounds our understanding of the individual, confounds treatment medically and clinically, and confounds research secondary to a conglomeration of factors which should not be considered a unitary concept.

As we have demonstrated, multiple issues remain unresolved. Within the realm of neural networks, we do not yet know whether or how damage to different components of the same system produces the same behavioral dysfunction, let alone how damage to the different parts of the same network produces disorders that differ slightly from each other. We do not yet know if we can repair or encourage repair of damaged white matter networks, and we have little knowledge of, other than practice, how to encourage neural plasticity in order to recover function. All of this contributes to the problem of classifying disruptions of motor coordination as representing apraxia or some separate condition.

Take for example a phenomenon labeled as swallowing apraxia (Daniels, 2000). Swallowing apraxia is a disorder of lingual, labial, and mandibular coordination, which has been observed before bolus transfer during the oral stage of swallowing. It is extensively discussed in the literature on dysphagia. To date, the possible mechanisms and neural networks of swallowing apraxia have not been identified, although similarities with other apraxia are evident. Daniels (2000), in a review of the literature, identified possible similarities as greater occurrence upon command, transitive nature of the action, and evidence of spatial errors. Differences such as hemispheric lateralization and multiple gesture assessment seem to exist between swallowing apraxia and more traditional forms of apraxia. The author concludes the review by noting "until discrete error patterns of swallowing apraxia are identified and precisely measured, the nature of this disorder and its relationship with the praxis system will continue to remain elusive" (pg. 159). Similarly, Van Der Merwe (2020) states that the complexity of speech motor control and the incomplete conceptualization of phases in the transformation of the speech code from linguistic symbols to a code amenable to a motor system tend to obscure the understanding of acquired apraxia of speech (AOS). Taken together, these comments state the case succinctly. Until now, all that was necessary is for the clinician to observe the speech or swallowing difficulty. That is clearly not enough to establish whether a particular disorder is a condition of praxis or not, probably because the exact neural network basis of apraxia has not been elucidated.

Problems for Neuropsychologists

One of our major concerns as far as the future of neuropsychology is that the current practice of neuropsychology has led to a diminishing role for neuropsychologists in the treatment of many disorders. It seems that the standard of care at the current time is that many practicing neuropsychologists want to conduct an evaluation to determine if the person meets the behavioral criteria. It the person does not meet the cutoffs, there is likely no formal intervention as there is not pathology deemed present. On the other hand, when a person meets the criteria, often the best we do is refer out; I have found out that the individual is apraxic and sent them to a qualified speech and language therapist or occupational therapist. I have done my job! The situation is analogous to diagnosing a reading disorder in a child sent to us for assessment of reading difficulties noted at home or in school. We test reading level, substantiate that the child is "behind" (the parents knew that anyway; that's why they brought the child to you in the first place), and then send the child to a reading specialist for treatment. This recommendation is often unaccompanied by any information regarding what type of reading difficulties or practices the child is engaging in, how their reading is impacted, which other cognitive or academic areas may be impacted, nor, other than generic recommendations, which interventions might be appropriate for that child and why. The schools have noticed this sort of circular reasoning and have, as Response To Intervention has shown, decided that they can do without our services in many instances. The current process would appear to represent clinical practice, not science. If we continue, without being able to offer meaningful treatment intervention advice, the result for instances of apraxia will be the same as for reading; people will decide that they don't need us. We are not alone in expressing the concern that the current behaviorally based process does not represent science (McLaren, 2010; Hofmann et al., 2016). We believe we have to do better. We need to be able to tell our clients if the identified disorder is associated with other areas of noted weakness, what are the implications, and which of the numerous treatment approaches available in the marketplace have been scientifically validated. We would profit from knowing and sharing what impact there may be in, for example, associated skills or activities of daily living and types of intervention which may be useful for the particular client we have assessed.

Staying in Our Lane

Historically, the domain of neuropsychology has been cognition. Many of our tests are designed to assess cognition directly. When there is a motor component, it is most often motor speed as a reflection of cognitive processing speed or a functional assessment of a skill like handwriting. Perhaps this focus on one particular domain made sense when we believed that we could reliably assess one domain independently of the impact on other domains. Since research clearly suggests that motor networks play a role in almost all human cognitive activity, sustaining this idea no longer corresponds with what the science is telling us. As we have seen, this has implications for the assessment of functionality related to acquired apraxic conditions in terms of comorbid conditions that should be investigated. The same motor basis of complex cognition has even greater implications for the assessment of a child with childhood apraxia of speech (CAS).

As regards CAS, what the science is telling us is that there is a complex and predictable relationship between early motor integrity and later cognitive performance. This relationship is impacted by numerous factors all worth of investigation. For example, Piek et al. (2008) demonstrated that socio-economic status (SES) predicted fine motor performance and three of four cognitive domains at school age in a typically developing population. After controlling for SES, fine motor trajectory information did not account for a significant proportion of the variance in school-aged fine motor performance or cognitive performance. However, gross motor trajectory did account for a significant proportion of the variance for cognitive performance once SES was controlled for. Analysis showed a significant predictive relationship for gross motor trajectory information and the subtests of working memory and processing speed on standard psychological tests. Similarly, research has indicated that attention, fine motor skills, and general knowledge are much stronger overall predictors of later math, reading, and science scores than early math and reading scores alone (Grissmer et al., 2010). More specifically, children with CAS are at risk for persistent reading and spelling disorders in addition to their spoken communication difficulties (Gillon & Moriarty, 2007). They identify four factors that increase the risk of written language disorder in this population: (1) the nature of the speech disorder, (2) the presence of phonological awareness difficulties, (3) genetic risk factors, and (4) the negative impact of early reading difficulty on later written language development. A complete diagnostic interview can assess for these factors and aid the neuropsychologist in establishing treatment protocols. It is true that these are not test scores, but the information is just as valid. Finally, there is evidence to suggest that speech-motor programming difficulties may also contribute to reading, writing, and spelling difficulties. Children lacking the motor control to pronounce a word, either aloud or covertly, may have difficulty with segmentation tasks. Children with CAS are generally poorer spellers than children with normal articulation. These spelling deficits of the CAS group could not be attributed to an inability to pronounce words or a difficulty with phoneme-grapheme correspondences (Lewis et al., 2004). Earlier in this volume, the associated impact was addressed from the perspective of dyslexia, academic difficulties, and neurodevelopmental disorders.

Collectively, this research suggests that life course circumstances in conjunction with early motor competence will impact later higher-order cognitive functioning. The research also suggests that neuropsychologists should be conversant in assessing motor functionality early on. This is because motor function is a core component of later higher-order cognitive activity. This research also suggests that the distinction between early "developmental" assessment and later cognitive or neuropsychological assessment is arbitrary at best, reflecting limitations of test construction rather than substantial differences in what is being assessed.

Understanding Disorders from a Neural Network Perspective

Given the increasing concerns regarding the scientific utility of the current behaviorally based nosologies, there have been suggestions for alternative systems. For example, Hofmann et al. (2016) offer a complex network approach to diagnoses as an alternative to the latent disease model. This model may offer better utility for understanding the neural network components of disorders such as apraxia. According to this model, symptoms do not indicate a solitary underlying latent disease that causes their appearance and co-occurrence. Rather, the disorders are manifestations of interrelated elements of networks. Symptoms are the actual components of, not reflective, of the disorder. A disorder constitutes a network of symptoms that interact in ways that tend to sustain and reinforce themselves. For example, a stressful event does not activate an underlying entity called anxiety, which then causes the emergence of symptoms. Stressful events activate certain elements that in turn activate other elements, and when a critical mass of these elements occur, an episode of disorder may be diagnosable. They posit that "Depending on the structure of the network, change can occur abruptly once the network reaches a critical threshold (the tipping point)." This model also provides a framework for therapeutic change as "Homogeneous and highly connected networks often recover more slowly from local perturbations when the network approaches the tipping point, potentially making it possible to predict treatment change, relapse, and recovery."

Network Theory and Complex Networks

Hofmann et al. (2016) offer a comprehensive contrast and comparison of latent disease vs. complex network theory. The latent disease model will not be reviewed here as the current authors assume the reader has both training in and experience with the current working model of latent disease. To understand the newer proposal, it is necessary to understand that the origins of network theory lie a branch of mathematics, specifically a subset of graph theory. This subset is concerned with the visual representation of a set of objects and the links connecting pairs of objects. As we have discussed in our discussions of the connectome, networks contain two components: nodes representing objects (e.g., individual persons, neurons, symptoms, nations) and edges – lines that connect these two objects, thereby representing the association between them (e.g., the relationship between apples and oranges in a network of fruit). An unweighted network depicts whether two nodes are connected. A weighted network also represents the strength of the connection.

Network theory permits the computation of the importance of a particular node in the operation of a network. This is known as centrality. "A highly central node is one, when activated, is likely to spread activation throughout the network via the multiple edges connecting it to other nodes. For example, a node high on degree centrality is one with many edges connected to it (e.g., a highly popular person in a social network). A node high on strength centrality in a weighted network is one having many edges connected to it that are great in terms of their magnitude of associations (e.g., the Pearson's r of each edge is large). A node high on betweenness centrality is one that often lies on the shortest pathway between two other)" (Hofmann et al., 2016, pg. 598).

Complex networks comprise many nodes whose connections are neither random nor uniform in their connectiveness with other nodes in the network. That is, the structure of the network varies; some nodes cluster in subgroups, whereas others have few or weak connections with other nodes. Complex networks are the empirical norm in sociology, neuroscience, and psychopathology.

This network perspective directs attention to the defining features of the pathology (nodes) and their functional interconnections (edges) and away from a search for an underlying common cause of the activated elements, expressed as a sum score designed to index severity. It intends a search for mechanisms (or biomarkers) causing specific elements (e.g., failure to coordinate movement of the tongue), instead of disorders (apraxia). It does not eliminate the need of categorical diagnosis but rather adds a scientific element to it.

This neural network model views symptom heterogeneity as patterns suggestive of causal links between features of a disorder. It would enable the clinician to understand that there may be core elements (symptoms) to every disorder of a certain class while acknowledging that different features may produce different patterns of related elements or symptoms. This analysis would produce a different form of differential diagnosis and related understanding. It would look at subtypes of the core disorder based on their associated features and perhaps provide an understanding of how the component neural networks are participating in the dysfunction. Finally, this would entail a different perspective on comorbidity in that comorbidity would be looked at as shared patterns of network contribution between various disorders. Instead of diagnosing depression and anxiety as discrete disorders, this method would look at their shared properties and perhaps, along the way, identify a latent class disorder that explains them both. This is at odd with the current diagnostic system which views the significant overlap between depression and anxiety as a confound that both complicates diagnosis and muddies research.

Research Domain Criteria (RDoC) (Insel, 2014)

RDoC is a research framework designed to improve research approaches regarding mental disorders. It emanates from a discussion and the research on precision medicine which deconstructs current diagnostic groups with specific biomarkers that predict and improve treatment methodology. It integrates many levels of information (from genomics and circuits to behavior and self-report) to explore basic dimensions of functioning that span the full range of human behavior from normal to abnormal.

RDoC is not meant to replace the current diagnostic system nor does it serve as diagnostic guide. The goal, as far as psychology and neuropsychology is concerned, is to understand the nature of mental health and illness in terms of variable degrees of dysfunction across and within psychological and biological systems.

The currently in use DSM and ICD systems are diagnostic manuals and are based upon behaviorally articulated classes. There are problems in this approach. One of the primary problems is that there are very significant limitations in the scientific application of heterogeneous syndromes where the defining psychopathologies are not unique to the diagnostic class and vary within categories between cases. RDoC seeks to avoid this problem. What RDoC does, instead, is to establish a set of principles for deriving and studying biobehavioral constructs implicated in psychiatric disorders (Carpenter, 2016). The issue is not whether RDoC is an alternative diagnostic approach but whether the paradigm will promote information that informs nosology and facilitates application of brain science in clinical diagnostic concepts. The RDoC framework attempts to alert investigators to the fallacy of methods that equate diagnosis with a specific disease. Rather, researchers are encouraged to focus on psychopathology in the context of hypothesized neural circuits and behavioral constructs (Cuthbert & Insel, 2013). Clearly this approach is very much in line with the focus of this book.

The RDoC model has been used to describe motor-based language deficiencies such as apraxia (Appendix 1). It describes the sensorimotor systems involved in language apraxia as a "multifaceted construct comprising the processes that must be engaged during the planning and execution of a motor action in a context-appropriate manner. Component processes include action planning and selection, sensorimotor dynamics, initiation, execution, and inhibition and termination. Each of these components have their associated networks identified and outlined. Of note, these processes will often be recruited in conjunction with motivational processes described in other domains, as when appetitive motivations drive approach behaviors (Wasserman & Wasserman, 2020). As for developmental apraxia, the construct explicitly includes the modulation and refinement of actions during development and learning" (National Institute of Mental Health, 2022).

Recently, other researchers seeking greater clarity have proposed alternative diagnostic models for some or all apraxic conditions. For example, Baumard and Le Gall (2021) note that the diagnosis of limb apraxia relies mainly on exclusion criteria (e.g., elementary motor or sensory deficits, aphasia). This is certainly true for most apraxic conditions. That points out that the plethora of apraxia definitions and assessment methods cause different diagnostic outcomes. Specifically, patients may or may not show apraxia depending on the chosen assessment method or theory, making the definition of apraxia somewhat arbitrary. They note that, as a result, "apraxia" may be diagnosed in patients with different cognitive impairments, hypothesizing that the current situation is the result of an evolution from a task-based approach toward a process-based approach. This process approach is based on the deconstruction of the conceptual or production systems of action into multiple cognitive processes: language, executive functions, working memory, semantic memory, body schema, body image, visual-spatial skills, social cognition, visual-kinesthetic engrams, manipulation knowledge, technical reasoning, structural inference, and categorical apprehension. The fact that both these systems of diagnosis coexist in the current literature represents, in their view, a major challenge that stands in the way of a scientific definition of apraxia. To eliminate this problem, they suggest a focus on symptoms and on two complementary definition criteria (in addition with traditional exclusion criteria): specifically, is apraxia explained by the alteration of cognitive processes specifically dedicated to gesture production and consistency, as in whether the gesture production impairment is consistent across tasks. They conclude that after a century of Liepmann's demonstration of the autonomy of apraxia toward language, the autonomy of this syndrome toward the rest of cognition remains an open question and that this lack of clarity continues to pose new challenges to apraxia studies.

Diagnosing Apraxia: Why Make It Complicated?

There is an argument to be made that clinical diagnosis is a process separate and distinct from the process of researching the underlying mechanisms of a disorder of any type. This argument is as follows: Clinical and research diagnostic criteria serve different purposes. Clinical criteria should be used to diagnose referred cases and to confirm suspected cases arising from screening tests. In these situations, appropriate diagnosis and labeling is a necessity for decisions related to access to things like special education, treatment, remedial teaching, and reimbursement of costs related to services rendered by medical insurance programs. On the other hand, the use of research diagnostic criteria ensures the selection of a sample that is optimally suited for answering the research question. The sample is as free of confounds as can be achieved and independent of the source from which children are selected, the main sources being clinical referrals and screening procedures. Research diagnostic criteria should be carefully tuned to the research questions addressed (Geuze et al., 2015). This view attempts to bridge the gap between the two processes arguing that each has its place in science.

We have taken notice of what seems to be a strategic tension between applied science and basic research science. This occurs in all areas of science where both possibilities exist, and it is certainly present in neuropsychology. Basically, basic research science increases the knowledge base of a field of research while applied science uses that knowledge to solve specific problems. As regards the etiology of disease process, both positions have their supporters. It would be fair to say that the authors of the present volume are split as to the wisdom of each approach. It would also be fair to say that we have argued in the past, and will continue to advocate, for the wisdom of having basic science to inform diagnostic process.

More than 100 years ago, Joseph Henery, in his presidential address to the American Association of Science, stated "The incessant call in this country for practical results and the confounding of mechanical inventions with scientific discoveries has a very prejudicial influence on science... A single scientific principle may include a thousand applications and is therefore, though if not of immediate use, of vastly more importance even in a practical view" (Trigilio, 2013). The other position could be stated thusly: applied science is important as it enables science to be more applicable in the real life. Without it, great scientific discoveries may be limited as human knowledge will increase, but be underutilized. Every invention, medicine, and even buildings are a result of applied science. Certainly, it can be argued that neuropsychology respects both positions, but, to a large extent, much of neuropsychology is an applied science. When it comes to apraxia, as in other topics but perhaps more so here, the divide is clear. We diagnose apraxia based on an observed dysfunction of a particular motor system. Nothing more is required. Once I know that the particular system is not working correctly, all I really want to know is how to fix it.

We have seen lots of examples of this sort of thinking, and we have come to believe that it has become detrimental to neuropsychology. For example, to diagnose dyslexia we give tests of phonetic reading and reading comprehension. We "discover" that the child is "behind" based on national norms. We really don't know why, but it is not necessary because all we are going to do is refer to a reading specialist for remediation. Job is done. The same happens with speech and language deficits and motor deficits when we refer to speech and language pathologists or occupational therapists. This process ignores the obvious. In almost every instance, the referral to us for assessment was made because the parents and the school already knew the child was "behind" and they wanted to know why, which is the one thing we often fail to explain and what the current diagnostic nosologies do not require of us to know. It is sort of like telling a parent whose child is crawling that the child is in the crawling phase. They already knew that. It was logic like this, we believe, that resulted in "Response to Intervention" and the diminished importance of psychological testing in the special education process.

We believe that neuropsychologists and others must be able to say why something is happening not simply that it is just happening. We often read professional chat room or conference discussions about how long a report should be or how much information should be provided to a parent, often advocating to "keep it simple." While we agree that "length of report" does not correlate with our professional value, we strongly believe that we must provide more and better etiological information to our clients and referral sources. This is so we can continue to provide current information on effective treatment. It is insufficient merely to say that something is wrong and go to another person to fix it without telling the client what they should ask for treatment wise and why. We must do this, or we become obsolete. For example, a recent evaluation feedback explained to a parent how their child's early gross motor oddities, their diagnosed dyslexia, and their child's attention issues and spelling issues and difficulty reading math equations and slow writing output speed (previously explained to her as slow processing) were all related, helped her to an "aha" moment.

While at the current time it might be very true that the only effective treatment for apraxia is to encourage neural plasticity by providing massed practice, more effective treatment options might be available if we look for them. For example, by understanding that neural networks are at the core of the disorder, are there more effective ways of encouraging the growth and repair to these networks than simply massed practice? Can we develop ways to target network growth? Can we discover how these networks become disrupted in the first place?

We believe that neuropsychology has the potential to do this. In his review Bunge (1985) examined the three main strategies for the study of behavior and mentation: behaviorism, mentalism, and psychobiology. "Behaviorism is found wanting for eschewing most of the problems that traditional psychology posed but left unsolved." Two kinds of mentalism are distinguished: traditional and cognitivist (or information-theoretic). Both are found wanting for ignoring the nervous system and begging the question, since they postulate the mind instead of explaining it. Only the psychobiological (or neuropsychological) approach, which regards the mind as a collection of brain functions, is found promising for studying that which guides behavior and does the mentation, namely, the brain. It is also shown to have the advantage of promoting the union of psychology with biology and of bridging psychiatry to neurology, neurophysiology, and neurochemistry. It is argued that this approach is the only fully "scientific" one (pg. 115). We could not agree more. To support this process, our applied branch must incorporate more basic science into their everyday work. We believe that this is essential to establish and maintain our credibility with our client and referral base.

Assess It All: Downstream and Upstream Impact of Network Disruption

We have suggested at several points that disruptions of a neural network affect not only the target or most observable behavior but potentially all other aspects of behavioral function dependent on that network component. That implies functions that are part of the network related to the target behavior (i.e., apraxia of speech) but also other functions that rely on recruiting the impacted network. So, let's provide an example to illustrate. Damage to dominant dorsolateral prefrontal cortex has been reported to cause disordered speech motor control because of disrupted planning and programming of articulatory performance (anarthria or apraxia of speech). However, more recent data provide some evidence that apraxia of speech may be caused by dysfunction of the dominant anterior insula (Riecker et al., 2005). So, it is clear that damage to this area causes disruption in the planning, pacing, and timing of speech to be sure, but what other cognitive functions might we reasonably expect to be impacted? It turns out that there are quite a few. Lesions of the dorsolateral PFC (DLPFC), consisting of Brodmann areas (BA) 9 and 46, can result in deficits across a wide range of functions, including working memory, rule-learning, planning, attention, and motivation (Szczepanski & Knight, 2014). In other words, if you are assessing for apraxia based on observation of speech production and you find it, you would be very judicious to consider the fact that your client may have had disruption of function, to some degree, in all those areas as well, and that treatment might be much more extensive than it initially appeared. Given the number of systems involved in most apraxic conditions (see Appendix 1 for an example), expectations like this should be the rule rather than the exception. Indeed, just diagnosing the apraxia may be doing an injustice to your client.

The Case for a Separate Diagnosis for Childhood Apraxia of Speech

As we have discussed, there are significant differences functionally and etiologically between childhood (developmental) apraxia of speech (CAS) and its adult counterpart. On an operational level, not initiating speech is not initiating speech; therefore they are both apraxia.

However, there is research that clearly indicates that the network operation that leads to the production of speech changes across the developmental course. There is also a lack of consensus as to what causes developmental apraxia in the first place. Indeed, multiple etiologies have been identified (Maassen, 2015). Whereas adult-onset apraxia conditions are caused by brain insult of identifiable origin, the great preponderance of childhood apraxia is not. Multiple genetic contributors, white matter developmental issues, and environmental issues have all been identified as contributing to the development of childhood apraxia of speech. A summary of the arguments describing the differences between adult and childhood apraxia has been provided by Maassen (2015). He notes that dissociation, or more importantly double dissociation, does not apply to developmental disorders. Double dissociation is the ideal neuropsychological/cognitive neuroscience evidentiary standard in the study of acquired disorders in adults. Double dissociation is when two related mental processes are shown to be functionally independent of each other. A clear example of double dissociation related to speech and language occurs when examining damage to the Broca's area and Wernicke's area in adults. When Broca's area is damaged, affected patients may still understand language, but be unable to speak fluently. They know what they want to say but are unable to say it. When Wernicke's area is damaged, patients may still speak fluently, but be unable to understand language. This results in properly constructed but nonsensical sentences (AlleyDog.com, 2022). There are multiple reasons for the failure to demonstrate double dissociation in children, but the primary one is that a disruption in language development in a developing child will affect the development and emergence of other functions and skills in the future that partly depend on this function being intact in the first place. In developmental disorders, it is more common to identify associations between functions rather than dissociations (Karmiloff-Smith et al., 2003).

A second difference between childhood and adult apraxia is that research suggests that speech and language production during infancy and early childhood can be characterized by a more simplified model, consisting of fewer processing stages than what is seen with the full-fledged adult system (Maassen, 2002). At the earliest stage of speech development, children have at their disposition a restricted set of articulatory forms the size of a syllable. At a later developmental stage, under the communicative pressure of the growing vocabulary, the phonological system expands and takes advantage of the more productive phonological combination rules of the adult system. As a result, a word forms lexicon and a phonological encoding system develops (Levelt et al., 1999). These differences have major implications for treatment planning and intervention purposes. In therapy for AOS in an adult population, higher-level psycholinguistic, phonological, skills have been acquired prior to the injury and can be utilized to facilitate treatment. As a result, use can be made of their linguistic knowledge, of written material, for instance, and the treatment can appeal to available syntactic, lexical, and phonological skills. In therapy with children, many of these skills have not yet developed, and as a result, no previously acquired or less stable higher-level knowledge is available. These very skills must be acquired by the child via the problematic speech production and perception networks. This implies that more explicit attention during therapy must be devoted to these higher-level skills, which otherwise do not emerge.

Genetics

Perhaps the most compelling argument for separating the diagnosis of childhood apraxia of speech from the other adult apraxia is the etiology argument. While adult-onset apraxia are almost entirely a function of brain insult, childhood apraxia is a neurodevelopmental disorder frequently caused by genetic mutations. Indeed, clinical MRI scans fail to reveal overt neural anomalies in individual cases with CAS (Morgan & Webster, 2018). Genetic causes include both de novo genetic conditions and familial inherited conditions. Research findings support the likelihood of heterogeneous genomic pathways associated with childhood apraxia of speech. In addition to the well-known FOXP2 mutation, at least ten chromosomes have been identified as involved in childhood apraxia, several of which have two or three candidate sites. In some instances, multiple copy variations occur on more than one chromosome in the same individual (Laffin et al., 2012).

CAS is a complex disorder, defined as a higher-order motor system deficit of motor planning and programming. More specifically, motor planning involves transforming abstract sound representations into speech-motor goals or commands, and it also involves further specifying the specific movement or acoustic parameters within each articulator for speech production. There is general consensus regarding three core diagnostic features for CAS: (I) inconsistent speech errors (e.g., producing the same syllable or word differently across repetitions of the same word), (2) lengthened and disrupted co-articulatory transitions (e.g., oral groping during speech; difficulty sequencing sounds and syllables, including frequent omissions of sounds in some cases; marked vowel errors; or hypernasality due to poor online planning and programming of velum (palatal) movements for denoting oral/nasal contrasts); and (3) inappropriate prosody (e.g., disrupted rhythm and intonation of speech, such as placing stress on a typically unstressed syllable of a word or placing equal stress across all syllables). A CAS diagnosis is based on differentiating the speech presentation from other developmental speech impairments of articulation disorder, phonological disorder, stuttering, or dysarthria. In addition, CAS often occurs in association with other neurodevelopmental conditions, such as epilepsy, intellectual disability, motor impairment, and autism.

There appear to be clear and significant differences between childhood and adult apraxia in etiology, network operation, and treatment methodology that would be obscured by incorporating them together under one general behaviorally based descriptor.

The Problem of Treatment

Currently, the treatment of all apraxic conditions is based on the idea that massed practice of the desired skill outcome will, by dint of neural plasticity, couple in the case of CAS with continued development and produce a repair or acquisition in the case of CAS of language function. When it comes to childhood apraxia of speech, statements like this are common: for children with suspected CAS, or children who have been identified with planning and sequencing issues, approaches that target motor learning principles such as mass and distributed practice, concrete stepped learning with high intensity, and functional lexicons that have noncomplex motor movements are now being recommended (Dale & Hayden, 2013). These approaches consider speech production to be a motor skill like any other human (fine) motor skill; it is learned following repeated practice under certain conditions. The authors go on to state that a wide range of treatment approaches have been proposed for CAS, although little rigorous evaluation research has been conducted and no comparative studies have been reported. The situation for most other apraxic conditions is the same.

It is difficult to believe that we have reached a permanent state of the art in terms of treatment for apraxia. It is likely that we will not reach beyond this condition if we retain the current diagnostic model and its implications. In fact, it is incumbent upon neuropsychologists, as well as other disciplines, to keep abreast and integrate information from these other disciplines. As mentioned throughout this volume, genetics and neuroimaging are fields with increasingly applicable findings. Much information from neuroimaging has been allowing for an increasing and more comprehensive understanding of how systems in the connectome interact and are impacted by disorders or trauma. Genetics may prove to be not only diagnostic but to have rehabilitative components. The information provided elsewhere in this volume is of specific relevance. That is, for example, research into using adult neural progenitor cells for clinical application, specifically as a source of autologous cell replacement for neurologic diseases such as Parkinson's, trauma such as stroke, and cell-based gene therapy for neurometabolic diseases (Xenia Lojewski, 2014).

"Testing" for Apraxia

Apraxia is diagnosed based on behavioral disorder, and, as a result, behavioral assessment is required. Specifically, assessment of motor functioning is required. Currently neuropsychological testing instruments are not designed to pick up apraxia. They may pick up comorbid conditions, and, from a network perspective, this would be a great step forward toward demonstrating the interplay of the various neural networks in a specific individual if the results were understood in this way.

This inability of current neuropsychological tests to assess apraxia should not be disconcerting to the practicing neuropsychologist. Neuropsychology practice is not synonymous with neuropsychological tests. It represents knowledge about how the brain functions to produce behavior, and this functioning can be assessed in many ways. Standard neurological assessment includes assessment of neural functioning based on specific behavioral responses to stimuli. We suggest that it would probably be wise to expand the training of neuropsychologists to include this methodology as part of their toolkit.

All of this presupposes that it is the neuropsychologist who is doing the observing of the responses. It should be clear that normative test data, as it is currently comprised, will not be able to assess for apraxia and that the diagnosis for the foreseeable future will be based on the assessment of observed behavior. To observe it, you have to be there, and by implication, that means that you do not allocate the assessment process to a technician. We have no wish to wade into the ongoing discussion about the wisdom of utilizing technicians to collect certain data. We will report to you that, especially because we are pediatric neuropsychologists, we do not use them. We passionately believe that the observations we make on the behavior of the children we assess provide a critical and irreplaceable source of information. It is our practice to meet the youngsters coming for evaluation in the waiting room. We walk behind them as they walk toward the clinician's office. This practice was how one of us caught the little boy somewhat dragging his right foot, not too blatantly, but enough for the parents to have reported that they had asked pediatrician about it. Ot the little boy who descending the stairs after the eval was noted to hold on to the bannister and use his foot to feel the edge of the steps before descending. In the case of apraxia, perhaps especially apraxia of speech, these observations are invaluable. As far as assessments for apraxia are concerned, observation of behavior is the only way that a neuropsychologist, neurologist, speech pathologist, or occupational therapist is going to do to obtain the data necessary to make the diagnosis.

To go a step further, we suggest that the clinician conducting the assessment understands the neural network implications of the behavior that they are observing. In this way, they are more likely to understand the extended network implications of what they are seeing and speak authoritatively helpfully about the various comorbid conditions that might reasonably be expected. And perhaps, that is the clearest point this volume aspired to.

References

Ahel, I., Rass, U., El-Khamisy, S., Katyal, S., Celements, P., Mckinnon, P., Caldecott, K. W., & West, S. (2006). The neurodegenerative disease protein aprataxin resolves abortive DNA ligation intermediates. *Nature, 443(7112)*, 713–716. https://doi.org/10.1038/nature05164

AlleyDog.com. (2022). *Double dissociation*. Retrieved from AlleyDog.com.: https://alleydog.com/glossary/definition.php?term=Double+Dissociation

Allison, K. C.-S. (2020). Differential diagnosis of apraxia of speech in children and adults: A scoping view. *Journal of Speech, Language, and Hearing Research, 63*(9), 2952–2994.

American Speech Hearing Association. (2022). Retrieved from Childhood Apraxia of Speech: http://ASHA.org

American Speech-Language-Hearing Association. (2007). *Childhood apraxia of speech (Position Statement)*. Retrieved from American Speech-Language-Hearing Association. Asha.org/policy

Andres, E. E. (2022). Family based whole exome Analysis of Specific Language Impairment identifies rare variants in BUD13, a component of the retention and splicing complex. *Brain Sciences, 12*, 47.

Armstrong, P. (2010). *Bloom's taxonomy*. Retrieved from Vanderbilt University Center for Teaching. https://cft.vanderbilt.edu/guides-sub-pages/blooms-taxonomy/.

ASHA. (2007). *Childhood apraxia of speech technical report*. American Speech and Language Association.

ASHA. (2021). *Childhood apraxia of speech*. Retrieved from ASHA/Practice Portal/Clinical Topics/. https://www.asha.org/practice-portal/clinical-topics/childhood-apraxia-of-speech/

Ayres, J. (1972). Types of sensory integrative dysfunction among disabled learners. *American Journal of Occupational Therapy, 26*(*1*), 13–18.

Bak, T. H. (2012). What wires together dies together: Verbs, actions and neurodegeneration in motor neuron disease. *Cortex, 48*(*7*), 936–944.

Baldassare, A., Lewis, C., Committeri, G., Snyder, A. Z., Romani, G. L., & Corbetta, M. (2012). Individual variability in functional connectivity predicts performance of a perceptual task. *Proceedings of the National Academy of Science U. S. A., 109*, 3516–3521.

Ballard, K., Tourville, J., & Robin, D. (2014, November 3). Behavioral, computational, and neuroimaging studies of acquired apraxia of speech. *Frontiers in Human Neuroscience*. https://doi.org/10.3389/fnhum.2014.00892

Bangert, M., Peschel, T., Schlaug, G., Rotte, M., Drescher, D., Hinrichs, H., Heinze, H. J., & Altenmüller, E. (2006). Shared networks for auditory and motor processing in professional pianists: Evidence from fMRI conjunction. *Neuroimage, 30*, 917–926.

Barrios, J., Weng, W., England, R., Reifenberg, E., & Douglass, A. (2020). Hypothalamic dopamine neurons control sensorimotor behavior by modulating brainstem premotor nuclei in zebrafish. *Current Biology, 30(23)*, 4606–4619. https://doi.org/10.1016/j.cub.2020.09.002

Basso, A., Luzzatti, C., & Spinler, H. (1980). Is ideomotor apraxia the outcome of damage to well-defined regions of the left hemisphere? *Journal of Neurology, Neurosurgery, and Psychiatry, 43*, 118–126.

Batista-García-Ramó, K., & Fernández-Verdecia, C. (2018). What we know about the brain structure–function relationship. *Behavioral Sciences, 8(4), 39*. https://doi.org/10.3390/bs8040039

Baumard, J., & Le Gall, D. (2021). The challenge of apraxia: Toward an operational definition? *Cortex, 141*, 55–80. https://doi.org/10.1016/j.cortex.2021.04.001

Belanger, S., Duffy, R., & Coelho, D. (1996). The Assessment of limb apraxia: An investigation of task effects and their cause. *Brain and Cognition, 32*(3), 384–404. https://doi.org/10.1006/brcg.1996.0072

Bernstein, N. (2003). *Contemporary studies on the physiology of the neural process*. Smysl.

Bickel, W. (2012). Are executive function and impulsivity antipodes? A conceptual reconstruction with special reference to addiction. *Psychopharmacology (Berl), 221*(3), 361–387. https://doi.org/10.1007/s00213-012-2689-x

Bieńkiewicz, M., Brandi, M. G., Hughes, C., & Hermsdörfer, J. (2014, April 23). The tool in the brain: Apraxia in ADL. Behavioral and neurological correlates of apraxia in daily living. *Frontiers in Psycholology*. https://doi.org/10.3389/fpsyg.2014.00353, online.

Binkofsky, F., Kunesch, E., Classen, J., Seitz, R., & Freund, H. (2001). Tactile apraxia: Unimodal apractic disorder of tactile object exploration associated with parietal lobe lesions. *Rain, 124*(1), 132–144. https://doi.org/10.1093/brain/124.1.132

Bootsma, J., Caljouw, S., Veldman, M., Maurits, N., Rothwell, J., & Hortobágyi, T. (2021). Neural correlates of motor skill learning are dependent on both age and task difficulty. *Frontiers in Aging Neuroscience, 22*. https://doi.org/10.3389/fnagi.2021.643132

Brazelton, T. B., & Nugent, J. K. (2011). *The neonatal behavioral assessment scale*. Mac Keith Press, Cambridge.

Brennan, B., Wang, D., Li, M., Perriello, C. R., Elias, J., Van Kirk, N., et al. (2019). Use of an individual-level approach to identify cortical connectivity biomarkers in obsessive-compulsive disorder. *Biological Psychiatry: Cognitive Neuroscience and Neuroimaging, 4*(1), 27–38. https://doi.org/10.1016/j.bpsc.2018.07.014

Bunge, M. (1985). From mindless neuroscience and brainless psychology to neuropsychology. In K. Madsen & L. Mos (Eds.), *Annals of theoretical psychology* (pp. 115–133). Springer. https://doi.org/10.1007/978-1-4613-2487-4_7

Bush, G. (2010). Attention-deficit/hyperactivity disorder and attention networks. *Neuropsychopharmacology, 35*(1), 278–300. https://doi.org/10.1038/npp.2009.120

Cabrero, F., & De Jesus, O. (2021, August 30). *Apraxia of lid opening*. Retrieved from National Library of Medicine: https://www.ncbi.nlm.nih.gov/books/NBK560542/

Cantagallo, A., Maini, M., & Rumiati, R. (2013). The cognitive rehabilitation of limb apraxia in patients with stroke. *Neuropsychological Rehabilitation, 22(3)*, 473–488.

Carpenter, W. (2016). The RDoC controversy: Alternate paradigm. *American Journal of Psychiatry, 173(6), 562*–563. https://doi.org/10.1176/appi.ajp.2016.16030347

Carrera, E., & Tononi, D. (2014). Diaschisis: Past, present, future. *Brain, 137*(9), 2408–2422. https://doi.org/10.1093/brain/awu101

Cassidy, A. (2016). The clinical assessment of apraxia. *Practical Neurology, 16*, 317–322.

Chatterjeea, D., Hegdeb, S., & Thaut, M. (2021). Neural plasticity: The substratum of music-based interventions in neurorehabilitation. *NeuroRehabilitation, 48*, 155–166. https://doi.org/10.3233/NRE-208011

Chaytor, N., & Schmitter-Edgecombe, M. (2003). The ecological validity of neuropsychological tests: A review of the literature on everyday cognitive skills. *Neuropsychology Review, 13*(4), 181–187.
Childhood Apraxia of Speech. (2022). Retrieved from American Speech-Language Hearing Association: ASHA.ORG
Churchland, M. M., & Shenoy, K. V. (2007). Temporal complexity and heterogeneity of single-neuron activity in premotor and motor cortex. *Journal of Neurophysiology, 97*, 4235–4257.
Chvatal, S., & Ting, L. (2012). Voluntary and reactive recruitment of locomotor muscle synergies during perturbed walking. *The Journal of Neuroscience, 32*(35), 12237–12250. https://doi.org/10.1523/JNEUROSCI.6344-11.2012
Cleaton, A. T.-S., Tal-Saban, M., Hill, E. L., & Kirby, A. (2021). Gender and age differences in the presentation of at-risk or probable Developmental Coordination Disorder in adults. *Research in Developmental Disabilities., 115*, 104010. https://doi.org/10.1016/j.ridd.2021.104010
Coe, B., Witherspoon, K., Rosenfeld, J., & al., e. (2014). Refining analyses of copy number variation identifies specific genes associated with developmental delay. *Nature Genetics, 46*, 1053–1017.
Cogan, D. (1952). A type of congenital ocular motor apraxia presenting jerky head movements. *Transactions - American Academy of Ophthalmology and Otolaryngology, 56*, 579–588.
Conterno, M., Kümmerer, D., Dressing, A., Glauche, V., Urbach, H., Weiler, C., & Rijntjes, R. (2021). Speech apraxia and oral apraxia: Association or dissociation? A multivariate lesion–symptom mapping study in acute stroke patients. *Experimental Brain Research*. https://doi.org/10.1007/s00221-021-06224-3
Cooper, R. (2007). Tool use and related errors in ideational apraxia: The quantitative simulation of patient error profiles. *Cortex, 43*(*3*), 319–337.
Cousins, M. S. (2003). Developmental coordination impairments in adulthood. *Human Movement Science, 22*, 433–459. https://doi.org/10.1016/j.humov.2003.09.003
Cunningham, A. C. (2019). Coordination difficulties, IQ and psychopathology in children with high-risk copy number variants. *Psychological Medicine, 51*, 290–299. https://doi.org/10.1017/S0033291719003210
Cuthbert, B., & Insel, T. (2013). Toward the future of psychiatric diagnosis: The seven pillars of RDoC. *BMC Medicine, 11*, 126–133.
Dabul, B. (2000). *Apraxia battery for adults - Second edition*. Pro-ed.
Dale, P., & Hayden, D. (2013). Treating speech subsystems in childhood: Apraxia of speech with tactual input: The PROMPT approach. *American Journal of Speech-Language Pathology, 22*, 644–661. https://doi.org/10.1044/1058-0360(2013/12-0055)
Dale, P., & Hayden, D. (2014). Treating speech subsystems in childhood apraxia of speech with tactual input: The PROMPT approach. *American Journal of Speech-Language Pathology*, 644–661. https://doi.org/10.1044/1058-0360(2013/12-0055)
Daniels, S. (2000). Swallowing apraxia: A disorder of the praxis system? *Dysphagia, 15*, 159–166. https://doi.org/10.1007/s004550010019
Darley, F. (1967). Lacunae and research approaches to them. In C. Miliken & F. Darley (Eds.), *Brain mechanisms underlying speech and language*. Grune & Stratton.
Davis, B., Jakielski, K., & Marquardt, T. (1998). Developmental apraxia of speech: Determiners of differential diagnosis. *Clinical Linguistics & Phonetics, 12*, 25–45. https://doi.org/10.3109/02699209808985211
De Renzi, E., & Faglioni, P. (1999). Apraxia. In G. Denes & L. Pizzamiglio (Eds.), *Handbook of clinical and experimental psychiatry*. Psychology Press. https://doi.org/10.4324/9781315791272
De Renzi, E., & Lucchelli, F. (1988). Ideational apraxia. *Brain, 111*(5), 1173–1185. https://doi.org/10.1093/brain/111.5.1173
Delaney, A. L., & Kent, R. D. (2004). Developmental profiles of children diagnosed with apraxia of speech. *The annual convention of the American-Speech-Language-Hearing Association. Poster.* American-Speech-Language-Hearing Association.

Dewey, D. T. (2019). Very preterm children at risk for developmental coordination disorder have brain alterations in motor areas. *Acta Paediatrica, 108*(9), 1649. https://doi.org/10.1111/apa.14786

Donkervoort, M.-S., & Deelman, B. (2000). Prevalence of apraxia among patients with a first left hemisphere stroke in rehabilitation centres and nursing homes. *Clinical Rehabilitation, 14*(2), 130–136.

Duffy, J. (2006). Apraxia of Speech in degenerative neurologic disease. *Aphasiology, 20*, 511–527.

Duffy, J. J. (2012). The diagnosis and understanding of apraxia of speech: Why including neurodegenerative etiologies may be important. *Journal of Speech, Language and Hearing Research, 55*(5), S1518–S1522. https://doi.org/10.1044/1092-4388(2012/11-0309)

Duménieu, M., Marquèze-Pouey, B., Russier, M., & Debanne, D. (2021). Mechanisms of plasticity in subcortical visual areas. *Cells, 10*(11), 3162. https://doi.org/10.3390/cells10113162

Dumont, C., Ska, B., & Joanette, Y. (2000). Conceptual apraxia and semantic memory deficit in Alzheimer's disease: Two sides of the same coin? *Journal of the International Neuropsychological Society, 6*(6), 693–703. https://doi.org/10.1017/S1355617700666079

Edelman, G., & Gally, J. (2001). Degeneracy and Complexity in Biological Systems. *Proceedings of the National Academy of Sciences, 98*(*24*), 13763–13768.

Einspieler, C. P. (2021). Fetal movements; the origin of human behaviour. *Developmental Medicine & Child Neurology, 63*(*10*), 1142–1148.

Evarts, E. V. (1868). Relation of pyramidal tract activity to force exerted during voluntary movement. *Journal of Neurophysiology, 31*, 14–27.

Farah, M. J., O'Reilly, R. C., & Vecera, S. P. (1993). Dissociated overt and covert recognition as an emergent property of a lesioned neural network. *Psychological Review, 100*(*4*), 571–588. https://doi.org/10.1037/0033-295X.100.4.571

Feldman, A. G., & Levin, M. F. (1995). Positional frames of reference in motor control: Their origin and use. *Behavioral and Brain Sciences, 18*, 723–806.

Fernandes, W. S.-P. (2016). Motor coordination correlates with academic achievement and cognitive function in children. *Frontiers in Psychology*. https://doi.org/10.3389/fpsyg.2016.00318

Fogassi, L., Ferrari, P., Gesierich, B., Rozzi, S., Chersi, F., & Rizzolatti, G. (2005). Parietal lobe: From action organization to intention understanding. *Science, 308*, 662–667.

Foki, T., Vanbellingen, C. T., Pirker, A. L., Bohlhalter, S., Nyffeler, T., Kraemmer, J., et al. (2016). Limb-kinetic apraxia affects activities of daily living in Parkinson's disease: A multi-center study. *European Journal of Neurology, 23*(8), 1301–1307. https://doi.org/10.1111/ene.13021

Fornito, A., Zalesky, A., & Breakspear, M. (2015). The connectomics of brain disorders. *Nature Reviews | Neuroscience, 16*, 150–172.

French, M., Cohen, M., Pohlig, R., & Reisman, D. (2021). Fluid cognitive abilities are important for learning and retention of a new, explicitly-learned walking pattern in individuals after stroke. *Neurorehabilitation Neural Repair, 35*(5), 419–430. https://doi.org/10.1177/15459683211001025

Friedman, N., Hatoum, A., Gustavson, D., Corley, R., Hewitt, J., & Young, S. (2020). Executive functions and impulsivity are genetically distinct and independently predict psychopathology: Results from two adult twin studies. *Clinical Psychological Science, 8*(3), 519–536. https://doi.org/10.1177/2167702619898814

Fu, X., Zhou, G., Zhuang, J., Xu, C., Zhou, H., Peng, Y., et al. (2021). White matter injury after intracerebral hemorrhage. *Frontiers in Neurology, 12, 562090*. https://doi.org/10.3389/fneur.2021.562090

Fulceri, F., Grossi, E., Contaldo, A., Narzisa, A., Apicella, F., Parrini, I., et al. (2019). Motor skills as moderators of core symptoms in autism spectrum disorders: Preliminary data from an exploratory analysis with artificial neural networks. *Frontiers in Psychology, 9, 2683*. https://doi.org/10.3389/fpsyg.2018.02683

Fuster, J. (1997). Network memory. *Trends in Neuroscience, 20*(10), 451–459. https://doi.org/10.1016/S0166-2236(97)01128-4

Gaines, R. C. (2008). Clinical expression of developmental coordination disorder in a large Canadian family. *Paediatrics and Child Health, 13*, 763–768.

Gainotti, G., & Trojano, L. (2018). Chapter 16 - Constructional apraxia. In G. Vallar & H. Coslett (Eds.), *Handbook of clinical neurology* (Vol. 151, pp. 331–348). Elsevier. https://doi.org/10.1016/B978-0-444-63622-5.00016-4

Gallego, J., Perich, M., Naufel, S., Ethier, C., Solla, S., & Miller, E. (2018). Cortical population activity within a preserved neural manifold underlies multiple motor behaviors. *Nature Communication, 9*, 4233. https://doi.org/10.1038/s41467-018-06560-z

Galvan, A. (2010). Neural plasticity of development and learning. *Human Brain Mapping, 31*(6), 879–890. https://doi.org/10.1002/hbm.21029

Ganguly, J., & Jog, M. (2020). Tauopathy and movement disorders—unveiling the chameleons and mimics. *Frontiers in Neurology: Movement Disorders, 11, 599384*. https://doi.org/10.3389/fneur.2020.599384

Garibotto, V., Scifo, P., Gorini, A., Alonso, C., Brambati, S., Bellodi, L., & Perani, D. (2010). Disorganization of anatomical connectivity in obsessive compulsive disorder: A multi-parameter diffusion tensor imaging study in a subpopulation of patients. *Neurobiology of Disease, 37*(2), 468–476. https://doi.org/10.1016/j.nbd.2009.11.003

Gerstner, W., Kistler, W., Naud, R., & Paninsk, L. (2014). Neuronal populations. In W. Gerstner, W. Kistler, R. Naud, & L. Paninsk (Eds.), *Neuronal dynamics from single neurons to networks and models of cognition* (pp. 291–322). Cambridge University Press.

Geuze, R., Shoemaker, M., & Smits-Engelsman, B. (2015). Clinical and research criteria for developmental coordination disorder—Should they be one and the same? *Current Developmental Disorders Reports, 2*, 127–130. https://doi.org/10.1007/s40474-015-0043-9

Gillon, G., & Moriarty, B. (2007). Childhood apraxia of speech: Children at risk for persistent reading and spelling disorder. *Seminars in Speech and Language, 28*(1), 48–57. https://doi.org/10.1055/s-2007-967929

Giovannetti, T., Libon, D., Buxbaum, L., & Schwartz, M. (2002). Naturalistic action impairments in dementia. *Neuropsychologia, 40*, 1220–1232.

Gold, L., & Lauritzen, M. N. (2002). Neuronal deactivisation explains decreased cerebellar blood flow in response to focal cerebral ischemia or suppressed neocortical function. *Proceedings of the National Academy of Science USA, 99*, 7699–7704.

Gomez, M., McCabe, P., & Purcell, A. (2022). A survey of the clinical management of childhood apraxia of speech in the United States and Canada. *Journal of Communication Disorders, 96*, 106193. https://doi.org/10.1016/j.jcomdis.2022.106193

Gonzales-Rothi, L., & Heilman, K. (1996). Liepmann (1900 and 1905): A definition of apraxia and a model of praxis. In I. C. Code, Y. Joanette, A. Roch- Lecours, & C. Wallesch (Eds.), *Classic cases in neuropsychology*. Psychology Press.

Goyen, T. (2005). Motor dysfunction in apparently normal high-risk children. *Academia.edu*. https://www.academia.edu/27667038/Motor_dysfunction_in_apparently_normal_high_risk_children

Green, D. C. (2008). Does subtype of developmental coordination disorder Count: Is there a differential effect on outcome following intervention? *Human Movement Science*. https://doi.org/10.1016/j.humov.2008.02.009

Grissmer, G., Grimm, K., Aiyer, S., Murrah, W., & Steele, J. (2010). Fine motor skills and early comprehension of the world: Two new school readiness indicators. *Developmental Psychology, 46*(5), 1008–1017. https://doi.org/10.1037/a0020104

Gross, R., & Grossman, M. (2008). Update on apraxia. *Current Neurology and Neuroscience Reports, 8*(6), 490–496. https://doi.org/10.1007/s11910-008-0078-y

Guyette, T. W., & Diedrich, W. M. (1981). A critical review of developmental apraxia of speech. *Speech and Language, 5*, 1–49.

Hale, J., Alfonso, V., Berninger, V., Bracken, B., Christo, C., Clark, E., et al. (2010). Critical issues in response-to-intervention, comprehensive evaluation, and specific learning disabilities identification and intervention: An expert white paper commodus. *Learning Disability Quarterly, 33*(*3*), 223–238.

Hamilton, J., Haaland, K., Adair, J., & Brandt, J. (1993). Ideomotor limb apraxia in Huntington's disease: Implications for corticostriate involvement. *Neuropsychologia., 41*, 614–621.

Handiru, V., Alivar, A., Hoxa, A., Saleh, S., Suviseshamuthu, E. S., Yue, G. H., & Allexandre, D. (2021). Graph-theoretical analysis of EEG functional connectivity during balance perturbation in traumatic brain injury: A pilot study. *Human Brain Mapping, 14(42)*, 4427–4447. https://doi.org/10.1002/hbm.25554

Harrowell, I. H. (2017). Mental health outcomes of developmental coordination disorder in late adolescence. *Developmental Medicine & Child Neurology, 59(9)*, 973–979.

Hayden, D., Eigen, J., Walker, A., & Olsen, L. (2010). Prompt: A tactually grounded model for the treatment of childhood in speech production disorders. In L. Williams, S. McCleod, & R. McCauley (Eds.), *Treatment for speech sound disorders in children* (pp. 453–474). Brooks.

Hazy, T. F. (2007). Towards an executive without a homunculus: computational models of the prefrontal cortex/basal ganglia system. *Philosophical Transactions of the Royal Society B: Biological Sciences, 362*, 1601–1613.

HealthLine. (2022). *What's the treatment for apraxia of speech?* Retrieved from Healthline: https://www.healthline.com/health/apraxia-of-speech#treatment

Heilman, K., Rothi, L., & Valenstein, E. (1982). Two forms of ideomotor apraxia. *Neurology, 32, 342–346.*

Heilman, K., Maher, L., Greenwald, M., & Rothi, L. (1997). Conceptual apraxia from lateralized lesions. *Neurology, 49(2)*, 457. https://doi.org/10.1212/WNL.49.2.457

van den Heuvel, M., & Sporns, O. (2013). Network hubs in the human brain. *Trends in Cognitive Sciences, 17*(12), 683–696. https://doi.org/10.1016/j.tics.2013.09.012

Hildebrand, M. J. (2020). Severe childhood speech disorder. *Neurology, 94*, 2148–2167.

Hofmann, S., Curtiss, J., & McNally, R. (2016). A complex network perspective on clinical science. *Perspectives in Psychological Science, 11*(5), 597–605. https://doi.org/10.1177/1745691616639283

Holtmaat, A., & Svoboda, K. (2009). Experience-dependent structural synaptic plasticity in the mammalian brain. *National Review Neuroscience., 10*, 647–658.

Honey, C. J., & Sporns, O. (2008). Dynamical consequences of lesions in cortical networks. *Human Brain Mapping, 29*, 802–809.

Honey, C., Sporns, O., Cammoun, G. X., Thiran, J., et al. (2009). Predicting human resting-state functional connectivity from structural connectivity. *Proceedings of the National Academy of Science USA, 106*, 2035–2040.

Hua, J. W. (2022). Early motor milestones in infancy and later motor impairments: A population-based data linkage study. *Psychiatry*. https://doi.org/10.3389/fpsyt.2022.809181

Humphrey, D. R., & Thompson, W. D. (1970). Predicting measures of motor performance from multiple cortical spike trains. *Science, 170(7)*, 758–762.

Huth, A., De Heer, W. A., Griffiths, T. L., Theunissen, F. E., & Gallant, J. L. (2016). Natural speech reveals the semantic maps that tile human cerebral cortex. *Nature, 532*(7600), 453–459. https://doi.org/10.1038/nature17637

Insel, T. (2014). The NIMH Research Domain Criteria (RDoC) project: Precision medicine for psychiatry. *The American Journal of Psychiatry, 171*(4), 395–397. https://doi.org/10.1176/appi.ajp.2014.14020138

Iuzzini, J. (2012a). *Inconsistency of speech in children with childhood apraxia of speech, phonological disorders and typical speech.* Indiana University.

Iuzzini, J. (2012b). *Inconsistency of speech in children with childhood apraxia of speech, phonological disorders, and typical speech.* Indiana University ProQuest Dissertations Publishing.

Iuzzini-Seigel, J. M. (2017). Speech assessment in children with childhood apraxia of speech. In *Perspectives of the ASHA Special Interest Groups* (pp. 47–60). American Speech Language Hearing Association.

Iuzzini-Siegel, J. H. (2017). Speech inconsistency in children with childhood apraxia of speech, language impairment and speech delay: Depends on the stimuli. *Journal of Speech, Language, and Hearing Research, 60*, 1194–1220.

Johansen-Berg, H., Dawes, H., Guy, C., Smith, S. M., Wade, D. T., & Matthews, P. M. (2002). Correlation between motor improvements and altered fMRI activity after rehabilitative therapy. *Brain, 125*, 2731–2742. https://doi.org/10.1093/brain/awf282

Johansson, B. (2004). Functional and cellular effects of environmental enrichment after experimental brain infarcts. *Restorative Neuroscience, 22*, 163–174.

Karmiloff-Smith, A., Scerif, G., & Ansari, D. (2003). Double dissociations in developmental disorders? Theoretically misconceived, empirically dubious. *Cortex, 39*, 161–163.

Kelley, A., Shiltz, C., & Landry, C. (2005). Neural systems recruited by drug- and food-related cues: Studies of gene activation in corticolimbic regions. *Physiology & Behavior, 86*(1–2), 11–14. https://doi.org/10.1016/j.physbeh.2005.06.018

Kertes, A., & Ferro, J. (1984). Lesion size and location in ideomotor apraxia. *Brain, 107(92)*, 1–33.

Kirrie, B., Granier, J., & Robin, D. (2008). Understanding the nature of apraxia of speech: Theory, analysis, and treatment. *Neuropsychological Trends, 4*, 7–44.

Kirst, C., Modes, C., & Magnasco, M. (2017). Shifting attention to dynamics: Self-reconfiguration of neural networks. *Current Opinion in Systems Biology, 3*, 132–140. https://doi.org/10.1016/j.coisb.2017.04.006

Koziol, L. B. (2009). *Subcortical structures and cognition*. Springe.

Koziol, L. (2014). *The myth of executive functioning: Missing elements in conceptualization, evaluation and assessment*. Springer.

Koziol, L., Budding, D., & Chidekel, D. (2012). From movement to thought: Executive function, embodied cognition, and the cerebellum. *Cerebellum, 11*(2), 505–525. https://doi.org/10.1007/s12311-011-0321-y

Kozubski, W., Ong, K., Waleszczyk, W., Zabel, M., & Dorszewska, J. (2021). Molecular factors mediating neural cell plasticity changes in dementia brain diseases. *Neural Plasticity, 2021*, 8834645. https://doi.org/10.1155/2021/8834645

Laffin, J., Raca, G., Jackson, C., Strand, E., Jakielski, K., & Shriberg, L. (2012). Novel candidate genes and regions for childhood apraxia of speech identified by array comparative genomic hybridization. *Genetic Medecine, 14*(11), 928–936. https://doi.org/10.1038/gim.2012.72

Langevin, L. M. (2015). Distinct patterns of cortical thinning in concurrent motor and attention disorders. *Developmental Medicine and Child Neurology, 3*, 257–264.

Latash, M. (2008). Evolution of motor control: From reflexes and motor programs to the equilibrium-point hypothesis. *Journal of Human Kinetics, 19*, 3–24.

Law, J. B. (2000). Prevalence and natural history. *International Journal of Language & Communication Disorders, 35*(2), *165*–188.

Leiguarda, R. (2001). Limb apraxia: Cortical or subcortical. *NeuroImage, 14*(1), 5137–5141. https://doi.org/10.1006/nimg.2001.0833

Leiguarda, C. D., & Marsden, C. (2000). Limb apraxias: Higher-order disorders of sensorimotor integration. *Brain, 123*(*Pt 5*), 650–879. https://doi.org/10.1093/brain/123.5.860

Lesny, I. (1980). Developmental dyspraxia-dysgnosia as a cause of congenital children's clumsiness. *Brain Development, 2, 69–71*. https://doi.org/10.1016/S0387-7604(80)80009-X

Levelt, C., Schiller, N., & Levelt, W. (1999). A developmental grammar for syllable structure in the production of child language. *Brain and language, 68*, 201–299.

Lewis, B., Freebairn, L., Hansen, A., Iyengar, S., & Taylor, H. (2004). School-age follow up of children with childhood apraxia of speech. *Language, Speech, and Hearing Services in Schools, 35*, 122–140.

Liepmann, S., & Mass, O. (1907). Fall von linksseitiger Agraphie und Apraxie bei rechtsseitiger Lahmung. *Journal of Psychology and Neurology, 10, 14*.

Long, C. J., & Kibby, M. Y. (1995). Ecological validity of neuropsychological tests: A look at neuropsychology's past and the impact. *Advances in Medical Psychotherapy, 8*, 59–78.

Luria, A. (1973). *The working brain*. Basic Books.

Luzzi, S., Piccirilli, M., Pessalacia, M., Fabi, K., & Provincialia, L. (2010). Dissociation apraxia secondary to right premotor stroke. *Neuropsychologia, 48*(1), 68–76. https://doi.org/10.1016/j.neuropsychologia.2009.08.010

Maasen, B. (2002). Issues contrasting adult acquired versus developmental apraxia of speech. *Semin Speech Language, 23*, 257–266.

Maassen, B. (2015). Developmental models of childhood apraxia of speech. In R. Barr & E. Sillimen (Eds.), *Routledge handbook of communication disorder* (pp. 124–133). Routledge.

Maleki, S., Chye, Y., Zhang, X., Parkes, L., Chamberlain, S., FFontenelle, L., et al. (2020). Neural correlates of symptom severity in obsessive-compulsive disorder using magnetization transfer and diffusion tensor imaging. *Psychiatry Research: Neuroimaging, 298*, 111046. https://doi.org/10.1016/j.pscychresns.2020.111046

Malkani, R., & Zadikoff, C. (2011). The apraxias in movement disorders. In N. Galvaez-Jimenez, P. Tuite, & K. Bhatia (Eds.), *Uncommon causes of movement disorders* (pp. 35–45). Cambridge University Press.

Martin, N. P. (2006). DCD and ADHD: A genetic study of their shared aetiology. *Human Movement Science*, 110–124.

Mayo Clinic. (2022). *Childhood apraxia of speech*. Retrieved from Mayo Clinic: https://www.mayoclinic.org/diseases-conditions/childhood-apraxia-of-speech/diagnosis-treatment/drc-20352051

McGinty, H., Phillips, K., Jim, H., Cessna, J., Asvat, Y., Cases, M., et al. (2014). Cognitive functioning in men receiving androgen deprivation therapy for prostate cancer: A systematic review and meta-analysis. *Supportive Care in Cancer, 22*(8), 2271–2280. https://doi.org/10.1007/s00520-014-2285-1

McLaren, N. (2010). The DSM-V project: Bad science produces bad psychiatry. *Ethical Human Psychology and Psychiatry, 12(3), 189–199*. https://doi.org/10.1891/1559-4343.12.3.189

McNeil, M. (2011). *Clinical management of sensorimotor speech disorders*. Thieme.

Menon, V. (2013). Developmental pathways to functional brain networks: Emerging principles. *Trends in Cognitive Sciences, 17*(12), 627–640. https://doi.org/10.1016/j.tics.2013.09.015

Merceron-Martinez, D., Ibaceta-Gonzalez, C., Salazr, C., Almaguer-Melian, W., Bergado-Rosado, J., & Palacios, A. (2021). Alzheimer's disease, neural plasticity, and functional recovery. *Journal of Alzheimer's Disease, 82*(s1), S37–S50. https://doi.org/10.3233/JAD-201178

Meyer, K., & Damasio, A. (2009). Convergence and divergence in a architecture for recognition and memory. *Trends in Neuroscience, 32*(7), 376–382. https://doi.org/10.1016/j.tins.2009.04.002

Middleton, F., & Strick, P. (2000). Basal ganglia output and cognition: Evidence from anatomical, behavioral, and clinical studies. *Brain and Cognition, 42*(2), 183–200. https://doi.org/10.1006/brcg.1999.1099

Mihailidis, A., Boger, J. N., Craig, T., & Hoey, J. (2006). The COACH prompting systems to assist older adults with dementia through handwashing: An efficacy study. *BMC Geriatrics, 8, 28. http://www.biomedcentral.com*. https://doi.org/10.1186/1471-2318-8-28

Miller, G. L.-H. (2019). Reading outcomes for individuals with histories of suspected childhood apraxia of speech. *American Journal of Speech Language Pathology, 28*, 1432–1447.

Mirabella, G. D. (2017). Developmental coordination disorder affects the processing of action relate verbs. *Frontiers in Human Neuroscience, 10*, 661. https://doi.org/10.3389/fnhum.2016.00661

Missiuna, C., Rivard, L., & Bartlett, D. (2003). Early identification and risk management of children with developmental coordination disorder. *Pediatric Physical Therapy: Spring, 15(1)*, 32–38.

Molloy, J., & Jagoe, C. (2019). Use of diverse diagnostic criteria for acquired apraxia of speech: A scoping review. *International Journal of Language and Communication Disorders, 54*(6), 875–893. https://doi.org/10.1111/1460-6984.12494

Moncrieff, J. C. (2022). The serotonin theory of depression: A systematic umbrella review of the evidence. *Molecular Psychiatry*. https://doi.org/10.1038/s41380-022-01661-0

Morgan, A., & Webster, R. (2018). Aetiology of childhood apraxia of speech: A clinical practice. *Journal of Paediatrics and Child Health, 54*, 1090–1095. https://doi.org/10.1111/jpc.14150

Morgan, A., Fisher, S., Scheffer, I., & Hildebrand, M. (2016). FOXP2-related speech and language disorders. In M. A. Adam (Ed.), *Gene reviews*. University of Washington.

Moruzzi, S. P.-G. (2010). Clumsiness and psychopathology: Causation or shared etiology? A twin study with the CBCL 6–18 questionnaire in a general school-age population sample. *Human Movement Science, 29*, 326–338. https://doi.org/10.1016/j.humov.2010.01.005

Mosca, S. L. (2016). Copy-number variations are enriched for neurodevelopmental genes in children with developmental coordination disorder. *Journal of Medical Genetics, 53*(12), 812–819. https://doi.org/10.1136/jmedgenet-2016-103818

Moser, D., Basilakos, A., Fillmore, P., & Fridriksson, J. (2016). Brain damage associated with apraxia of speech: Evidence from case studies. *Neurocase, 22*(4), 346–356. https://doi.org/10.1080/13554794.2016.1172645

Moss, A. G. (2012). Interarticulatory coordination of the lips and jaw in childhood apraxia of speech. *Journal of Medical Speech-Language Pathology, 20*(4), 127–132.

Mountford, H. B. (2022). The genetic and molecular basis of developmental language. *Children, 9*, 586.

Murray, E., McCabe, P., & Ballard, K. (2015a). Differential diagnosis of children with suspected childhood apraxia of speech. *Journal of Speech, Language, and Hearing Research, 58(1)*, 43–60. https://doi.org/10.1044/2014_JSLHR-S-12-0358

Murray, E., McCabe, P., & Ballard, K. J. (2015b). A randomized controlled trial for children with childhood apraxia of speech comparing Rapid Syllable Transition treatment and the Nuffield. *Journal of Speech, Language, and Hearing Research, 58*, 669–686. https://doi.org/10.1044/2015_JSLHR-S-13-0179

Mutha, P., Sainburg, R., & Haaland, K. (2010). Coordination deficits in ideomotor apraxia during visually targeted reaching reflect impaired visuomotor transformations. *Neuropsychologia, 48*(13), 3855–3867. https://doi.org/10.1016/j.neuropsychologia.2010.09.018

Nasios, G., Dardiostis, E., & Messinis, L. (2019). From Broca and Wernicke to the neuromodulation era: Insights of brain language networks for neurorehabilitation. *Behavioural Neurology, 2019*. https://doi.org/10.1155/2019/9894571

National Institute of Deafness and Other Communication Disorders. (2022). *Home page*. Retrieved from National Institute of Deafness and Other Communication Disorders: https://www.nidcd.nih.gov/

National Institute of Mental Health. (2022). *Motor actions*. Retrieved from National Institute of mental Health National Research Design Criteria Initiative: https://www.nimh.nih.gov/research/research-funded-by-nimh/rdoc/constructs/motor-actions

Naxarro, X. (2009). Chapter 27 Neural plasticity after nerve injury and regeneration. *International Review of Neurobiology, 87*, 483–505. https://doi.org/10.1016/S0074-7742(09)87027-X

Newbury, D. W. (2009). CMIP and ATP2C2 Modulate phonological short term memory in language impairment. *The American Journal of Human Genetics, 85*, 264–272.

Norbury, C. F. (2016). The impact of nonverbal ability on prevalence and clinical presentation of and clinical presentation of language disorder: Evidence from a population study. *Journal of Child Psychology and Psychiatry, 57*, 1247–1257.

NORD. (2021). *Ocular Motor Apraxia, Cogan Type*. Retrieved from National Organization of Rare Disorders: https://rarediseases.org/rare-diseases/ocular-motor-apraxia-cogan-type/

Ochipa, C., Rothi, L. J., & Heilman, K. M. (1992). Conceptual apraxia in Alzheimer's disease. *Brain, 115(Pt 4)*, 1061–1071.

Ogar, J., Slama, H., Dronkers, N., Amici, S., & Gorno-Tempini, M. (2005). Apraxia of Speech: An overview. *Neurocase, 11*, 427–432. https://doi.org/10.1080/13554790500263529

Ogar, J., Willock, S., Baldo, J., Wilkins, D., Ludy, C., & Dronkers, N. (2006). Clinical and anatomical correlates of apraxia of speech. *Brain and Language, 97(3)*, 343–350. https://doi.org/10.1016/j.bandl.2006.01.008Get

Ogar, J. M., Dronkers, N. F., Brambati, S. M., Miller, B. L., & Gorno-Tempini, M. L. (2007). Progressive nonfluent aphasia and its characteristic motor speech deficits. *Alzheimer Disease and Associated Disorders, 21*, S23–S30.

Park, J. (2017). Apraxia: Review and update. *Journal of Clinical Neurology, 13*(4), 317–324. https://doi.org/10.3988/jcn.2017.13.4.317

Park, E., Velumian, A., & Fehlings, M. (2004). Mechanisms of spinal cord injury: A review with an emphasis on the implications for white matter degeneration. *Journal of Neurotrauma, 21*(6), Reviews. https://doi.org/10.1089/0897715041269641, online.

Pazzaglia, M., Pizzamiglio, L., Pes, E., & Aglioti, S. (2008a). The sound of actions in apraxia. *Current Biology, 18*(22), 1766–1772. https://doi.org/10.1016/j.cub.2008.09.061

Pazzaglia, M., Smania, N., Corato, E., & Aglioti, S. (2008b). Neural underpinnings of gesture discrimination in patients with limb apraxia. *The Journal of Neuroscience, 28*(12), 3030–3041. https://doi.org/10.1523/JNEUROSCI.5748-07.2008

Piek, J. P., Dawson, L., Smith, L. M., & Gasson, N. (2008). The role of early fine and gross motor development on later motor and cognitive ability. *Human Movement Science, 27*(5), 668–681.

Pinson, A. X. (2022). Human TKTL1 implies greater neurogenesis in frontal neocortex of modern humans than Neanderthals. *Science, 377*, eabl6422. https://doi.org/10.1126/science.abl6422

Poore, M. B. (2009). Suck predicts neuromotor integrity and developmental outcomes. *Perspective on Speech and Orofacial Disorders*. https://doi.org/10.1044/ssod19.1.44

Pramstaller, P., & Marsden, C. (1996). The basal ganglia and apraxia. *Brain, 119*(1), 319–340. https://doi.org/10.1093/brain/119.1.319

Ramus, F. (2003). Developmental Dyslexia: Specific phonological deficit or general sensorimotor dysfunction. *Current Opinion in Neurobiology, 13*, 212–218.

Rehme, A. K., & Grefkes, C. (2012). Cerebral network disorders after stroke: Evidence from imaging-based connectivity analyses of active and resting brain states in humans. *Journal of Physiology, 591*, 17–51.

Renzi, D. E., Faglioni, P., & Sorgato, P. (1982). Modality specific and supramodal mechanisms of apraxia. *Brain, 105*, 301–312.

Riecker, A., Mathiak, K., Wildgruber, D., Erb, M., Hertfich, I., Grodd, W., & Ackermann, H. (2005). fMRI reveals two distinct cerebral networks subserving speech motor control. *Neurology, 64*, 700–706.

Roig, M., Gratacòs, M., Vazquez, E., del Toro, M., Foguet, A., Ferrer, I., & Macaya, A. (2003). Brainstem dysgenesis: Report of five patients with congenital hypotonia, multiple cranial nerve involvement and ocular motor apraxia. *Developmental Medicine & Child Neurology, 45*, 489–493.

Rosenzopf, H., Wiesen, D., Basilakos, A., Yourganov, G., Bonilha, L., Fridriksson, J., et al. (2022). Mapping the human praxis network: An investigation of white matter disconnection in limb apraxia of gesture production. *Brain Communications, 4(1)*, 1–14. https://doi.org/10.1093/braincomms/fcac004

Rosenzoph, H., Weisen, D., Basilakos, A., Yourganov, G., Bonilha, L., Rorden, C., et al. (2020, April 17). *Mapping the Human Praxis Network: An investigation of white matter disconnection in limb apraxia.* Retrieved from bioRxiv.org: https://doi.org/10.1101/2020.04.14.041442

Salo, V. F. (2019). The role of the motor stem in action understanding and communication: Evidence from human infants and non human primates. *Developmental Psychobiology, 61(3)*, 390–401.

Salvi, R., Wang, J., & Ding, D. (2000). Auditory plasticity and hyperactivity following cochlear damage. *Hearing Research, 147*, 261–274.

Sato, J. R., Biazoli, C. E., Jr., Zugman, A., Pan, P. M., Bueno, A. P. A., Moura, L. M., et al. (2021). Long-term stability of the cortical volumetric profile and the functional human connectome throughout childhood and adolescence. *European Journal of Neuroscience, 54*, 6187–6201. https://doi.org/10.1111/ejn.15435

Saxena, S., & Caroni, P. (2011). Selective neuronal vulnerability in neurodegenerative diseases: From stressor thresholds to degeneration. *Neuron, 71*, 35–48.

Scott, S. H., & Kalaska, J. F. (1997). Reaching movements with similar hand paths but different arm orientations. I. Activity of individual cells in motor cortex. *Journal of Neurophysiology, 77*, 826–852.

Seven, Y., Mantilla, C., & Sieck, G. (2014). Recruitment of rat diaphragm motor units across motor behaviors with different levels of diaphragm activation. *Journal of Applied Physiology, 117*(11), 1308–1316. https://doi.org/10.1152/japplphysiol.01395.2013

Shandley, S. C. (2021). Abnormal nutritive sucking as an indicator of neonatal brain injury. *Frontiers in Pediatrics*. https://doi.org/10.3389/fped.2020.599633

Sharma, V., & Wong, L. (2022). Middle cerebral artery disease. In J. Grotta, G. Albers, J. Broderick, S. Kasner, R. Sacco, A. Day, et al. (Eds.), *Stroke (Seventh edition) pathophysiology, diagnosis, and management* (pp. 317–346). Elsevier. https://doi.org/10.1016/B978-0-323-69424-7.00024-7

Sharma, N., Classen, J., & Cohen, L. (2013). Neural plasticity and its contribution to functional recovery. *Handbook of Clinical Neurology, 110*, 3–12. https://doi.org/10.1016/B978-0-444-52901-5.00001-0

Shriberg, L. D. (2019). Estimates of prevalence of speech and motor speech disorders in persons with complex neurodevelopmental disorders. *Clinical Linguistics & Phonetics, 33*(8), 707–736.

Shriberg, L. D., Fourakis, M., Hall, S. D., Karlsson, H. B., Lohmeier, H. L., McSweeny, J. L., Potter, N. L., Scheer-Cohen, A. R., Strand, E. A., Tilkens, C. M., & Wilson, D. L. (2010). Extensions to the speech disorders classification system (SDCS). *Clinical Linguistics & Phonetics, 24*, 795–824.

Shriberg, L., KwiatkowskiI, J., & Mabie, H. (2019). Estimates of the prevalence of motor speech disorders in children with idiopathic speech delay. *Clinical Linguistics & Phonetics, 33*, 679–706. https://doi.org/10.1080/02699206.2019.1595731

Singer, W. (1993). Synchronization of cortical activity and its putative. *Annual Review of Physiology, 55*, 349–374.

Soliveri, P., Piacentini, S., & Girotti, F. (2005). Limb apraxia in corticobasal degeneration and progressive supranuclear palsy. *Neurology, 64*, 448–453.

Sonuga-Barke, E. (2003). The dual pathway model of AD/HD: An elaboration of neuro-developmental characteristics. *Neuroscience Biobehavioral Review, 27*, 593–604.

Sonuga-Barke, E., Bitsakou, P., & Thompson, M. (2010). Beyond the dual pathway model: Evidence for the dissociation of timing, inhibitory and delay-related impairments in Attention Deficit/Hyperactivity disorder. *Journal of Child and Adolescent Psychiatry, 49*, 345–355. https://doi.org/10.1016/j.jaac.2009.12.018

Sporns, O., Tononi, G., & Kötter, R. (2005). The human connectome: A structural description of the human brain. *PLOS Computational Biology*. https://doi.org/10.1371/journal.pcbi.0010042

Stackhouse, J. W. (1997). *Children's speech and literacy difficulties 1: A psycholinguistic framework*. Wurr.

Steward, M., Sridhar, A., & Meyer, J. (2013). Neural regeneration. *Current Topics in Microbiology and Immunology, 367*, 153–191. https://doi.org/10.1007/82_2012_302

Stoll, G., & Muller, H. (1998). Nerve injury, axonal degeneration and neural regeneration: Basic insights. *Brain Pathology, 9*, 313–325. https://doi.org/10.1111/j.1750-3639.1999.tb00229.x

Strand, E. (2019, January 9). *Diagnosis and management of CAS*.

Sunderland, A., & Shiner, C. (2007). Ideomotor apraxia and functional ability. *Cortex, 43*(3), 359–367. https://doi.org/10.1016/S0010-9452(08)70461-1

Sweatt, D. (2016). Neural Plasticity and Behavior- sixty years of conceptual advances. *Journal of Neurochemistry, 139*(2), 179–199. https://doi.org/10.1111/jnc.13580

Szczepanski, S., & Knight, R. (2014). Insights into human behavior from lesions to the prefrontal cortex. *Neuron., 83*(5), 1002–1018. https://doi.org/10.1016/j.neuron.2014.08.011

Tal Saban, M. O. (2014). Executive function and attention in young adults with and without Developmental Coordination Disorder – A comparative study. *Research in Developmental Disabilities., 35*, 2644–2650.

Tal-Saba, M. Z. (2012). The functional profile of young adults with suspected developmental coordination disorder (DCD). *Research in Developmental Disabilities, 33*, 2193–2202. https://doi.org/10.1016/j.ridd.2012.06.005

Tarsy, D. (2012). *Movement disorders: A video atlas*. Humana Press.

Terband, H. M. (2019). A psycholinguistic framework for diagnosis and treatment planning of developmental speech disorders. *Folia Phoniatrica et Logopaedica, 71*(5–6), 216–227.

Tettamanti, M., Buccino, G., Saccuman, M., Gallese, V., Danna, M., Scifo, P., et al. (2005). Listening to action-related sentences activates fronto-parietal motor circuits. *Journal of Cognitive Neuroscience, 17*, 273–281.

Teverovsky, E., Bickel, J., & Feldman, H. (2009). Functional characteristics of children diagnosed with Childhood Apraxia of Speech. *Disability and Rehabilitation, 31*(2), 94–102. https://doi.org/10.1080/09638280701795030

The Health Jade Team. (2022). *Brain plasticity*. Retrieved from Health Jade: https://healthjade.net/brain-plasticity/

The Medical Dictionary. (2021). *Apraxia*. Retrieved from The Medical Dictionary: http://the-medical-dictionary.com/apraxia_article_2.htm

Thomason, M., Hect, J., Waller, R., Manning, J., Stacks, A., Beeghly, M., et al. (2018). Prenatal neural origins of infant motor development: Associations between fetal brain and infant motor development. *Developmental Psychopathology, 30*(3), 763–772. https://doi.org/10.1017/S095457941800072X

Trigilio, M. (2013, December 3). *A Smithsonian dilemma: Pure scientific research, "A thousand applications," or both?* Retrieved from National Museum of American History. https://americanhistory.si.edu/blog/2013/12/a-smithsonian-dilemma-pure-scientific-research-a-thousand-applications-or-both.html

Tse, M. (2012). Double duty of tail caudate nucleus neurons. *Nature Reviews Neuroscience, 13*, 11005–11016. https://doi.org/10.1038/nrn3342

Tuttolomondo, A., Pecoraro, R., & Pinto, A. (2014). Studies of selective TNF inhibitors in the treatment of brain injury from stroke and trauma: A review of the evidence to date. *Drug Design, Development and Therapy, 8*, 2221–2238. https://doi.org/10.2147/DDDT.S67655

Van Der Merwe, A. (2020). New perspectives on speech motor planning and programming in the context of the four-level model and its implications for understanding the pathophysiology underlying apraxia of speech and other motor speech disorders. *Aphasiology*. https://doi.org/10.1080/02687038.2020.1765306, online.

Wang, M. L. (2014a). Co-occurring development of early childhood communication and motor skills: Results from a population based longitudinal study. *Child: Care, Health and Development, 40*, 77–84.

Wang, M. L. (2014b). The developmental relationship between language and motor performance from 3 to 5 years of age: A prospective longitudinal population study. *BMC Psychology, 2, 34*. https://doi.org/10.1186/s40359-014-0034-3

Waring, R., & Knight, R. (2013). How should children with speech sound disorders be classified? A review and critical evaluation of current classification systems. *Journal of Language & Communication Disorders, 48(1)*, 25–40. https://doi.org/10.1111/j.1460-6984.2012.00195.x

Wasserman, T., & Wasserman, L. (2013). Towards a unifying model of executive function. *Applied Neuropsychology: Child, 2*(2), 88–96. https://doi.org/10.1080/21622965.2013.748394

Wasserman, T., & Wasserman, L. (2016). *Depathologizing Psychopathology*. Springer.

Wasserman, T., & Wasserman, L. (2017). Touching the elephant: The search for fluid intelligence. *Applied Neuropsychology Child, 6*(3), 228–236. https://doi.org/10.1080/21622965.2017.1317489

Wasserman, T., & Wasserman, L. (2020). *Neural network series: Motivation, effort and the neural network system*. Springer Nature.

Watemberg, N. W.-S. (2007). Developmental coordination disorder in children with attention-deficit–hyperactivity disorder and physical therapy intervention. *Developmental Medicine & Child Neurology, 49*(12), 920–925.

Watson, R., & Heilman, K. (1983). Callosal apraxia. *Brain, 106*(2), 391–403. https://doi.org/10.1093/brain/106.2.391

Weintraub, S. (2000a). Neuropsychological assessment of mental state. In M. Mesulam (Ed.), *Principles of behavioral and cognitive neurology* (pp. 135–136). Oxford University Press.

Weintraub, S. (2000b). Neuropsychological assessment of mental state. In M. Mesulam (Ed.), *Principles of behavioral and cognitive neurology* (p. 121). Oxford University Press.

Wessel, J., & Aron, A. (2017). On the globality of motor suppression: Unexpected events and their influence on behavior and cognition. *Neuron, 93*(2), 259–280. https://doi.org/10.1016/j.neuron.2016.12.013

West, C., Bowen, A., Hesketh, A., & Vail, A. (2008). Interventions for motor apraxia following stroke. *Cochrane Database of Systematic Reviews*. https://doi.org/10.1002/14651858.CD004132.pub2

Wheaton, L., & Hallet, M. (2007). Ideomotor apraxia: A review. *Journal of the Neurological Sciences, 260*, 1–8. https://doi.org/10.1016/j.jns.2007.04.014

Whiteside, S., Dyson, L., Cowell, P., & Varley, R. (2015). The relationship between apraxia of speech and oral apraxia: Association or dissociation? *Archives of Clinical Neuropsychology, 30*(7), 670–682. https://doi.org/10.1093/arclin/acv051

Wielock, T., & Nikolich, K. (2006). Mechanisms of neural plasticity following brain injury. *Current Opinion in Neurobiology, 2(16)*, 1–7.

Wilson, P. M. (1998). information processing deficits associated with developmental coordination disorder: A meta-analysis of research findings. *Journal of Child Psychology, 39*, 829–840.

World Health Organization (WHO). (1993). *The ICD-10 classification of mental and behavioural disorders*. World Health Organization (WHO).

Worthington, A. (2016). Treatments and technologies in the rehabilitation of apraxia and action disorganisation syndrome: A review. *Neurorehabilitation, 39(1)*, 163–174. https://doi.org/10.3233/NRE-161348

Xenia Lojewski, L. X.-B.-E. (2014). Human adult white matter progenitor cells are multipotent neuroprogenitors similar to adult hippocampal progenitors. *Stem Cells Translational Medicine, 3(4)*, 458–469.

Yadegari, F., Azimian, M., Rahgozar, M., & Shekarchi, B. (2014). Brain areas impaired in oral and verbal apraxic patients. *Iranian Journal of Neurology, 13*(2), 77–82.

Yun, J., Shin, S., & Son, S. (2021). Clinical utility of repeated urimal test of articulation and phonation for patients with childhood apraxia of speech. *Children, 8*(12), 1–7. https://doi.org/10.3390/children8121106

Yuste, R. (2015). From the neuron doctrine to neural networks. *Nature Reviews Neuroscience, 16*, 487–497. https://doi.org/10.1038/nrn3962

Zadikoff, C. L., & Lang, A. (2005). Apraxia in movement disorders. *Brain, 128*(7), 1480–1497. https://doi.org/10.1093/brain/awh560

Zang, Z., Ping, L., Zhai, A., & Zhou, Z. (2021). Microstructural white matter abnormalities in obsessive-compulsive disorder: A coordinate-based meta-analysis of diffusion tensor imaging studies. *Asian Journal of Psychiatry, 55*, 102467. https://doi.org/10.1016/j.ajp.2020.102467

Zohary, E., Shadlen, M., & Newsome, W. (1994). Correlated neuronal discharge rate and its implications for psychophysical performance. *Nature, 370*, 140–143.

Zwicker, J. M. (2009). Neural correlates of developmental coordination disorder: A review of hypotheses. *Child Neurology, 24*, 1273–1281.

Appendix I: Network Properties Breakdown of Ideational Apraxia

Research Domain Criteria

The following is extrapolated from the Research Domain Initiative of the National Institute of Mental Health (National Institute of Mental Health, 2022). It is presented here to give the reader an idea of the complexity of networks and interactions and the potential magnitude of effect a disruption of one or several components can produce in one type of apraxia, in this example, an ideational apraxia.

Ideational Apraxia

Type of Element Behavior

Domain Sensorimotor Systems

Sensorimotor systems are primarily responsible for the control and execution of motor behaviors and their refinement during learning and development.

Construct Motor Actions

A multifaceted construct is comprised of the processes that must be engaged during the planning and execution of a motor action in a context-appropriate manner. Component processes include action planning and selection, sensorimotor dynamics, initiation, execution, and inhibition and termination. Of note, these processes will often be recruited in conjunction with motivational processes described in other domains, as when appetitive motivations drive approach behaviors. This construct explicitly includes the modulation and refinement of actions during development

T. Wasserman, L. D. Wasserman, *Apraxia: The Neural Network Model*, Neural Network Model: Applications and Implications,
https://doi.org/10.1007/978-3-031-24105-5

and learning. The list of subconstructs is not intended to imply a specific order or sequence.

Subconstruct Action Planning and Selection

Processes whereby an individual engages a plan for spatial and temporal components of possible purposeful movements, which match internal and external constraints to achieve a goal. This may also include cost-benefit calculations in the development and selection of motor plans.

Circuits Involved

Inferior Parietal Cortex

Posterior Parietal Cortex: Goal Selection

Goal selection refers to the cognitive process of choosing among potential outcomes, actions, or behaviors and can be considered as a component process of cognitive control.

Goal updating involves refreshing the cognitive content related to specific potential outcomes, actions, or behaviors and can be considered a component process of cognitive control.

Circuits Involved in Goal Selection
Frontopolar/Anterior LPFC (BA10)
Inhibition of the Default Mode Network (DMN)
The DMN is a set of brain regions that exhibit strong low-frequency oscillations coherent during resting state and is thought to be activated when individuals are focused on their internal mental state processes, such as self-referential processing, interoception, autobiographical memory retrieval, or imagining future events.

Premotor Cortex

The premotor cortex is an area of the motor cortex lying within the frontal lobe of the brain just anterior to the primary motor cortex. The premotor cortex, as might be expected, is involved in a number of apraxic conditions including conceptual apraxia, ideational apraxia, limb kinetic apraxia, and ideomotor apraxia. Within it lies Broca's area a region in the frontal lobe of the dominant hemisphere, usually the left, of the brain with functions linked to speech production.

Superior Temporal Sulcus

Involved in motor apraxic conditions such as conceptual apraxia, ideational apraxia, limb kinetic apraxia, and ideomotor apraxia. This circuit contains mirror neurons which are involved in the sense that one is initiating, executing, and in control of their volitional actions and their sensory consequences and the sense that one's body or body parts belong to oneself. This may include the comparison of the predicted and actual sensory consequences of one's action, *awareness of the intention to move*, temporal binding of self-generated action and their immediate effects, and attenuation of sensory consequences of self-generated actions. These mirror neurons are components of numerous other circuits.

Supplementary Motor Area

Participates in the control of processes involved in the initiation of a selected action plan, which often includes timing of movement onset. Associated circuits include the basal ganglia and the dorsal cingulate.

Construct: Initiation

Processes involved in the initiation of a selected action plan; this may include timing of movement onset.

Circuits Involved

Basal Ganglia

The basal ganglia are a group of structures linked to the thalamus in the base of the brain and involved in coordination of movement. The main components of the basal ganglia are the striatum, consisting of both the dorsal striatum (caudate nucleus and putamen) and the ventral striatum (nucleus accumbens and olfactory tubercle), the globus pallidus, the ventral pallidum, the substantia nigra, and the subthalamic nucleus.

Processes involved in the specification/parameterization of an action plan and program based on integration of internal or external information, such as sensations and urges and modeling of body dynamics. This process is continuously and iteratively refined via sensory information and reward-reinforced information. This circuit is also involved in processes involved in the inhibition of motor plans, either before or after an action is initiated, and the sense that a motor plan has been successfully completed. The inhibition subconstruct is commonly operationalized as motor response inhibition and has conceptual overlaps with the inhibition/suppression subconstruct of the cognitive control construct within the cognitive systems domain.

Dorsal Cingulate

Also involved with the initiation of a selected action plan.

Construct: Execution

These are processes involved in the actualization and adaptation of action implementation.

Circuits Involved

Efferent and Afferent Spinal and Peripheral Pathways

Afferent and efferent pathways are two types of nerves in the peripheral nervous system. Afferent pathways bring information from the body to the central nervous system, and efferent pathways bring information from the central nervous system to the body.

Motor Cortex

The motor cortex is an area within the cerebral cortex of the brain that is involved in the planning, control, and execution of voluntary movements. The motor cortex is often divided into the primary motor cortex and the nonprimary motor cortex. The primary motor cortex is critical for initiating motor movements.

Construct: Inhibition and Execution

Processes involved in the inhibition of motor plans, either before or after an action is initiated, and the sense that a motor plan has been successfully completed. The inhibition subconstruct is commonly operationalized as motor response inhibition and has conceptual overlaps with the inhibition/suppression subconstruct of the cognitive control construct within the cognitive systems domain.

Circuits Involved

Basal Ganglia

Previously described

Supplementary Motor Area

Previously described

Posterior Cingulate Gyrus

A central node of the default mode network (DMN), it is a set of brain regions showing strongly correlated neural activity and a reliable deactivation in activity during many cognitive tasks.

Inferior Frontal Gyrus

The inferior frontal gyrus is a part of the articulatory network involved in motor syllable programs. The articulatory network also contains the premotor cortex and the anterior insula. These areas are interrelated but have specific functions in speech comprehension and production. The articulatory network acts mostly when the vocal tract moves to produce syllables. The inferior frontal gyrus contains the Broca's area, which is involved in language processing and speech production.

Dorsolateral Prefrontal Cortex

The dorsolateral prefrontal cortex has been found to be involved in superordinate control functions for various cognitive tasks such as decision-making, novelty detection, working memory, conflict management, mood regulation, theory of mind processing, and *timing*.

Inferior Parietal Cortex

The inferior parietal lobe (IPL) is a key neural substrate underlying diverse mental processes, from basic attention to language and social cognition, that define human interactions.

Lateral Premotor Cortex

Contributes to the overall control of movement

Medial Prefrontal Cortex

The medial prefrontal cortex plays an important regulatory role in numerous cognitive functions, including attention, inhibitory control, habit formation and working, and spatial or long-term memory.

Things that are unclear are the following:

1. It is unclear whether a disruption of any of the component networks would produce the same outcome.
2. It is unclear as to just what combination of networks must be disrupted in order to produce an ideational apraxia.
3. Can the same network disruption that produces ideational apraxia also produce something else depending on where in the network configuration the disruption occurs? This is not clear.
4. It is unclear whether multiple sets of networks that can be disrupted would produce the same outcome.
5. As each of the networks outlined above participates in other functional behaviors and outcomes, it seems likely that disruptions of those networks would also produce comorbid conditions. This area of research is poorly investigated and resultingly unclear. It seems logical to suggest that if the initiation networks are dysfunctional, any downstream behavior or associated network would be impacted.

Index

T. Wasserman, L. D. Wasserman, *Apraxia: The Neural Network Model*, Neural Network Model: Applications and Implications,
https://doi.org/10.1007/978-3-031-24105-5